Biomechanics and Medicine in Swimming

Biomechanics and Medicine in Swimming

Swimming Science VI

EDITED BY
D. MacLaren, T. Reilly
and
A. Lees

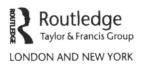

Routledge
Taylor & Francis Group

LONDON AND NEW YORK

First Published 1992
by Taylor & Francis

Published 2014 by Routledge
2 Park Square, Milton Park, Abingdon, Oxfordshire OX14 4RN
711 Third Avenue, New York, NY 10017

Transferred to Digital Printing 2006
First issued in paperback 2014

Routledge is an imprint of the Taylor & Francis Group, an informa business

ISBN 978-0-419-15600-0 (hbk)
ISBN 978-1-138-88047-4 (pbk)

A catalogue record for this book is available from the British Library.

Library of Congress Cataloguing-in-Publication data available

Publisher's Note
The publisher has gone to great lengths to ensure the quality of this reprint
but points out that some imperfections in the original may be apparent

Sixth International Symposium on Biomechanics and Medicine in Swimming
Liverpool, 7–11th September 1990

Organized from Liverpool Polytechnic and held at the
Britannia Adelphi Hotel, Liverpool

Organizing Committee

S. Colebrook
D. Jameson
A. Lees
M. Hughes
D. Robinson
C. Sharkey

Symposium Organizers

D. MacLaren and T. Reilly
School of Health Sciences
Liverpool Polytechnic
Byrom Street
Liverpool L3 3AF

Contents

PART THREE   ELECTROMYOGRAPHY

PART FOUR   SWIM TECHNIQUE

PART FIVE   TRAINING

PART EIGHT   MEDICAL CONSIDERATIONS

PART NINE   KINANTHROPOMETRY

PART TEN   PSYCHOLOGICAL FACTORS

Symposium organization

Liverpool Polytechnic hosted the VIth International Symposium on Bio-mechanics and Medicine in Swimming at the Britannia Adelphi Hotel, 7–11th September, 1990. The Symposium was attended by about 170 delegates from 30 different countries. The programme consisted of 60 oral communications, 27 posters, four keynote addresses, four workshops and one seminar. A half-day was set aside for demonstrations pool-side. These included electromyography during swimming using the techniques developed by Jan Cabri, Jan Clarys and colleagues at Brussels; measurement of active drag using the MAD system shown by Peter Hollander, Huub Toussaint and co-workers from Amsterdam; and a two-speed 'lactate test' orchestrated by Malcolm Robson and Ralph Marsh (Analox Instruments, UK).

The scientific programme of the symposium was of a high standard and all keynote addresses were outstanding. David Costill related lactate metabolism to swimming and outlined the variety of factors influencing the interpretation of lactate concentation values. Huub Toussaint explained the most important factors determining swimming performance and placed his own work on efficiency in context. Kurt Wilke provided a systematic analysis of sprint swimming, while Terry Denison gave the audience an insight into the redoubtable tasks associated with coaching an Olympic champion.

The workshops provided a forum for debate about broader aspects relating science and swimming than those covered in the formal sessions. Topics included hydrodynamics and swimming (Mike Hughes and Bodo Ungerechts), the child swimmer (Diane Jameson, Deryk Snelling and Kurt Wilke), biological rhythms and swimming (Claire Dickenson and Tom Reilly) and nutrition (Don MacLaren). The seminar on 'Coach education: the links between theory and practice' chaired by Jan Clarys and sponsored by British Coal Enterprise included expositions from Terry Dennison and Deryk Snelling covering the UK and Canadian scenes, respectively.

The prestigious Archimedes award, presented to new, outstanding researchers every four years at this Symposium was shared for the first time. The prize went to Delia Roberts (University of Calgary) for her paper on 'Serum erythropoietin (EPO) training at moderate altitude' and to Veronique Colman (Leuven University) for her work on 'Relation between physical characteristics and the degree of undulation in the breaststroke'.

A special ambience was created during the Symposium by the social events. These included a competitive swim round the Albert Dock (organised by Liverpool City Swimming Club), a Beatles Tour, an evening of sea-shanties and Liverpool songs, and a 'pub crawl'. At the Symposium Banquet, Professor T. Reilly paid tribute to the work of Jan Clarys for coordinating the series of Symposia on behalf of the World Commission of Sport Biomechanics. Special awards were presented to members who were at the First Symposium in Brussels in 1970 and at the Sixth in Liverpool – John Atha, Jan Clarys, Jurgen Klauck, Mitsamasa Miytashita, Ulrich Persyn and Bob Stallman.

For promotion and administration of the Symposium we are indebted to David Robinson, Colette Sharkey and Joanne Lunt from the National Coaching Foundation Centre based at Liverpool Polytechnic, and for the marketing initiatives from Sandra Colebrook of Jack Stopforth Associates. The Secretariat was supported during the Symposium by students and staff from the Centre for Sport and Exercise Sciences at Liverpool Polytechnic. Their cheerful helpfulness was much appreciated by all the delegates. Finally, we wish to extend our grateful thanks to Professor Peter Toyne, Rector and Chief Executive of Liverpool Polytechnic, who officially opened the Symposium and whose wholehearted support ensured that the event took place in Liverpool.

The closing address by Jan Clarys and John Troup looked forward to the Seventh Symposium which will be held at the US Swimming Centre (Colorado) in 1994. We are confident that the continued excellence in swim research will be borne out yet again at that meeting. Until then these Proceedings provide a compendium of contemporary research.

Don MacLaren and Tom Reilly
Symposium Organisers

Preface

This volume contains papers presented at the Sixth International Symposium on Biomechanics and Medicine in Swimming at Liverpool, September 7–11, 1990. The Symposium itself saw four keynote addresses, four workshops, 27 posters and 60 oral communications. Manuscripts of the presentations were subjected to 'peer review', and where necessary revised and edited. For various reasons it was not possible to publish all of the papers, but those that have been included do provide a flavour of the Symposium programme, and highlight the wealth of good quality research being undertaken in the field of swimming throughout the world.

The contents are organized into parts; these are based on the various disciplines contributing to the science of swimming. The nature of some of the papers presented was such that they transcended disciplinary boundaries and their placement in a certain section was based on compatibility with others in that section.

The editors are indebted to the contributors who responded promptly and indeed to those individuals who acted as our referees. Finally, but not least, a great debt of thanks must go to our extremely competent and patient typist, Sue Abraham, who has painstakingly prepared the typescript of all the papers within these Proceedings.

D.MacLaren
T. Reilly
A. Lees

PART ONE

KEYNOTE ADDRESSES

LACTATE METABOLISM FOR SWIMMING

D.L. Costill
Human Performance Laboratory, Ball State University, Indiana, USA

Abstract
During swimming, lactic acid production results from the breakdown of
muscle glycogen stores via the process of glycolysis. In short
intensive bouts of swimming the large production and accumulation of
lactic acid in muscle leads to an increase in acidity and results in
fatigue. The latter occurs as a consequence of an increase in
hydrogen ions (H^+) linked with lactic acid dissociation and a reduction in reduces muscle pH below 6.9. Such increases in H^+ and the
concomitant reduction in pH are the likely causes of fatigue.
Recovery from exhaustive high intensity exercise takes approximately
20 to 30 min during which time muscle pH returns to pre-exercise
levels. Coaches and sport physiologists use measurements of blood
lactate to gauge the intensity and volume of training needed to
produce an optimal training stimulus despite the fact that a variety
of factors influence blood lactate levels, thus bringing into
question the validity of this method. This paper examines the
factors associated with blood lactate concentrations, methods of
assessing blood lactate levels, and briefly considers other estimates
of assessing the anaerobic capacity of the swimmer.
Keywords: Lactate, Metabolism, Anaerobic Capacity, pH.

1 Introduction

Success or failure in swimming competition depends to a large extent
on the ability of active muscles to generate the energy needed to
propel the body through the water. The energy referred to here is
that produced from the foods we eat (i.e. carbohydrates, fats and
proteins). When broken down by the body these fuels yield low levels
of energy that are inadequate for muscular activity. Instead, the
cells convert these low energy sources into a "high-energy" compound,
adenosine triphosphate (ATP) that provides the immediate energy for
muscule action. In turn, the energy stored within the ATP molecule
is released when the third phosphate is separated from the structure.
   The muscles have four possible sources of ATP:

   (a) that stored within the muscle;
   (b) that generated from another phosphate compound (i.e. ATP-PCr
system);
   (c) ATP produced from the breakdown of muscle sugar (i.e.
glycolytic system), and

(d) the ATP generated with the aid of oxygen (i.e. oxidative system).

This paper focuses not on the processes of energy production, but on lactate, the by-product of the glycolytic system.

Glycolysis is the breakdown of muscle sugar, glycogen, in the absence of oxygen, resulting in the production and accumulation of lactic acid. Thus, glycolysis provides ATP when there is inadequate oxygen being supplied to the system. Unfortunately, this process is relatively inefficient, providing only a small, but essential, part of the ATP needed during competitive swimming. In the presence of oxygen, aerobic energy production can generate 13 times more ATP than can be generated by glycolysis. Thus the glycolytic system supplements the ATP-PCr system in providing energy for highly intense muscular effort when the oxygen supply is inadequate.

As noted in Fig. 1, the demands of the glycolytic system are highest during events that range from 50 to 200 m, causing lactic acid levels in muscle to rise from a resting value of about 1 mmol/kg of muscle to over 25 mmol/kg. The high acid content of the muscle fibres inhibits further breakdown of glycogen and may interfere with the muscle's contractile process. Thus, extended reliance on glycolysis for energy will result in muscular fatigue and exhaustion as the fibres become acidic.

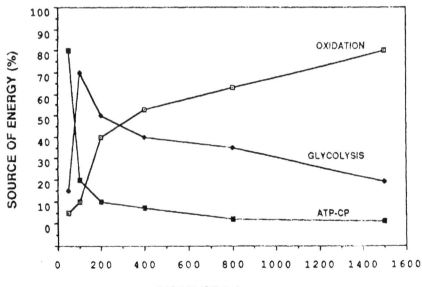

Fig. 1.   Relative energy sources for varying distances swum.

The association between fatigue and lactic acid accumulation in the blood has been recognized since the early 1930's. During strenuous exercise, some energy is provided with the formation of lactic acid in the cytosol of the muscle fibres. Since lactic acid is an acid, it dissociates to some degree, resulting in an accumulation of hydrogen ions and a decrease in pH. Though it is commonly believed that lactic acid is responsible for fatigue and exhaustion in all types of exercise, it is only during relatively short-term, highly intense muscular effort that lactate accumulates within the muscle fibre and alters its pH. Long distance swimmers (e.g. 5 km), for example, may have near resting lactate and pH levels at the end of the race despite their exhaustion. As noted earlier, the cause of their fatigue is inadequate energy supply, not an excess of lactate. Sprint swimming results in a large accumulation of lactate, the result of energy production via glycolysis. It should be realized, however, that it is not lactate per se that should be blamed for the feeling of fatigue. Hydrogen ion concentration that accompanies lactate and other acid accumulation within the cells may decrease muscle pH from 7.1 at rest to 6.4 at exhaustion, a value that is incompatible with normal cell function.

Such changes in pH have a negative effect on energy production and the contraction process within the muscle. A reduction in intra-cellular pH to less than 6.9 has been shown to inhibit the action of phosphofructokinase (PFK), an important glycolytic enzyme, thereby slowing the rate of glycolysis and ATP production. At a pH of 6.4 the influence of free H^+ is strong enough to stop any further breakdown of glycogen, resulting in a rapid drop in ATP and exhaustion. In addition, H^+ may act to displace calcium within the fibre, thereby interfering with the coupling of the crossbridges and a concomitant decline in the muscle's contractile force. It is generally agreed, therefore, that a decrease in pH within the muscle is the major factor limiting maximal sprint swimming.

As noted in Fig. 2, recovery from an exhaustive sprint exercise bout takes approximately 20 to 30 min. At that point, muscle pH has returned to the pre-exercise level, although blood and muscle lactate may still be quite elevated. Experience has shown that athletes can continue to exercise at relatively high intensities even when their muscle pH is below 7.0, with lactate levels above 6 or 7 mM, which is 4 to 5 times the resting value. Currently, coaches and sports physiologists are attempting to use measurements of blood lactate to gauge the intensity and volume of training needed to produce an optimal training stimulus. Although such measurements provide an index of the training intensity, they may not be related to the anaerobic processes or the state of acidosis within the muscles. As lactate and H^+ are generated within the muscles, they diffuse out of the cells, are diluted in body fluids, are transported to other areas of the body, and are metabolized. Consequently, blood values for lactate are dependent on their rate of production, diffusion and oxidation. Since there is a variety of factors that can influence this management of lactate and H^+, the validity of their use in evaluating training is questionable.

Although the stopwatch provides the best method of assessing the swimmer's adaptation to training, it offers few insights regarding the changes in the swimmer's physiology. As a result there have been numerous attempts to use physiological tests to objectively gauge the swimmer's improvements and to assist in planning the training pro-gramme. Such tests include measurements of blood lactate, heart rates, and the rating of perceived exertion (RPE). Although the validity and sensitivity of these tests as indices of one's adapta-tion to training are open to some debate, it is generally agreed

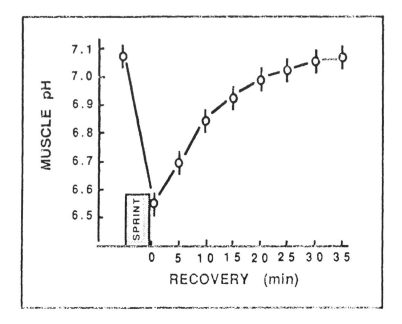

Fig. 2. Changes in muscle pH during sprint cycling to exhaustion
         and during 30 minutes of recovery. Note the slow rate
         of recovery for pH.

that they do correlate well with the swimmer's performance improvements during the early stages of training (Sharp et al., 1984).
**There is, however, no evidence to support the concept that these
tests provide sufficient information on which to base the swimmer's
training regimen.**

2 Blood lactate

The "lactate threshold" has been defined as that point in an exercise
of increasing intensity at which lactate starts to accumulate in the
blood. It has been suggested that the lactate threshold is an
indicator of the anaerobic processes of energy production within the
muscle. This is not the case. Rather, the measurements of blood
lactate accumulation simply provide a means of gauging the severity
of the exercise relative to the subject's physiological limits.
During easy swimming lactate remains only slightly above the resting
level, showing a significant rise only when the swimmer's muscles
produce more lactate than is being removed by other body tissues. At
that level of effort lactate begins to accumulate in the blood, and
this can be referred to as the "lactate threshold". An illustration

of the lactate response at various swimming speeds is shown in
Fig. 3. The lactate threshold can be expressed in terms of the
percent $\dot{V}O_2$max at which it occurs. An individual with a lactate
threshold that occurred at 60% $\dot{V}O_2$max, for example, would have a
greater endurance and performance potential than someone with a
lactate threshold at 45% $\dot{V}O_2$max. The higher percentage indicates
that the individual can exercise at relatively higher levels of
effort before experiencing the physiological stresses associated with
the onset of fatigue and ultimately exhaustion.

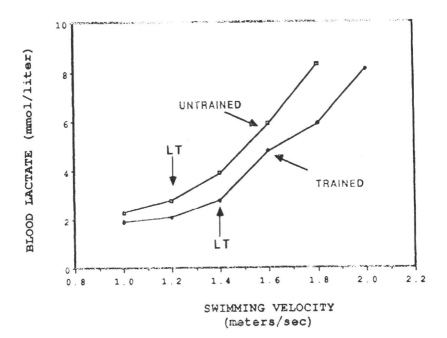

Fig. 3. The relationship between swimming speed and blood lactate
accumulation for two swimmers. The arrow notes the
"lactate threshold" for each swimmer.

It should be pointed out that the accumulation of lactate in the
blood is the combined result of (1) lactate production in the
muscles, (2) lactate diffusion from the muscles into the blood, and
(3) the rate of oxidation and removal of lactate from the blood.
Thus, the amount of lactate measured in a blood sample may reflect
both production and removal of lactate while telling us little about
the energetics of swimming. **The results of blood lactate values must
be viewed cautiously, since there are many potential interpretations
and few valid applications of such data to our understanding of
training and performance.**
   Nevertheless, when swimmers are required to perform a standard
swim at a relatively high intensity ($\sim$ 80–100% $\dot{V}O_2$max), blood lactate
is a reasonable indicator of swimming stress and can be used as one
index of their adjustment to training. When required to perform a

standardized 200 or 400 metre swim at a set speed, swimmers show a dramatic decline in post-exercise blood lactate during the first 6 to 10 weeks of training. Then, like $\dot{V}O_2$max, there is little additional improvement, despite additional weeks and months of intense training. Thus, such testing is most useful during the early period of adjustment.

2.1 Lactate testing procedures
In most studies of lactate, blood is drawn from the arm, ear, or finger tip within 1 to 3 min after the standardized swim. Although venous forearm blood better represents the lactate production in the forearm muscles, samples taken with a needle and syringe are often perceived by the swimmers as being more traumatic. Capillary blood samples can be obtained from a puncture wound to the finger tip or earlobe. However, the size of the sample is usually small (~ 25 microlitres, μl) and is often more difficult to obtain if the wound fails to bleed sufficiently. Application of a vasodilator to the skin of the earlobe will increase blood flow to that area, making it easier to collect a blood sample. For that reason the earlobe is the preferred site for sampling approximately 75 microlitres of blood.

Once the blood sample has been obtained, there are several methods for determining its lactate concentration. Although this technique requires a modestly equipped biochemistry laboratory, it offers the advantage of accuracy and low cost. As an alternative method, automatic analyzers have been developed which make lactate determinations fast, easy and reasonably accurate. The primary advantage of these analyzers is that they can be used at the pool, the results being available for the coach within minutes after the trials.

In order to determine the swimmer's lactate threshold it is necessary to have him/her perform a series of three or four 200 or 400 m swims at increasing speeds. If attempts are made to do all of the swims on the same day, at least 30 min must separate the swims to allow blood lactate to return to resting levels before starting the next swim. However, at the higher velocities, where more lactate is produced, even 30 minutes will not be sufficient time to normalize blood lactate. For that reason, some investigators recommend that the lactate swims be performed on certain days, which, unfortunately, takes additional time away from training and reduces the sensitivity of the test.

The swimmer's adaptation to training can also be gauged with a single, standardized swim performed at about 95% of his/her best time for 200 or 400 m. This intensity is sufficient to produce a relatively high blood lactate when the swimmer is poorly trained, and reflects the gains in conditioning during subsequent trials. Such testing can be performed at 3 to 4 week intervals, using the same swimming velocity. A series of computer-controlled lights can be placed along the bottom of the swimming pool or a pace clock should be used to help the swimmer gauge the correct pace for each swim. As shown in Fig. 4, the results from these tests can be graphed to illustrate the swimmer's adaptation to training. Lower blood lactates after these standardized swims suggest that the swimmer has become more efficient, has improved aerobic power ($\dot{V}O_2$max), produces less lactate, and/or is able to remove lactate faster.

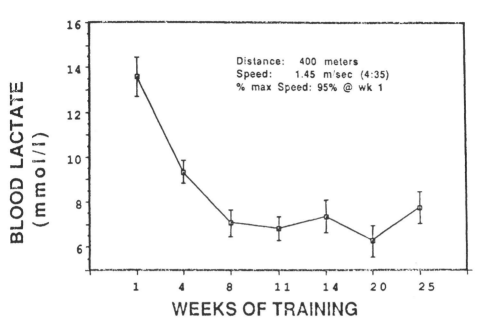

Fig. 4. Changes in blood lactate after a standardized 200 m front crawl swim during 24 weeks of training.

3 Estimates of anaerobic capacity

Since a large portion of the energy used during sprint swimming is derived from anaerobic metabolism, a test to assess this capacity should prove helpful in determining the swimmer's potential for success in events from 50 to 400 m. Unlike the aerobic power ($\dot{V}O_2$max), there are no direct methods to measure one's anaerobic capacity. Several estimates have been developed for this purpose, though they are time consuming and generally provide little more information than we might obtain from the stopwatch during an all-out swim test or a set of maximal sprint intervals. Nevertheless, the following discussion is offered as an alternative method for estimating anaerobic capacity, using measurements of oxygen uptake and tests of interval sets.

One method used to estimate the anaerobic capacity is to calculate the difference between one's estimated oxygen demand during all-out exercise and the maximal oxygen uptake (Medbo et al., 1988). When the swimmer's oxygen uptake is determined at three or four different submaximal swimming speeds, it is possible to extrapolate a line to estimate the oxygen uptake at other swimming speeds above and below the $\dot{V}O_2$max. The oxygen required above the $\dot{V}O_2$max is referred to as the oxygen deficit and is assumed to represent the anaerobic capacity during a maximal sprint swim. It is assumed, but not proven, that the swimmers with the greatest anaerobic capacity will have the largest O_2 deficit.

It is possible to calculate the swimmer's oxygen deficit or anaerobic capacity for the 100 m swim by the following equations:

$$O_2 \text{ deficit} = [(100 \text{ m time}) \times (\text{Est. } \dot{V}O_2)] - [100 \text{ m time}) \times (\dot{V}O_2\text{max})$$

Example:
$$= [0.92 \text{ min}) \times (78 \text{ ml/kg/min}$$
$$- [(0.92 \text{ min}) \times (58 \text{ ml/kg/min})]$$
$$= [71.8 \text{ ml/kg}] - [53.4 \text{ ml/kg}]$$
$$= 18.4 \text{ ml/kg} = O_2 \text{ deficit}$$

A second but less complex index of the swimmer's capacity for anaerobic effort can be obtained from a series of repeated short sprints with a reasonably long rest interval between bouts. Examples of such "anaerobic test sets" are as follows:

10 × 50 m with 90 s rest
or
5 × 100 m with 3 min rest

The average times for these maximal swims can be used as an index of the swimmer's tolerance for an anaerobic-sprint effort. Unlike the aerobic capacity, however, the swimmer's maximal O_2 deficit and changes in the anaerobic test sets show only small improvements with training. It is interesting to note that most of the adaptations occur during the first eight weeks of training, a surprising finding, since the swimmers generally continue to show improvements in performance throughout the final 16 weeks of training. This would suggest that either the tests for anaerobic and aerobic fitness are not sensitive to performance changes or that the improvements in performance are related to factors such as swimming skill.

Prior to puberty children have only limited ability to perform anaerobic types of activities. This fact is demonstrated by the child's inability to achieve the same blood or muscle lactate levels as observed in adults during submaximal and maximal rates of exercise. It has been shown that some of the key enzymes of glycolysis are lower in prepubescent boys than in adults. As a result, the child's muscle fibres are unable to generate large amounts of ATP by the anaerobic breakdown of glycogen, resulting in less lactate production and a more rapid depletion of available ATP and PCr. This diminished anaerobic capacity seems to be similar in both boys and girls, though it can be improved with training. From a coaching point of view, it should be realized that, although these young swimmers lack anaerobic capacity, their ability to perform aerobically does not appear to be diminished as a consequence of their age.

In conclusion, the use of blood lactate testing to gauge the training adaptations and for use as a tool in planning training regimens is still open to debate. Blood lactate measurements do not directly reflect the anaerobic activity of capacity of the muscle. When used in combination with other measurements, such as heart rate, perceived exertion (Borg, 1982) and training performance, blood lactate may provide an indication of the physiological stress imposed on the swimmer and his/her adaptations to training.

4 References

Borg, G.A.V. (1982) Psychophysical bases of perceived exertion. **Med. Sci. Sports Exerc.**, 14, 377-381.

Costill, D.L., Kovaleski, J., Porter, D., Kirwan, J., Fielding, R. and King, D. (1985) Energy expenditure during front crawl swimming: predicting success in middle-distance events. **Int. J. Sports Med.**, 6, 266-270.

Eriksson, B.O. (1972) Physical training, oxygen supply and muscle metabolisj in 11 to 13 year-old boys. **Acta Physiol. Scand.** (Suppl. 384).

Mader, A.H., Heck, H. and Hollmann, W. (1976) Evaluation of lactic acid anaerobic energy contribution by determination of post-exercise lactic acid concentration of ear capillary blood in middle distance runners and swimmers, in **Exercise Physiology** (eds F. Landry and W. Orban), Symposia Specialists Inc., Florida, pp. 187-189.

Medbø, J.I., Mohn, A-C., Tabata, I., Bahr, R., Vagge, O. and Sejersted, O.M. (1988) Anaerobic capacity determined by maximal accumulated O_2 deficit. **J. Appl. Physiol.**, 64, 50-60.

Sharp, R.L., Vitelli, C.A., Costill, D.L. and Thomas, R. (1984) Comparison between blood lactate and heart rate profiles during a season of competitive swim training. **J. Swimming Res.**, 1, 17-20.

PERFORMANCE DETERMINING FACTORS IN FRONT CRAWL SWIMMING

H.M. TOUSSAINT
Faculty of Human Movement Studies, Vrije Universiteit and
Universiteit van Amsterdam, Amsterdam, The Netherlands

Abstract
A biomechanical analysis of swimming taking into account the physiological basis of performance leads to the identification of several
performance determining factors. Swimming velocity (v) is related to
drag (A), power input (P_i, the rate of energy liberation via the
aerobic/anaerobic metabolism), the gross efficiency (e_g), propelling
efficiency (e_p), and power output (P_o) according to:

$$v = \sqrt[3]{\frac{e_g \cdot e_p \cdot P_i}{A}} \quad \text{or} \quad v = \sqrt[3]{\frac{e_p \cdot P_o}{A}}$$

Based on the research available at present it is concluded that:
- drag in groups of elite swimmers, homogeneous with respect to
  swimming technique, is determined by anthropometric dimensions
- aerobic power is only of moderate importance, since most races do
  not last long enough to make it a major concern
- gross efficiency is not different for groups differing in performance level
- propelling efficiency seems to be important since it is much higher
  in elite swimmers (61%) compared to triathletes (44%)
- total mechanical power output (P_o) is important since improvement
  in performance is related to increased P_o. Furthermore, it shows
  dramatic changes with training and possibly reflects the size of
  the 'swimming engine'.
Keywords: Power Output, Power Input, Propelling Efficiency, Gross
Efficiency, Distance Per Stroke, Training.

1 Introduction

An analysis of the demands which a particular swimming event places
on the body should form the basis for determining the training
programme, taking into consideration whatever deficiencies there may
be in the swimmer's resources or capabilities to meet these demands
(Åstrand and Rodahl, 1977). These capabilities or performance
factors can be improved with training; however, they are not all
equally important in the training process. Certain of these factors
are "weak links" in the performance chain and therefore assume a
position of greater concern. That is, they represent the phase of
the process where the performance system first becomes insufficient.

13

These are known as limiting or determining factors, because they are the first to reduce, and hence determine, performance (Maglischo, 1982). This could lead to the conclusion that the best form of swim training is competitive swimming, because then the greatest stress is put on the weakest factor needing the most improvement. However, it could be argued that training these factors in a somewhat isolated manner and overloading them maximally without interference from other processes, might improve each separately to a greater extent and then contribute more to performance when integrated with the other factors during a race. This makes it necessary to identify and assess the relative importance of the performance determining factors.

In a very broad sense the swimming performance is determined by the swimmer's capacity for energy output (aerobic and anaerobic processes), neuromuscular function (capacity of the muscle to generate force, to do work, and deliver power, coordination, and technique), joint mobility, and psychological factors (Åstrand and Rodahl, 1977). In this paper attention will be focussed on the first two factors as determinants of performance in **front crawl** swimming. Furthermore, since it is generally agreed that the arms provide more than 85% of the total thrust in the crawl stroke (Bucher, 1975; Faulkner, 1966; Hollander et al., 1988; Toussaint et al., 1990; Watkins and Gordon, 1983), attention will be focussed on the arms. An analysis of swimming from a biomechanical standpoint taking into account the physiological basis of performance will help to identify several performance determining factors.

2 Force, work, power and efficiency in swimming

2.1 Force
The success of a swimmer will be determined by the ability to gene-rate propulsive force while reducing the resistance to forward motion. This resistance or drag (F_d in N) is related to the square of the swimming velocity (v in m/s) (Clarys, 1979; Karpovich, 1933) according to:

$$F_d = A \cdot v^2 \tag{1}$$

where A is a constant of proportionality, being ±30 for males and ±24 for females in front crawl swimming (Karpovich, 1933; Toussaint et al., 1988b). To be able to swim at a constant speed the swimmer has to generate a propulsive force (F_p) to balance the drag force:

$$F_p = F_d \tag{2}$$

The maximal swimming velocity is attained when the maximal propulsive force is balanced by the opposing drag force. How this propulsive force depends on stroke technique and especially the use of lift forces has been explored by Schleihauf (Schleihauf, 1979; Schleihauf et al., 1983; Schleihauf et al., 1988). From this work it appears that the capacity to generate lift forces seems to distinguish the better swimmers from the poorer ones (Reischle, 1979; Schleihauf et al., 1988).

Although there is a direct relation between the mean propulsive force and the swimming speed, swimming, and especially swimming fast, is not just a matter of generating high propulsive forces. Swimming is a form of exercise in which the capacity of aerobic and anaerobic processes also determines success. So the question is not simply how to maximize the propulsive force, but rather how to achieve a high propulsive force with a finite metabolic capacity.

2.2 Work, power and propelling efficiency
When analyzing the energetics of swimming it is tempting to think that the work (J) the swimmer has to deliver is simply the drag force (F_d) times the distance (d) covered, or if we consider the time derivative of work, the mechanical power output of the swimmer has to be equal to the drag force times the swimming velocity. However, contrary to most on-land activities, where the push-off is performed against the earth, which for all practical purposes is not accelerated, the push off in swimming is made against water, which indeed will be accelerated (van Ingen Schenau and Cavanagh, 1990). The principle is illustrated in Fig. 1.

To generate a propulsive force, the swimmer gives a mass of water Σm_i a velocity change Δv_i in time T. The mean propulsive force will equal:

$$F_p = \frac{1}{T} \int_0^T F_p \, dt = \frac{1}{T} \Sigma m_i \cdot \Delta v_i \qquad (3)$$

where T equals the cycle time. The masses of water pushed away (Σm_i) have acquired a kinetic energy (E_k) in time T equal to:

$$E_k = \frac{1}{2} \Sigma m_i (\Delta v_i)^2 \qquad (4)$$

This energy is transferred from the swimmer to the water. It implies

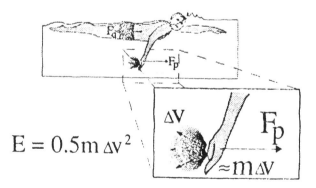

Fig. 1.   In swimming a fixed point to push off from is not available. The propulsive force is generated by pushing off against masses of water and will equal the impulse (mΔv) of the water that is pushed away. During the push off energy ($\frac{1}{2}$mΔv^2) is transferred from the swimmer to the water.

that part of the mechanical work the swimmer delivers during the push-off is expended in moving water (Charbonnier et al., 1975; Holmér, 1975; Miyashita, 1974). Hence, only a proportion of the total mechanical energy the swimmer delivers is used beneficially to overcome body drag. As was pointed out in the literature on the swimming of fish (Alexander and Goldspink, 1977; Bone, 1975; Webb, 1971a,b), and the design of swim fins (Lewis and Lorch, 1979; McMurray, 1977) the energy flow to the accelerated water should be included in the power 'book-keeping'. Hence, the total mechanical power (P_o) produced by the swimmer equals not only power to overcome drag (P_d) but also power expended in giving pushed away masses of water a kinetic energy change (P_k):

$$P_o = P_d + P_k \tag{5}$$

The ratio of the useful power (to overcome drag) to the total power output has been defined as the propelling efficiency (e_p) (Alexander and Goldspink, 1977; de Groot and van Ingen Schenau, 1988; Huijing et al., 1983; van Ingen Schenau and Cavanagh, 1990; Toussaint, 1990; Toussaint et al., 1988a):

$$e_p = \frac{P_d}{P_o} = \frac{P_d}{P_d + P_k} \tag{6}$$

Another approach to elucidate this phenomenon is to examine a free body diagram of a swimmer (see Fig. 2). The swimmer has to produce mechanical power to overcome the power he loses due to the drag force. This power lost to drag equals:

$$P_d = F_d \cdot v_b \cdot \cos(180°) \tag{7}$$

where v_b represents the velocity of the body, and cos 180° accounts for the opposite directions of the force and velocity vector. Since

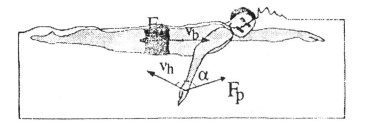

Fig. 2. Free body diagram of a swimmer at time t. F_p represents the propulsive force acting on the hand. F_d represents the drag force acting on the swimmer, v_h and v_b represent the respective velocities of the point of application of the forces. See text for further explanation.

$\cos(180°) = -1$, P_d will be negative, indicating the loss of power the swimmer has to compensate. The same principle holds for the propulsive force; again it can be observed that the force and velocity vector have approximate opposite directions. Hence, the swimmer also loses power to the water during the push-off (as was explained in the above) equal to:

$$P_k = F_p \cdot v_h \cdot \cos(\alpha) \tag{8}$$

where v_h is the velocity of the hand and α the angle between the force and velocity vector. It is interesting to observe that when the push-off is made using only 'drag propulsion', α will be 180° and hence $\cos(\alpha)$ will be -1. As more 'lift propulsion' is used, α will approach 90°, resulting in $\cos(\alpha)$ nearing zero. This implies that more lift propulsion should lead to decreasing values of P_k, hence increasing the propelling efficiency (de Groot and van Ingen Schenau, 1988).

The mechanical power output (P_o) of the swimmer is dependent on the rate at which aerobic and anaerobic metabolism liberate energy from the storage compounds. This latter is the power input (P_i) of the 'swimming engine'. If the total power input is fixed then the swimming velocity will depend on three major factors:

1. The rate of energy liberation (P_i) necessary to generate mechanical power output (P_o). This can be expressed in terms of a ratio, which is the gross efficiency (e_g):

$$e_g = \frac{P_o}{P_i} \quad \text{Hence,} \quad P_o = e_g \cdot P_i \tag{9}$$

2. The effective apportionment of this power output to power to overcome drag (the propelling efficiency):

$$P_d = e_p \cdot P_o \tag{10}$$

3. The relation between the swimming velocity (v) and the power required to overcome drag (P_d):

$$P_d = F_d \cdot v \text{ with } F_d = A \cdot v^2 \tag{11}$$

Hence,

$$P_d = e_g \cdot e_p \cdot P_i \tag{12}$$

and

$$v = \sqrt[3]{\frac{e_g \cdot e_p \cdot P_i}{A}} \quad \text{or} \quad v = \sqrt[3]{\frac{e_p \cdot P_o}{A}}$$

As a result of this analysis it seems as if the swimming velocity is determined by five major factors: the drag (A), the power input (P_i) (aerobic/anaerobic metabolism), the gross efficiency (e_g), the propelling efficiency (e_p), and the power output (P_o). This is visualised in Fig. 3.

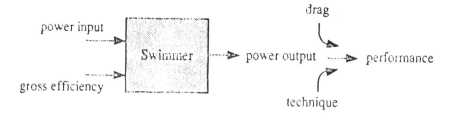

Fig. 3. Diagram indicating five performances determining factors of
swimming.

3.1 Drag

A high propulsive force will not in itself lead to a high swimming
velocity. The drag force retards the motion of the swimmer and
several authors have suggested that these resistive forces must be
reduced by improving swimming technique (Bober and Czabanski, 1975;
Counsilman, 1968; Maglischo, 1982). This leads to the hypothesis
that elite swimmers have lower resistive forces at high swimming
velocities than poorer ones. To verify this hypothesis it is
necessary to determine the resistive forces to which the swimmer is
exposed while stroking. For the measurement of this so-called **active
drag,** different methods have been used; for reviews and discussions
of these methods see Clarys (1979), Hay (1988), Miller (1975) and
Vaart et al. (1987). Recently the MAD–system has been introduced as
a system to measure active drag; for an extensive description see
Hollander et al. (1986) and Toussaint et al. (1988a). Although the
application and possible limitations of the MAD system to the
measurement of active drag in front crawl swimming are still open to
discussion (Hay, 1988), it is, in the author's view, the best of
several alternatives available for the estimation of drag force
during front crawl swimming.

In one of the first experiments using the MAD–system attention was
paid to the proposed hypothesis and the relationship between drag and
maximal swimming performance was investigated (Hollander et al.,
1985). Active drag was determined in both a group of 12 female and
12 male elite swimmers at high velociites (1.63 and 1.86 m/s respectively). As no significant correlations were found (males $r = -0.27$,
females $r = 0.77$, see Fig. 4) it was concluded that drag per se is
not a performance determining factor of the maximal swimming speed.

In the literature, however, it has often been claimed that good
swimmers have an advantageous body build with respect to drag. For
instance Cureton (1975) reported that the "tall slim type has been
shown to glide better through the water". In addition several others
noted that swimmers are taller than the mean population, suggesting a
performance advantage with increasing height (Andrew et al., 1972;
Faulkner, 1968; Marconnet et al., 1978; Nomura, 1983). Furthermore,
Kunski et al. (1988) observed in a longitudinal study that a relation
exists between growth rate and the improvement in performance. These
observations warranted further research into the relation between
drag and morphology, although the first extensive studies in this
area by Clarys (1979) yielded few relations between human morphology
and active drag.

In cooperation with Clarys and using the MAD system the relation

18

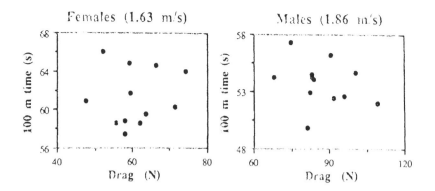

Fig. 4. Performance expressed as 100 m time is presented dependent
on drag measured at a velocity of 1.63 m/s for females
(n = 12) and 1.86 m/s for males (n = 12).

between morphology and active drag was re-evaluated (Huijing et al.,
1988). This time significant correlations were shown to exist
between selected anthropometric variables and active drag.
Especially notable was the high degree of correlation of the maximal
body cross-section (r = 0.87) and active drag. In another study
using the MAD-system the drag values for male and female swimmers
were compared (Toussaint et al., 1988b). The higher drag values in
the males ($F_d = 30$ v^2 versus $F_d = 24$ v^2 for the females) could be
related to a larger body cross-section (0.091 m^2 males versus 0.075
m^2 females. However, in that study the observed groups were
homogeneous with respect to height. Therefore, a longitudinal study
(2.5 years, Toussaint et al., 1990b) of a group of growing children
was undertaken (mean age at the start 12.9 years). In this study the
hypothesis was tested that an increase in body dimensions (especially
the body cross-sectional area) as occurs during growth would result
in a corresponding increase of drag during swimming. However, while
the body cross-sectional area of the chlldren increased in size by
16%, no differences in total drag were detected (1985; 30.1 $\pm$ 2.37 N
vs 1988: 30.8 $\pm$ 4.50 N).

This unexpected result was explained by the fact that the total
drag force (F_d) in swimming is not only determined by the pressure
drag (F_p) but consists of two more components: friction drag (F_f) and
wave-making resistance (F_w). Hence:

$$F_d = F_p + F_f + F_w \qquad (14)$$

The first component (F_p) which dominates at the prevailing high
Reynold's number R_e of 22 $\times$ 10^6 - 2.5 $\times$ 10^6 (Clarys, 1979) will be
determined mainly by the body cross-sectional area.

The friction drag (F_f) will be dependent on the friction between
skin and water and will theoretically increase somewhat since the
total skin surface will increase (but see also Toussaint et al.,
1989). Hence this component could not explain the unchanged total
drag value.

The wave making resistance (F_w) is the result of the deformation
of the surface in which the water tends to pile up in front of the

swimmer and form hollows behind, thus initiating a wave system. At higher velocities a significant bow-wave develops (Alley, 1952), which could indicate the wave drag contributes considerably to total drag (Miller, 1975). This seems especially the case when one is swimming near the 'hull speed', a concept used in shipbuilding introduced into human swimming by Miller. It is the maximum speed that is reached when the wavelength of the bow wave and the water-line length of the hull are equal (Miller, 1975). A longer hull (increased height) would make a higher swimming speed possible.

The suggested relation between height and wave drag finds its expression in the Froude number (F_r) which depends in human swimming on the height of the swimmer as shown in equation 15.

$$F_r = \frac{v}{\sqrt{g \cdot l}} \tag{15}$$

where v represents swimming velocity, l height of the swimmer, and g represents the acceleration due to gravity (9.81 m s^{-2}).

This implies that a decrease in F_r will lower the wave making resistance. Thus in the growing children the increase in height (from 1.52 to 1.69 m) resulted in a decrease in F_r (from 0.324 to 0.308 at a swimming velocity of 1.25 m/s) and hence in a decrease in wave making resistance. In Fig. 5 the mean drag curves for the whole group are related to speed. Again it is clear that the drag has not changed. When the same drag data are presented with respect to the Froude number (Fig. 5), hence correcting for a change in height, it appears that the drag had increased. If the drag is calculated for a Froude number of 0.324 (1985: v = 1.25 m/s) it gives a drag of 20.1 N in 1985 and a value of 34.6 N in 1988. The increase of 15% is about the increase in size of the body cross-sectional area. The suggestion that the increase in pressure drag was compensated by a decrease in wave making resistance is in line with the common notion that taller swimmers seem to have an advantage for a good (front crawl) swimming performance. Furthermore, form indices derived from ship-building technology, demonstrated changes that indicated a more 'streamlined' body form. Therefore, it was concluded that during growth a complex process takes place in which different factors determining drag, such as height, body shape and body cross-sectional area, change in directions that have opposite effects on drag.

To these conclusions should perhaps be added that an improved technique could result in lower drag values. Support for this latter idea was obtained in an experiment in which triathletes were compared to swimmers (Toussaint, 1990). A considerable difference in performance was found and, among other performance determining factors, this difference was attributed to a difference in the coefficient A (formula $F_d = A \cdot v^2$, see equation 1), which was 30.5 for the competitive swimmers and 41.6 for the triathletes. This could be explained as being a result of the poorer technique of the triathletes causing more body movements in the vertical and horizontal plane perpendicular to the swimming velocity (Bober and Czabanski, 1975; Counsilman, 1968; Maglischo, 1982). In other words the competitive swimmers were able to use a more symmetrical stroking pattern which gives a more stable body position and hence smaller A.

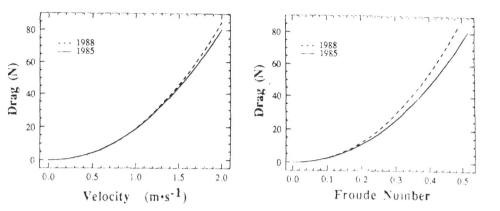

Fig. 5. Drag is presented for the whole group dependent on velocity
         (left panel) and dependent on the Froude Number (right
         panel).

The question of whether drag is a major performance determining
factor cannot be finally resolved on the basis of the research at
present available. It seems as if drag in groups of elite swimmers,
homogeneous with respect to swimming technique, is determined by
anthropometric dimensions (e.g. body cross-sectional area and
height). Probably a small reduction in drag can be achieved by
stretching the arm in the glide-phase of the stroke, as was suggested
by Holmér (1979a). The body cross-sectional area is especially
reduced when the shoulder is 'stretched behind the arm'. Furthermore, stretching 'elongates the body', possibly resulting in reduced
wave resistance (Larsen et al., 1981).
    Most importantly, the poorer swimmer should concentrate on
developing a symmetrical stroking pattern in which body movements
perpendicular to the swimming direction are minimized.

3.2 Power input
Swimming is a form of exercise in which the capacity to generate
mechanical power seems to be an important performance determining
factor. This power is generated by the liberation of energy in
aerobic and anaerobic processes. An overview of the power 'book-
keeping' is presented in Fig. 6.
    It will be obvious that in swimming events of longer duration, the
ability to consume oxygen will be an important determinant of the
swimming velocity. It is therefore not surprising that elite
swimmers are distinguished by high rates of oxygen uptake ($\dot{V}O_2max$)
(Holmér, 1979b; Holmér et al., 1974). Charbonnier et al (1975) found
correlations between the $\dot{V}O_2max$ (arm cranking) and the cubed swimming
velocity for the 400 and 1500 m of r = 0.9 and 0.91 respectively.
Costill et al. (1985b) reported a correlation of 0.80 between $\dot{V}O_2max$
(swimming) and swimming velocity during a 365.8 m (400 yard) swim;
however, no statistical difference in $\dot{V}O_2max$ was found between the
significantly slower recreational swimmers and the competitive
swimmers.

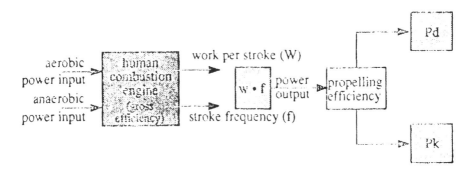

Fig. 6. Overview of the power book-keeping during swimming.

The fact that 50, 100 and 200 m events dominate competitive swimming events might be the basis for the common notion that $\dot{V}O_2$max is unrelated to swim performance in elite homogeneous groups (Handel et al., 1988) and that performance determining aspects in swimming should be sought in factors other than oxygen uptake (Kipke, 1978).

In a retrospective study Gullstrand and Holmér (1983) observed that the maximal oxygen uptake of top athletes today is no higher than that of athletes 20 years ago; nevertheless, there is an obvious difference in performances (see also Holmér, 1983). In this context Maglischo (1982) concluded: "Although optimizing maximal aerobic capacity is important, most races do not last long enough to make this a major concern.

3.3 Gross efficiency
Differences in performance might be due to differences in the rate of metabolic energy production (power input, P_i) necessary for a **measured** mechanical power output (P_o). The gross efficiency (e_g) quantifies this process and has been defined as the mechanical power output (P_o) with respect to the rate of energy expenditure or power input (P_i) (van Ingen Schenau and Cavanagh, 1990; Miller, 1975; Toussaint et al., 1990a):

$$e_g = \frac{P_o}{P_i} \qquad (16)$$

The measurement of the true gross efficiency requires both the measurement of P_i and P_o. At submaximal swimming speeds the power input of the swimmer is reflected by the power equivalence of the oxygen uptake. The quantification of the power output in swimming is rather complicated. As was explained in an earlier section, some energy is transferred to the water with each stroke. To circumvent this problem the MAD-system (Hollander et al., 1986) was used. The MAD-system allows the swimmer to push off from fixed push-off points at each stroke. Hence, no power is expended in giving water a kinetic energy change as in normal free swimming and so $P_o = P_d$. The MAD-system is equipped to measure P_d. This method (see for details Toussaint, 1990; Toussaint et al., 1988a; Toussaint et al., 1990a) was used to evaluate the significance of the gross efficiency as a performance determining factor in swimming.

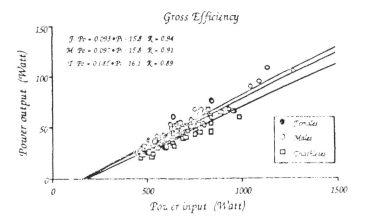

Fig. 7.   The power output is given in relation to the power input for
           for females, males and triathletes. The regression
           equations and coefficient of correlation (r) are given.

Three highly trained groups - a group of male competitive
swimmers, a group of female competitive swimmers and a group of
triathletes (Toussaint, 1990; Toussaint et al., 1990a) - were
compared. The results of the simultaneous measurement of P_o and P_i
for the three groups are presented in Fig. 7. No differences in
regression equations were found between the three groups. This in
accordance with the results of Charbonnier et al. (1975), who
reported no difference in gross efficiency between swimmer and non-
swimmers. These results seem to be in contrast to previous work
where differences were found between swimmers of different
performance level (Adrian et al., 1966; Anderson, 1960; Holmér, 1972;
Karpovich and Millman, 1944; Pendergast et al., 1977; di Prampero et
al., 1974). However, in these studies the mechanical power output
used in the calculation of efficiency was only that power used to
overcome drag, ignoring the power expended in moving water (see for
detailed discussion Toussaint et al., 1988a; Toussaint et al.,
1990a). Thus the lower efficiency values observed were probably due
to the additional P_k produced by the subjects. The differences
between good and poor swimmers might be due to a difference in the
amount of P_k spent by good and bad swimmers, hence to a difference in
propelling efficiency.

3.4 Propelling efficiency
A first attempt was made to evaluate the significance of the
propelling efficiency in swimming (Toussaint, 1990). Two highly
trained endurance groups - competitive swimmers (N = 6); and
triathletes (N = 5, one of them the European champion and world
record holder) - were compared. With the aid of individual
determined regression equations the groups were compared at equal
levels of energy expenditure representing a power input of
1000 Watt ($\pm$ 2.861 l O_2/min). Hence every subject of both groups was
provided with an equal amount of power input into the 'swimming
engine' (see Table 1).

Table 1. Competitive swimmers compared to triathletes when both
exercise at a power input level of 1000 Watt
(± 2.861 1 O_2/min), see Toussaint (1990).

		Competitive swimmers		Triathletes		t-value	p
		X	sd	X	sd		
Power input	(Watt)	1000	(-)	1000	(-)	-	-
Swimming velocity	(m/s)	1.17	(0.08)	0.95	(0.11)	3.87	0.004
Power output	(Watt)	81.3	(9.4)	80.4	(14.5)	0.13	n.s.
Power to drag	(Watt)	49.1	(3.4)	35.3	(8.2)	3.76	0.004
Power to water	(Watt)	32.3	(8.1)	45.1	(6.6)	-2.83	0.020
Propelling efficiency	(%)	60.8	(6.1)	43.6	(3.4)	5.61	0.00
Gross efficiency	(%)	8.13	(0.94)	8.04	(1.45)	0.13	n.s.
Distance per stroke	(m)	2.46	(0.42)	1.84	(0.46)	2.33	0.045
Stroke frequency	(s)	0.48	(0.09)	0.53	(0.13)	-0.82	n.s.
Work per stroke	(J)	172	(38.2)	152	(28.4)	0.96	n.s.

What can be observed from the results in Table 1 is that at an
equal level of power input (oxyen uptake) the triathletes could swim
at a velocity of 0.95 m/s. At this same level of power input the
competitive swimmers did 1.17 m/s, 23% faster. This difference could
not be explained by a difference in gross efficiency, stroke frequency, or work per stroke. But there was a difference in distance per
stroke (2.46 vs 1.894 m). This was due to a difference in the propelling efficiency, 44% for the triathletes and 61% for the swimmers.
In other words, the competitive swimmers used 61% of the work per
stroke to overcome drag, while only 39% was converted into kinetic
energy of the water during the push-off. Therefore, the competitive
swimmers were able to cover a greater distance per stroke compared to
the triathletes who in contrast wasted 56% of the available energy
per stroke in moving water.

These results do underline the importance of the propelling efficiency as a possible performance determining factor in swimming.
However, before this conclusion can be drawn with confidence, the
study should be replicated using a more homogeneous group of competitive swimmers. Furthermore, research must be focussed on the relation between technique and propelling efficiency, where special
attention should be paid to the notion that wasted power associated
with generating lift forces is considerably less than the power in
generating drag forces (Alexander and Golspink, 1977; de Groot and
van Ingen Schenau, 1988; van Ingen Schenau and Cavanagh, 1990). The
development of training programmes to improve propelling efficiency
seems to have great practical relevance.

3.4.1 Distance per stroke
Since a close relation was observed between propelling efficiency and
distance per stroke it is interesting to elaborate this relation
mathematically. Using equation (10) ($P_d = e_p \cdot P_o$) and (11) ($P_d = F_d \cdot v$ with $F_d = A \cdot v_2$) it can be derived that:

$$A \cdot v^3 = e_p \cdot P_o \qquad (17)$$

The velocity (v) equals the stroke frequency (f) times the distance per stroke (d), hence:

$$d^3 \cdot f^3 = \frac{e_p \cdot P_o}{A} \qquad (18)$$

The power output P_o equals work per stroke (W) times stroke frequency (f), giving:

$$d^3 = \frac{e_p \cdot W \cdot f}{A \cdot f^3} \qquad (19)$$

yielding the relation for distance per stroke:

$$d = \sqrt[3]{\frac{e_p \cdot W}{A \cdot f^2}} \qquad (20)$$

The distance per stroke seems to be related to the propelling efficiency and the work per stroke the swimmer delivers. This is interesting since the notion that the better swimmer distinguishes himself from the poorer one by a greater distance per stroke is widely accepted (Costill et al., 1985b; Craig et al., 1979; Craig and Pendergast, 1979; Craig and Pendergast, 1980; Craig et al., 1985; East, 1971; Hay and Guimaraes, 1983; Reischle, 1979; Swaine and Reilly, 1983; Toussaint et al., 1983). Also, the difference in speed between male and female swimmers is mainly due to a bigger distance per stroke (East, 1971; Letzelter and Freitag, 1983; Pai et al., 1984). Furthermore, the increase in speed with increasing age depends mainly on the increase in the distance covered during each stroke (Miyashita, 1975; Saito, 1982). In theory (de Groot and van Ingen Schenau, 1988), both propelling efficiency and distance per stroke are improving when the propulsion is mainly based on 'lift propulsion'. Indeed several researchers have provided experimental evidence that lift is the preferred source of propulsion (Barthels and Adrian, 1974; Schleihauf, 1974; 1979; Schleihauf et al., 1983; Schleihauf et al., 1988), while Reischle (1979) has reported that better swimmers do actually rely more on lift propulsion. Although the exact relationship between propelling efficiency, distance per stroke and lift propulsion remains to be determined, it seems reasonable to conclude that the distance per stroke gives an indication of the propelling efficiency, and can be used to evaluate individual progress in technical ability.

3.5 Power output

The 'human combustion engine' converts the power input (aerobic and anaerobic) into mechanical power output (see Fig. 6). The importance of the power output of the arms is outlined in studies in which improvements in swimming performance were associated with increased power output (Charbonnier et al., 1975; Costill et al., 1983; Costill et al., 1985a; Sharp et al., 1982; Toussaint and Vervoorn, 1990). Although in this section power output is discussed, it is interesting to come back to the discussion concerning the $\dot{V}O_2$max in the context of competitive swimming. In some studies it was observed that the $\dot{V}O_2$max swimming arms only, did change with training, whereas the

$\dot{V}O_2$max determined in the same subjects using conventional methods (treadmill, bicycle) remained the same (Holmér, 1974; Holmér and Åstrand, 1972). Gergley et al. (1984) compared the effects of swim exercise versus treadmill exercise. The results support the specificity of aerobic improvement with training and suggest that local adaptations contribute significantly to improvements in peak $\dot{V}O_2$. As pointed out earlier, the major part of the propulsion in front crawl swimming is produced by the arms. Therefore, it is reasonable to assume that the 'combustion engine' of the swimmer is mainly 'located' in the trunk and arm muscles. This could imply that the **maximum capacity** ($\dot{V}O_2$max) of the specific 'swimming combustion engine' is not determined by central circulatory factors, as may be the case in treadmill running, but rather by the amount and quality of the muscle mass used in swimming. Conversely this could imply that the limiting factor in the production of **mechanical power output** is the quantity and quality of the 'propelling muscles' rather than the capacity to transport oxygen to the working muscles (Holmér, 1974).

The results of a study concerning the effects of a year's training on different performance determining factors (Toussaint et al., in preparation) might substantiate this idea. In a group of elite swimmers (N = 11, see Table 2) the effect of training was evaluated approximately every six weeks (June–June). Maximal oxygen uptake while swimming, maximal power output (Watts) of the arms (MAD-system), and stroke characteristics (indicating propelling efficiency) were measured.

Table 2. Anthropometric and performance data of elite swimmers.

	Males (N = 6)	Females (N = 5)
Height (m)	1.85 ± 0.08	1.85 ± 0.02
Weight (kg)	79.6 ± 9.8	72.6 ± 8.6
$\dot{V}O_2$max (l/min)	4.83 ± 0.5	4.01 ± 0.2
100 m time (s)	53.4 ± 1.4	56.7 ± 1.3

The maximal power output of the arms showed significant ($P < 0.05$) changes during the season, which seemed to be related to training volume. The overall increase in power output was 18% ($P < 0.01$). The maximal oxygen uptake increased 4% ($P < 0.05$) over the period December to June. The stroke characteristic showed no change.

Expressed in percentage of change, the power output of the arms demonstrated the greatest response to training, 18% increase in one year. In this group of highly trained swimmers (among them three Olympic medal winners) this was a surprising result. It underlines the importance of the capacity of the arms to generate power output in relation to swimming performance.

The design of the experiment was such that it was not possible to relate the increase in $\dot{V}O_2$max while swimming directly to the size and quality of the arm musculature (the propelling engine). However, it was noticeable that during the 'aerobic phase' of the training (September/December) the $\dot{V}O_2$max did not change significantly, and showed a tendency to get lower. In the training period in which more high intensity work was done (January–March) and especially in the

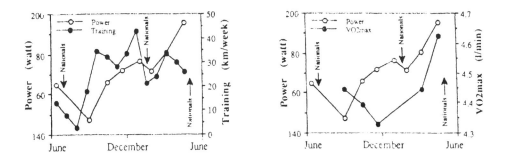

Fig. 8. Power output of the arms measured during one year of
training, in relation to training volume (left panel)
and the power output in relation to the $\dot{V}O_2$max
measured while swimming (right panel).

period after the short course Nationals (April–June), in which period
the training intensity was strongly increased at the expense of
training volume, both $\dot{V}O_2$max and power output did significantly
increase. This is in line with Neufer et al. (1987) who observed
increased values for $\dot{V}O_2$max after five months of training which were
no longer elevated when training was reduced. This was associatd
with a reduction in swim power and distance per stroke.

4 Conclusion

Swimming velocity is determined by the drag (A), the power input (P_i)
(aerobic/anaerobic metabolism), the gross efficiency (e_g), the propelling efficiency (e_p) and the power output (P_o). The gross efficiency seems to be of relatively little importance, since no differences in e_g were observed between three groups differing in performance level. With respect to drag and aerobic power, a distinction
must be made between young inexperienced and elite swimmers. While
training, the young swimmers should try to reduce drag by reducing
body movements perpendicular to the swimming direction. Furthermore,
they should optimize their maximal aerobic power. In groups of elite
swimmers, homogeneous with respect to swimming technique, drag is
determined by anthropometric dimensions. The aerobic power seems to
be of less concern. This is in contrast to both propelling
efficiency and power output. Considerable differences in values for
propelling efficiency were observed between groups differing in
swimming performance, suggesting that considerable training time
should be devoted to technique training. The distance per stroke can
be helpful in this respect, since it gives an indication of the
propelling efficiency, and can be used to evaluate individual
progress in technical ability. Furthermore, the capacity of the arms
to generate power output is possibly the most important factor
determining performance. It shows considerable improvement with
training and decline with detraining. Hence, training should focus
on the improvement of the power output of the 'swimming engine'. The
application of a recently developed water based training device
(Toussaint and Vervoorn, 1990) could help to achieve this objective.

5 Acknowledgement

Grateful acknowledgement is given to Michiel P. de Loose, A. Peter Hollander, Gerrit Jan van Ingen Schenau, and Tony Sargeant for their critical reading of the manuscript.

6 References

Adrian, M.J., Singh, M. and Karpovich, P.V. (1966) Energy cost of leg kick, arm stroke, and whole crawl stroke. **J. Appl. Physiol.**, 21, 1763-1766.

Alexander, R.M. and Goldspink, G. (1977) **Mechanics and Energetics of Animal Locomotion.** Chapman and Hall, London.

Alley, L.E. (1952) An analysis of water resistance and propulsion in swimming the crawl stroke. **Res. Quart.**, 23, 253-270.

Andersen, K.L. (1960) Energy cost of swimming. **Acta Chir. Scand. Suppl.**, 253, 169-174.

Andrew, G.M., Becklake, M.R., Glueria, J.S. and Bates, D.V. (1972) Heart and lung functions in swimmers and nonathletes during growth. **J. Appl. Physiol.**, 32, 245-251.

Åstrand, P.O. and Rodahl, K. (1977) **Textbook of Work Physiology.** McGraw-Hill, New York.

Barthels, K. and Adrian, M.J. (1974) Three dimensional spatial hand patterns of skilled butterfly swimmers, in **Swimming II** (eds J.P. Clarys and L. Lewillie), University Park Press, Baltimore, pp. 154-160.

Bober, T. and Czabanski, B. (1975) Changes in breaststroke techniques under different speed conditions, in **Swimming II** (eds J.P. Clarys and L. Lewillie), University Park Press, Baltimore, pp. 188-193.

Bone, Q. (1975) **Muscular and energetic aspects of fish swimming.** Plenum Press, New York.

Bucher, W. (1975) The influence of the leg kick and the arm stroke on the total speed during the crawl stroke, in **Swimming II** (eds J.P. Clarys and L.P. Lewillie), University Park Press, Baltimore, pp. 180-187.

Charbonnier, J.P., Lacour, J.R., Riffat, J. and Flandrois, R. (1975) Experimental study of the performance of competition swimmers. **Eur. J. Appl. Physiol.**, 34, 157-167.

Clarys, J.P. (1979) Human morphology and hydrodynamics, in **Swimming III** (eds J. Terauds and E.W. Bedingfield), University Park Press, Baltimore, pp. 3-43.

Costill, D.L., King, D.S., Holdren, A. and Hargreaves, M. (1983) Spring speed vs swimming power. **Swimming Technique**, 20, 20-22.

Costill, D.L., King, D.S., Thomas, R. and Hargreaves, M. (1985a) Muscle strength and the taper. **Swimming Technique**, 22, 23-26.

Costill, D.L., Kovaleski, J., Porter, D., Kirwan, J., Fielding, R. and King, D. (1985b) Energy expenditure during front crawl swimming; predicting success in middle-distance events. **Int. J. Sports Med.**, 6, 266-270.

Counsilman, J.E. (1968) **Science of Swimming.** Prentice-Hall, Englewood Cliffs, N.J.

Craig, A.B., Boomer, W.L. and Gibbons, J.F. (1979) Use of stroke rate, distance per stroke, and velocity relationships during training for competitive swimming, in **Swimming III** (eds J. Terauds and E.W. Bedingfield), University Park Press, Baltimore, pp.

265-274.

Craig, A.B. and Pendergast, D.R. (1979) Relationships of stroke rate, distance per stroke, and velocity in competitive swimming. **Med. Sci. Sports Exerc.**, 11, 278-283.

Criag, A.B. and Pendergast, D.R. (1980) Relationships of stroke rate, distance per stroke, and velocity in competitive swimming. **Swimming Technique,** 17, 23-29.

Craig, A.B., Skehan, P.L., Pawelczyk, J.A. and Boomer, W.L. (1985) Velocity, stroke rate, and distance per stroke during elite swimming competition. **Med. Sci. Sports Exerc.**, 17, 625-634.

Cureton, T.K. (1975) Factors governing success in competitive swimming: A brief review of related studies, in **Swimming II** (eds J.P. Clarys and L. Lewillie), University Park Press, Baltimore, pp. 9-39.

East, D.J. (1971) Stroke frequency, length and performance. **Swimming Technique,** 8, 68-73.

Faulkner, J.A. (1966) Physiology of swimming. **Res. Quart.,** 37, 41-54.

Faulkner, J.A. (1968) Physiology of swimming and diving, in **Exercise Physiology** (ed H.B. Falls), Academic Press, New York, pp. 415-446.

Gergley, T.J., McArdle, W.D., DeJesus, P., Toner, M.M., Jacobowitz, S. and Spina, R.J. (1984) Specificity of arm training on aerobic power during swimming and running. **Med. Sci. Sports Exerc.**, 16, 349-354.

Groot, G. de and Ingen Schenau, G.J. van (1988) Fundamental mechanics applied to swimming: Technique and propelling efficiency, in **Swimming Science V** (eds B.E. Ungerechts, K. Wilke and K. Reischle), Human Kinetics Books, Champaign, Ill., pp. 17-30.

Gullstrand, L. and Holmér, I. (1983) Physiological characteristics of champion swimmers during a five-year follow-up period, in **Biomechanics and Medicine in Swimming** (eds A.P. Hollander, P.A. Huijing and G. de Groot), Human Kinetics Publishers, Champaign, Ill., pp. 258-262.

Handel, P.J. van, Katz, A., Morrow, J.R., Troup, J.P., Daniels, J.T. and Bradley, P.W. (1988) Aerobic economy and competitive perform-ance of U.S. elite swimmers, in **Swimming Science V** (eds B. Ungerechts, K. Wilke and K. Reischle), Human Kinetics Books, Champaign, Ill., pp. 219-227.

Hay, J.G. (1988) The status of research on the biomechanics of swimming, in **Swimming Science V** (eds B.E. Ungerechts, K. Wilke and K. Reischle), Human Kinetics Books, Champaign, Ill., pp. 3-14.

Hay, J.G. and Guimaraes, A.C.S. (1983) A quantitative look at swimming biomechanics. **Swimming Technique,** 20, 11-17.

Hollander, A.P., Groot, G. de, Ingen Schenau, G.J. van, Kahman, R. and Toussaint, H.M. (1988) Contribution of the legs to propulsion in front crawl swimming, in **Swimming Science V** (eds B.E. Ungerechts, K. Wilke and K. Reischle), Human Kinetics Books, Champaign, Ill., pp. 39-43.

Hollander, A.P., Groot, G. de, Ingen Schenau, G.J. van, Toussaint, H.M., Best, H. de, Peeters, W., Meulemans, A. and Schreurs, A.W. (1986) Measurement of active drag forces during swimming. **J. Sports Sci.,** 4, 21-30.

Hollander, A.P., Toussaint, H.M., Groot, G. de and Ingen Schenau, G.J. van (1985) Active drag and swimming performance. **New Zealand J. Sports Med.,** 13, 110-113.

Holmér, I. (1972) Oxygen uptake during swimming in man. J. Appl. Physiol., 33, 502-509.

Holmér, I. (1974) Physiology of swimming man. Acta Physiol. Scand. Suppl., 407c.

Holmér, I. (1975) Efficiency of breaststroke, and freestyle swimming, in Swimming II (eds J.P. Clarys and L. Lewillie), University Park Press, Baltimore, pp. 130-136.

Holmér, I. (1979a) Analysis of acceleration as a measure of swimming proficiency, in Swimming III (eds J. Terauds and E.W. Bedingfield), University Park Press, Baltimore, pp. 118-125.

Holmér, I. (1979b) Physiology of swimming man, in Exercise and Sport Sciences Reviews (eds R.S. Hutton and D.I. Miller), The Franklin Institute Press, Philadelphia, pp. 87-123.

Holmér, I. (1983) Energetics and mechanical work in swimming, in Biomechanics and Medicine in Swimming (eds A.P. Hollander, P.A. Huijing and G. de Groot), Human Kinetics Publishers, Champaign, Ill., pp. 154-164.

Holmér, I. and Åstrand, P.-O. (1972) Swimming training and maximal oxygen uptake. J. Appl. Physiol., 33, 510-513.

Holmér, I., Lundin, A. and Eriksson, B.O. (1974) Maximum oxygen uptake during swimming and running by elite swimmers. J. Appl. Physiol., 36, 711-714.

Huijing, P.A., Hollander, A.P. and Groot, G. de (1983) Efficiency and specificity of training in swimming: an editorial, in Biomechanics and Medicine in Swimming (eds A.P. Hollander, P.A. Huijing and G. de Groot), Human Kinetics Publishers, Champaign, Ill., pp. 1-6.

Huijing, P.A., Toussaint, H.M., Clarys, J.P., Groot, G. de, Hollander, A.P., Vervoorn, K., Mackay, R. and Savelberg, H.H.C.M. (1988) Active drug related to body dimensions, in Swimming Science V (eds B.E. Ungerechts, K. Wilke and K. Reischle), Human Kinetics Books, Champaign, Ill., pp. 31-37.

Ingen Schenau, G.J. van and Cavanagh, P.R. (1990) Power equations in endurance sports. J. Biomech., 23, 865-881.

Karpovich, P.V. (1933) Water resistance in swimming. Res. Quart., 4, 21-28.

Karpovich, P.V. and Millman, N. (1944) Energy expenditure in swimming. Am. J. Physiol., 142, 140-144.

Kipke, L. (1978) Dynamics of oxygen intake during step-by-step loading in a swimming flume, in Swimming Medicine IV (eds B. Eirksson and B. Furberg), University Park Press, Baltimore, pp. 137-142.

Kunski, H., Jegier, A., Malankiewicz, A. and Rakus, E. (1988) The relationship of biological factors to swimming performance in top Polish junior swimmers aged 12 to 14 years, in Swimming Science V (eds B.E. Ungerechts, K. Wilke and K. Reischle), Human Kinetics Books, Champaign, Ill., pp. 109-113.

Larsen, O.W., Yancher, R.P. and Bear, C.L.H. (1981) Boat design and swimming performance. Swimming Technique, 18, 38-44.

Letzelter, H. and Freitag, W. (1983) Stroke length and stroke frequency variations in men's and women's 100 m freestyle swimming, in Biomechanics and Medicine in Swimming (eds A.P. Hollander, P.A. Huijing and G. de Groot), Human Kinetics Publishers, Champaign, Ill., pp. 315-322.

Lewis, E.R. and Lorch, D. (1979) Swim fin design utilizing principles of marine animal locomotion, in Swimming III (eds J. Terauds and

E.   :rgfield), University Park Press, Baltimore, pp. 289-297.

Maglischo, E.W. (1982) **Swimming Faster**. Mayfield Publishing Co., Palo Alto.

Marconnet, P., Spinel, W., Gastaud, M. and Ardisson, J.L. (1978) Evaluation of some physiological parameters in swimming school students during a two year period, in **Swimming Medicine IV** (eds B. Eriksson and B. Furberg), University Park Press, Baltimore, pp. 161-169.

McMurray, R.G. (1977) Comparative efficiencies of conventional and super-swimfin designs. **Human Factors**, 19, 495-501.

Miller, D.I. (1975) Biomechanics of swimming, in **Exercise and Sport Sciences Reviews** (eds J.H. Wilmore and J.F. Keogh), Academic Press, New York, pp. 219-248.

Miyashita, M. (1974) Method of calculating mechanical power in swimming the breast stroke. **Res. Quart.**, 45, 128-137.

Miyashita, M. (1975) Arm action in the crawl stroke, in **Swimming II** (eds J.P. Clarys and L. Lewillie), University Park Press, Baltimore, pp. 167-173.

Neufer, P.D., Costill, D.L., Fielding, R.A., Flynn, M.G. and Kirwan, J.P. (1987) Effect of reduced training on muscular strength and endurance in competitive swimming. **Med. Sci. Sports Exerc.**, 19, 486-490.

Nomura, T. (1983) The influence of training and age on $\dot{V}O_2$max during swimming in Japanese elite age group and Olympic swimmers, in **Biomechanics and Medicine in Swimming** (eds A.P. Hollander, P.A. Huijing and G. de Groot), Human Kinetics Publishers, Champaign, Ill., pp. 251-257.

Pai, Y.C., Hay, J.G. and Wilson, B.D. (1984) Stroking techniques of elite swimmers. **J. Sports Sci.**, 2, 225-239.

Pendergast, D.R., di Prampero, P.E., Craig, A.B., Wilson, D.R. and Rennie, D.W. (1974) Quantitative analysis of the front crawl in men and women. **J. Appl. Physiol.**, 43, 475-479.

Prampero, P.E. di, Pendergast, D.R., Wilson, D.W. and Rennie, D.W. (1974) Energetics of swimming in man. **J. Appl. Physiol.**, 37, 1-5.

Reischle, K. (1979) A kinematical investigation of movement patterns in swimming with photo-optical methods, in **Swimming III** (eds J. Terauds and E.W. Bedingfield), University Park Press, Baltimore, pp. 127-136.

Saito, M. (1982) The effect of training on the relationships among velocity, stroke rate, and distance per stroke in untrained subjected swimming the breaststroke. **Res. Quart.**, 53, 323-329.

Schleihauf, R.E. (1974) A biomechanical analysis of freestyle. **Swimming Technique,** 11,89-96.

Schleihauf, R.E. (1979) A hydrodynamic analysis of swimming propulsion, in **Swimming III** (eds J. Terauds and E.W. Bedingfield), University Park Press, Baltimore, pp. 70-109.

Schleihauf, R.E., Gray, L. and deRose, J. (1983) Three-dimensional analysis of swimming propulsion in the sprint front crawlstroke, in **Biomechanics and Medicine in Swimming** (eds A.P. Hollander, P.A. Huijing and G. de Groot), Human Kinetics Publishers, Champaign, Ill., pp. 173-184.

Schleihauf, R.E., Higgins, J.R., Hinrichs, R., Luedtke, D., Maglischo, C., Maglischo, E.W. and Thayer, A. (1988) Propulsive techniques: Front crawl stroke, butterfly, backstroke and breaststroke, in **Swimming Science V** (eds B.E. Ungerechts, K. Wilke and K. Reischle), Human Kinetics Books, Champaign, Ill., pp. 53-59.

Sharp, R.L., Troup, J.P. and Costill, D.L. (1982) Relationship between power and sprint freestyle swimming. **Med. Sci. Sports Exerc.**, 14, 53-56.

Swaine, I. and Reilly, T. (1983) The freely-chosen swimming stroke rate in a maximal swim and on a biokinetic swim bench. **Med. Sci. Sports Exerc.**, 15, 370-375.

Toussaint, H.M. (1990) Differences in propelling efficiency between competitive and triathlon swimmers. **Med. Sci. Sports Exerc.**, 22, 409-415.

Toussaint, H.M., Beelen, A., Rodenburg, A., Sargeant, A.J., Groot, G. de, Hollander, A.P. and Ingen Schenau, G.J. van (1988a) Propelling efficiency of front crawl swimming. **J. Appl. Physiol.**, 65, 2506-2512.

Toussaint, H.M., Bruinink, L., Coster, R., Looze, M. de., Rossem, B. van, Veenen, R. van and Groot, G. de (1989) Effect of a triathlon wet suit on drag during swimming. **Med. Sci. Sports Exerc.**, 21, 325-328.

Toussaint, H.M., Groot, G. de, Savelberg, H.H.C.M., Vervoorn, K., Hollander, A.P. and Ingen Schenau, G.J. van (1988b) Active drag related to velocity in male and female swimmers. **J. Biomech.**, 21, 435-438.

Toussaint, H.M., Helm, F.C.T. van de, Elzerman, J.R., Hollander, A.P., Groot, G. de and Ingen Schenau, G.J. van (1983) A power balance applied to swimming, in **Biomechanics and Medicine in Swimming** (eds A.P. Hollander, P.A. Huijing and G. de Groot), Human Kinetics Publishers, Champaign, Ill., pp. 165-172.

Toussaint, H.M., Hollander, A.P., Groot, G. de, Kahman, R. and Ingen Schenau, G.J. van (1990) Power of leg kicking in front crawl swimming, in **Biomechanics of Human Movement** (eds N. Berme and A. Capozzo), Bertec Corporation, Wortington, Ohio, pp. 87-91.

Toussaint, H.M., Knops, W., Groot, G. de and Hollander, A.P. (1990a) The mechanical efficiency of front crawl swimming. **Med. Sci. Sports Exerc.**, 22, 402-408.

Toussaint, H.M., Looze, M. de, Rossem, B. van, Leijdekkers, M. and Dignum, H. (1990b) The effect of growth of drag in young swimmers. **J. Sport Biomech.**, 6, 18-28.

Toussaint, H.M., Veenen, R. van and Vervoorn, K. (in preparation) Effect of a year of training on competitive swimmers.

Toussaint, H.M. and Vervoorn, K. (1990) Effects of specific high resistance training in the water on competitive swimmers. **Int. J. Sports Med.**, 11, 228-233.

Vaart, A.T.M. van der, Savelberg, H.H.C.M., Groot, G. de, Hollander, A.P., Toussaint, H.M. Ingen Schenau, G.J. van (1987) An estimation of active drag in front crawl swimming. **J. Biomech.**, 20, 543-546.

Watkins, J. and Gordon, A.T. (1983) The effect of leg action on performance in the front crawl stroke, in **Biomechanics and Medicine in Swimming** (eds A.P. Hollander, P.A. Huijing and G. de Groot), Human Kinetics Publishers, Champaign, Ill., pp. 310-314.

Webb, P.W. (1971a) The swimming energetics of trout I: Thrust and power output at cruising speeds. **J. Exp. Biol.**, 55, 489-520.

Webb, P.W. (1971b) The swimming energetics of trout II: Oxygen consumption and swimming efficiency. **J. Exp. Biol.**, 55, 521-540.

ANALYSIS OF SPRINT SWIMMING: THE 50 m FREESTYLE

K. WILKE, Deutsche Sporthochschule Köln, Germany

Abstract
This report presents an overview of research into 50 m freestyle
swimming. It also highlights the lack of information as international 50 m sprint contests are still relatively young. It
considers swim technique, energy supply, body structure, muscular
strength and kinematic profiles pertaining to sprint swimming.
Keywords: Sprint Swimming, Freestyle, Kinematic Profile, Technique.

1 Introduction

In order to achieve maximal performance in any sport there is a need
to optimize efficiency. This fact can be realised by observing the
various components which lead to efficient performance in elite
athletes. This paper examines such components in the elite performance of 50 m freestyle sprinting. This event has been chosen
because successful 50 m freestyle sprint performance, more than any
other distance (or stroke), is the result of inter-individual
differences in technique.

2 Swimming technique and sprint swimming

The achievement of 50 m freestyle swimming basically consists of two
components, which differ from each other in terms of motor-technique:
the start and the actual swimming-distance. In the case of the 25 m
length pool the turn adds a third component.

Thayer and Hay (1984) determined the start and the subsequent
gliding phase of 7.5 m as contributing 10.5% of the total racing
time, and the turn with a gliding-distance of 9.5 m as 20.5% in the
somewhat shorter 50 yards (46 m) distance. This means that one third
of the time in a 50 yard race using the short course depends on the
qualities of start and turn. Maglischo (1988) stated that the start
and gliding phase of the 50 m freestyle accounts for 18% of the total
time. He concluded that improvements of 0.5 to 1.0 s would be
possible by optimizing the starting technique. Therefore a fast
reaction time, a great jumping power, and a low resistance during
gliding should be the primary requirements for a good start.

Research on the start, especially in sprint swimming, is limited.
There is also little known about the sprint turn. For the "No-Touch-
Turn" generally, a correlation between power and the initial gliding

speed of 2.78 m/s was found with highly trained swimmers (Takahashi et al., 1983). The high impulse of 250 N allowed the conclusion that there is a similar degree of importance for the explosive force of the leg extensors in the turn as for the starting dive. Suitable training includes eccentric-concentric muscle contraction cycles as in drop jumps, and very fast muscular contractions by means of jumping supported by the pull of a bungee as a spring expander.

The turn is an influencing factor in the way speed is achieved in a 25 m or 50 m pool. Higher velocities of the turn section in a 25 m pool cannot be maintained to the end of the race (Büsken, 1986; Petzer, 1990). The 50 m shows the more constant velocity of motion and Büsken (1986) offered as an explanation a break in motivation after the turn in contrast to the motivation for a "final sprint" in a 50 m pool. There is still a need to examine the turn with respect to the muscular, energetic and coordination requirements and its effects on the second 25 m.

Racing the 50 m usually requires a higher stroke frequency (SF) than the other freestyle distances. An increase of frequency produces a temporal change of the phase of the arm motion (Table 1). The non-propulsive phases in particular are found to decrease and this negatively influences the relation of muscle contraction and relaxation. Therefore there is a limit to the increase in SF. Underwater recordings of sprint swimmers have shown a relatively small crook of the arm during the pull. The angle between upper arm and lower arm of the best German sprinters was more than 120 degrees, their arms being almost straight. Exact measurements with a representative number of sprinters were not available.

The same is true for the leg kick. Observations by eye, confirmed by video recordings of different championship finals, established that almost all of the 50 m swimmers performed a six beat kick. This would confirm the biomechanical results of Zaciorskij and Safarjan (1972) showing the dependence of the swimming speed at 50 m and 100 m on the propulsive power of the legs. In their understanding this dependence questions some authors' and coaches' assertion that the propelling force of the legs does not account for the total propelling force as the swimming velocity of a freestyle swimmer is faster than 1.5 m/s.

Watkins and Gordon (1983) came to similar conclusions. They divided the effect of the leg kick on the propulsion in the sprint into direct and indirect components. They took their results to suggest that leg action contributes indirectly to propulsion by (a) stabilizing the trunk which accounts for about 9% of the full stroke speed for both males and females, and (b) streamlining the body which

Table 1. Effect of stroke frequency on factors affecting the freestyle arm-stroke

Frequency	Catch	Pull-push	Leaving the water	Recovery
(S/min)	(s)	(s)	(s)	(s)
44	0.26	0.38	0.10	0.62
50	0.22	0.38	0.10	0.50
58	0.16	0.35	0.08	0.44

accounts for about 11 and 6% of the full stroke speed for males and females respectively. Maglischo (1988) agreed with this inter-pretation, stating that sprinters should maximize the propulsion from their kick, because saving energy is not nearly so important as attaining a fast swimming velocity.

Any meaningful analysis must consider that both the propelling and the stabilizing function of a strong flutter kick strengthens the significance of muscular bridges between legs, trunk and arms. Hence such an aspect belongs to the topic "muscular strength and sprint swimming".

All authors who have mentioned the breathing patterns during the 50 m freestyle sprint underline a minimal number of breaths (Table 2). This is compatible with the biomechanical advantages associated with reduced resistance due to body shape, and the lack of a need for breathing throughout the whole distance. Breathing patterns of this type require an ability to withstand the "drive" to breathe that is brought on by increased CO_2 resulting from restricted breathing. According to Maglischo (1988) hypoxic training and sprints of 25 and 50 m with 0 to 1 breaths are excellent for this purpose.

Newes and Brown (1977) substituted the reduced or missing respiration during swimming with the hyperventilation before the start. The intensified elimination of CO_2 should raise the pH value and delay the breathing stimulus. In their opinion this would be a psychological advantage for the sprinter, who knows before the race starts that he is not going to experience difficulty in breathing. Nevertheless Patton (1979) did not notice an improvement in performance over 50 yards after 10 weeks of hypoxic or controlled-breath training with 38 university swimmers.

3 Energy supply and sprint swimming

Investigations of the energy supply on the main energy resources, their flow and their eventual exhaustion during the 50 m freestyle sprint are unpublished. In contrast, there are many investigations concerning maximum efforts of short durations (up to 30 s) in other sports, such as running and cycling (Hultman and Sjöholm, 1986). Results from data gathered on other sports cannot simply be trans-ferred to 50 m sprint swimming since there are differences in motor recruitment patterns, in body position and in the fact that these other sports do not take place in the medium of water.

Torma and Szekely (1978) stated that swimming for 50 m represents the transitional range between alactacid and lactacid-anaerobic

Table 2. Amount of respiration and distribution on the 50 m freestyle

Authors	Total number of breaths	Distribution
Newes and Brown (1977)	0	Hyperventilation before
Ryan (1980)	1	Between 37–45 m
Maglischo (1982)	1	30 m
Maglischo (1988)	1–2	–

energy supply. The lactacid-anaerobic capacity is not fully
exhausted by a single swimming bout of 50 m. According to some
estimates, the prompt chemical reactions of the phosphagens enable
exercise to be continued for as long as 20 s. Maglischo (1988)
pointed out that the capacity for producing high levels of lactic
acid was to be considered for training. There is a lack of knowledge
of the physiological consequences of decreasing stroke frequency and
reducing stroke length over the 50 m distance.

4 Anthropometry and sprint swimming

Body height and body build are very important for sprint swimming.
The swimming distance becomes shorter for a tall swimmer because he
starts his turn and touches the finish wall earlier than a small
person with the same swimming speed. This advantage particularly
favours performances over short distances, where the energy supply
does not play a dominant role. Stroup et al. (1967) reported that
the tallest and heaviest swimmers preferred the 50 yard and 100 yard
freestyle distances.

Counsilman (1976) considered the tall and heavy swimmers to be at
an advantage because they accelerate a greater mass during the
starting dive and push-off after turning. In contrast Smith (1978)
did not find a measurable influence of body mass, height and length
of extremities on the 25 m sprint results using 40 male and female
swimmers without a push-off. During the 1989 European Championships
at Bonn we measured 40 swimmers (male: 23; female 17) who took part
in the 50 m races or were close to the qualification level. Their
body mass and height were examined and related to their actual 50 m
time. The results showed a significant correlation between body mass
and 50 m time ($r = 0.79$; $P < 0.001$), and between height and 50 m time
($r = 0.68$; $P < 0.001$). The correlation became stronger with the
older participants (22 years and older), especially for body mass (r
$= 0.87$; $P < 0.001$), and height ($r = 0.75$; $P < 0.001$).

It is also well known that body mass increases with age, even in
sports performers. That may be one of the reasons why older swimmers
often tend to change from the longer to the shorter race distances.
The relationship between of age and increasing weight was also
confirmed in the group of sprinters swimming faster than 23.5 s ($r =$
0.61; $P < 0.001$). Grimston and Hay (1986) and Montpetit and Smith
(1988) examined anthropometric measurements such as length of the
upper and lower extremities, cross-sectional and frontal areas of
trunk and limbs in order to include them in the frame of biomechanical models. Grimston and Hay (1986) considered the stroke
frequencies (SF) and stroke lengths (SL) to be dependent on the
anthropometric data. They established standard values for the
optimum stroke structure on 50 y, 100 y, 200 y and so on. The
competitors whom we measured during the European Championship showed
significant correlations between 50 m time and their limbs in the
following order:-

arm length   n 20 $r = 0.78$, $P < 0.001$
leg length   n 20 $r = 0.50$, $P < 0.05$
interior hand area n 28 $r = 0.76$, $P < 0.001$
interior foot area n 26 $r = 0.56$, $P < 0.001$.

These results correspond to those of Zaciorskij and Safarjan (1972)

in that arm length showed a greater correlation to the velocity in 50
m swimming than leg length. Furthermore these authors revealed the
stronger relationship between body mass and speed ($r = 0.59$), despite
the correlation between body mass and hydrodynamic resistance ($r = 0.84$). They considered the resistance in the sprint distance which
increased with increasing body mass to be easily overcome if the
force of the propulsive muscles was relatively greater. They
mentioned the girth of the upper arm as an indicator of the anthropometric value which correlated with swimming speed over the short
distance ($r = 0.67$). Grimston and Hay (1986) argued in a similar
manner. They assigned the axilla cross-sectional area of the trunk
to be an important function of the swimming speed because a large
axilla cross-section was an indication of the propelling muscles.
The results of our examinations during the European Championship
confirmed the relationship between the 50 m sprint velocity and the
trunk girth ($r = 0.63$, $P < 0.001$), and the girth of the upper arm,
respectively ($r = 0.72$, $P < 0.001$).

5 Muscular strength and sprint swimming

There is a logical connection between a swimmer's muscular strength
and freestyle swimming speed. As speed increases, the water
resistance which is to be overcome increases at almost the square of
the speed. The propelling muscles have to produce the necessary
force during 21-26 s if the period of the start phase is subtracted.
    Costill (1978) stated that the huge improvement in the short
distance records during the period from 1957-1977 was mainly due to
the gain of strength which developed in the propulsive muscles of
swimmers. Zaciorskij and Safarjan (1972) found a close connection
between the sprint speed over 50 m and the dynamic strength of the
main muscles initiating the pull motion.
    Costill et al. (1980) and Sharp et al. (1982) reported significant
correlations between the power-per-arm-pull on a biokinetic swim
bench and the time over 25 y using 41 non-elite swimmers ($r = 0.93$)
whereas national and international swimmers revealed a reduced
correlation ($r = 0.62$) and sprinters swimming at a velocity higher
than 2.1 m/s showed no relationship ($r = 0.25$). Sharp et al. (1982)
concluded that above a power output of 500 W the quality of swimming
technique and not strength is the factor limiting performance.
Additionally the relation between the force dispersion throughout the
pulling pattern and the strength endurance become evident when the
total work performed during a fatigue test was found to be closely
related to the subject's peak power in a single pull ($r = 0.96$).
    Hopper et al. (1983) showed a relation between power of arm pull
and 50 m time in semi-tethered swimming ($r = 0.80$). Christensen and
Smith (1987) found the correlation between arm power and 25 m time
differed for men ($r = 0.68$, $P < 0.005$) and women ($r = 0.57$, $P < 0.01$)
in a study of tethered swimming.
    Counsilman (1976) believed that sprinters possess a greater
proportion of FT muscle fibres than ST fibres. This is supported by
the results of a maximum vertical jump test by Bosco et al. (1983).
The mechanical capacity had a significant correlation with the
proportion of FT fibres ($r = 0.86$). The correlation lost its
significance if high power output was required for longer than 30 s.

Sharp (1986) summarised his research on swimming and strength with the contention that strength, per se, may be relatively unimportant to the performance of competitive swimmers whereas the power of swim-specific movements were more closely related to performance. However, no significant relationships were established between power and performance at a national championship. The latter may have been due to the fact that above a certain level of power, further improvements do not lead to faster sprint speed.

During the 1989 European Championships at Bonn the 50 m freestyle competitors, as well as some German candidates who were just below the qualification level, were asked to quantify both the number of strength training sessions performed per week during 1988 and 1989 (Table 3) and the mean duration of the strength sessions (Table 4). In principle, the view of Sharp (1986) was confirmed in that there were no significant differences between sprinters and non-sprinters with respect to the frequency and duration of the strength training. The female sprinters had an average increase ($P < 0.05$) from 1988 to 1989 not only in the number of their strength sessions per week but also the duration per session (Table 4). In addition, female sprinters performed significantly more stretching in connection with strength training than female non-sprinters. Furthermore, 62.7% of

Table 3. Mean number of strength training sessions per week for participants preparing for the 1989 European Championships

Year of preparation	Sex	Sprinters	Non-sprinters
1988	Male and female	3.1 (n = 24)	3.5 (n = 29)
	Male	3.8 (n = 14)	3.9 (n = 16)
	Female	2.1 (n = 10)	2.9 (n = 13)
1989	Male and female	3.1 (n = 24)	3.5 (n = 29)
	Male	3.4 (n = 14)	3.8 (n = 16)
	Female	2.8 (n = 10)	3.0 (n = 13)

Table 4. Mean duration of strength training units (min) for participants preparing for the 1989 European Championships

Year of preparation	Sex	Sprinters	Non-sprinters
1988	Male and female	61.1 (n = 24)	55.9 (n = 29)
	Male	65.4 (n = 14)	64.7 (n = 16)
	Female	55.0 (n = 10)	45.0 (n = 13)
1989	Male and female	59.8 (n = 24)	61.6 (n = 29
	Male	55.4 (n = 14)	70.3 (n = 16)
	Female	66.0 (n = 10)	50.8 (n = 13)

all swimmers being questioned practised strength training before swim training and only 15.7% after swim training. A quarter of the sprinters preferred the dry land workout after swimming.

A further speciality of sprint swimming lies in the time taken in which the arm pull produces maximum force and in the capability of achieving this maximum force in a very short period. This is a problem of neuromuscular coordination which concerns recruitment and synchronization of the muscle fibres. Rasulbekov et al. (1986) speculated that the augmentation of explosive power must lead to maximum strength exertion in the main propulsive phase. Electromyographical research of Clarys and Olbrecht (1983) and Clarys et al. (1988) has shown that the deployment of maximum force normally takes too much time and cannot be realized during the pull-push phase. Strass and Haberer (1987) applied the training method of maximum strength exertions of short duration, i.e. bench-pressing of a free moveable barbell, whereby the load was increased weekly according to individual improvement. The participants were asked to lift the barbell as fast as possible over the full range of motion, and after a training period of six weeks the correlation between maximum dynamic strength and speed for 50 m freestyle became stronger (from r = 0.57 to r = 0.80). The mean swim velocity at 50 m was significantly increased and was accompanied by a negligible reduction of SF and an enlarged d/S. Explosive power also showed a significant increase which resulted in an increase in the force-time ratio.

Pfeifer (1988) emphasised the necessity for 50 m sprinters to enhance maximum strength under conditions compatible for speed and the specialisation of the stroke pattern. Our studies in 1989 found that even more sprinters than non-sprinters used free weights for strength training (P < 0.05). A training study by Toussaint and Vervoorn (1990) conducted on elite male and female Dutch swimmers over a 10 week period of swim-specific strength training resulted in significant increases in force (91 N to 94N; 3.3%), in velocity (1.75 m/s to 1.81 m/s; 3.4%), and in power (160 W to 172 W; 7%) as measured by the measurement of active (MAD) system. Furthermore, an increase was found in distance per stroke (d/S) in free swimming. The training group also showed a significant improvement in time for 50 m sprint swimming. It appears that over short distances the power output of the arms is the predominant factor influencing performance. In longer events the capacity of the arms to generate maximum mechanical power may be relatively less important than the ability to sustain a high level of aerobic power.

The POP-system is an unusual apparatus for strength training in the water. According to our questioning of swimmers at the 1989 European Championship the following equipment was usual: paddles, fins, T-shirts, resistance belts and trousers, swimming against a rubber tube, and towing a partner. Both sprinters and non-sprinters used these methods of resistance training.

6 Kinematic profiles of the 50 m sprint swimming

East (1971) published measurements and calculations on the relation of swimming velocity, stroke frequency and stroke length, but not especially for sprint swimming. Reischle (1988) constructed a nomogram in which each branch of a hyperbola represented a certain

swim velocity. If pure swim time and SF were known, d/S could be
established directly. The nomogram accommodated 50 m distances based
on the observation that the swim time over a certain distance was the
product of SF and distance travelled per stroke (d/S) where $v = SF \times d/S$. Under conditions of steady velocity the increase in SF resulted
in a decrease in d/S and vice versa.

Ballreich (1979) described the 50 m freestyle sprint distance in
the form of two schemes in order to empirically comprehend the
complex performance by kinematic values (Fig. 1). Profiles of single
athletes and average profiles of selected groups can be calculated
using such an analytical framework. In this way profiles for
different age groups can be established and compared with each other.

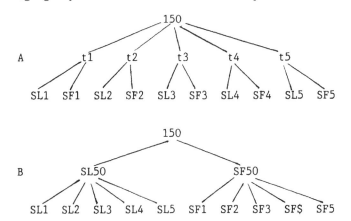

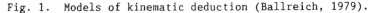

Fig. 1. Models of kinematic deduction (Ballreich, 1979).

The methodology of documentation and measurement can be explained
on examination of Fig. 2. Essentially it consists of video recording
by cameras which are fixed and adjusted at 10 m intervals along the
pool. The tapes can be evaluated later. The Olympic finals were the
only exceptions. They were analysed from existing video documents by
a complicated treatment in order to exclude the parallax error.

Firstly the total 50 m time is related to the five partial times
t1 to t5. In this case the subjects examined were participants in
the European Championships (1989) in Bonn, of the German Championship
(1989), and from video analysis of the 1988 Seoul Olympic Games
(Table 5). Comparison of the male to female mean differences in the
50 m times was 2.91 s. Males were 0.23 m/s or 12.9% faster than
females. Each 10 m section highlighted the advantage of the males
(Table 6). The men's advantage in velocity in sections 1 and 2 was
greater because of the more explosive dive start. The women achieved
their highest speed in the third section, not suffering as much loss
before the finish as observed for the men (Fig. 3). Their loss of
speed from 30 m proceeds far more steadily.

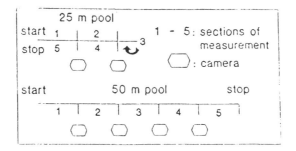

Fig. 2.   Scheme of video documentation.

Table 5.   Mean time for 50 m freestyle events at European and German
            Championships (1989) and Olympic Games (1988)

Sex	n	Range (s)	x̄	SD
Male	72	22.14-25.95	23.80	± 0.68
Female	45	25.49-28.14	26.71	± 0.73

Table 6.   Split times (s) of the 177 athletes for each 10 m section
            (mean ± standard deviation)

Sex	t1	t2	t3	t4	t5
Male	3.58 ± 0.15	4.88 ± 0.17	5.04 ± 0.19	5.08 ± 0.15	5.19 ± 0.23
Female	4.31 ± 0.27	5.52 ± 0.14	5.50 ± 0.24	5.72 ± 0.22	5.64 ± 0.16

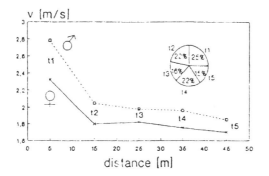

Fig. 3.   Differences in the velocity profile of the 50 m freestyle.

A differentiation according to level 2 reveals that the men showed
a stroke length 17 cm larger than the women, the mean difference
being highly significant (P < 0.001) whilst sex differences in mean
stroke frequency did not exist. Differences in performance were due
to the larger distance per stroke for males.

41

Table 7. Distance/stroke (m) and stroke frequency of 117 athletes
(mean ± standard deviation)

Sex	Distance per stroke	Stroke frequency
Male	2.04 ± 0.11	58.7 ± 3.7 min
Female	1.87 ± 0.15	58.1 ± 4.2 min

In order to find out which particular kinematic profiles could characterize the faster 50 m sprinters, the 117 participants of the championships mentioned above were divided into groups of faster and slower 50 m swimmers for both sexes according to competitive results (Table 8).

Table 8. Time (s) of the faster and slower groups for 50 m freestyle (variation, mean ± SD)

Sex/Performance		n	Variation	X̄	SD
Male	Faster	35	22.14–23.80	23.24	0.38
	Slower	37	23.90–25.95	24.32	0.44
Female	Faster	20	25.49–26.69	26.01	0.33
	Slower	25	26.70–28.14	27.27	0.41

The velocity profiles of the faster and the slower group did not proceed uniformly. The males' results in all five sections contributed to the higher velocity of 0.09 m/s or 4.5% for the faster group. The contributions differed per section (Fig. 4). The third section and the finish had the strongest influence on the total performance. Weak points occurred in gaining speed steadily and maintaining it to the end.

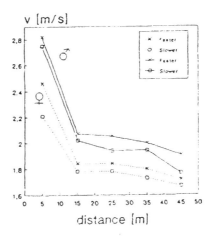

Fig. 4. The velocity of the 50 m freestyle.

The women's results showed a similarity between the total time and t3, t4, t5 in both groups whereas the start and the following section differentiated the female athletes in the two groups. The capabilities of jumping and accelerating were much less developed in the group of slower women than in the faster women swimmers.

The profiles of SF showed similar trends to the velocity profiles. They declined from the start in both men and women and in both faster and slower groups with 62 cycles/min at the start to 54 cycles/min at the finish representing a 13% loss of frequency. Therefore the velocity difference between males and females could only be explained by the larger d/S of 17 cm in men.

The faster male group exhibited a reduced stroke frequency during the second 10 m section compared to the slower group (Fig. 5). The difference was significant at the beginning (P < 0.05) and increased to section 5 (P < 0.001). This was the main cause of the difference in performance between the two male groups.

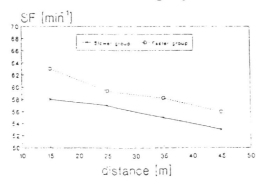

Fig. 5.   Stroke frequency profile of the 50 m freestyle (men).

The faster groups in both sexes may be distinguished by harmonic profiles of d/S (Fig. 6) whereas the curve of d/S of the slower males and females follows a zig-zag course. There is a stronger mean correlation between the stroke lengths per section in women (r = 0.78) than in men (r = 0.63).

7. Conclusions

To sum up the results for the 117 participants of the 1989 German and European Championships and of the 1988 Olympic Games, it can be stated that:
   (i) The velocity profiles of men and women, of the faster and slower group, broadly proceeded in parallel. The largest difference between men and women resulted from sections 1, 2 and 4.
   (ii) The faster swimmers, both males and females, surpassed the slower ones in each section. Sections 3 and 5 differentiated most of all between the faster and slower male group, whereas the starting section differentiated between the female groups.
   (iii) The main reason for the difference in performance between male and female athletes originated from the highly significant difference in d/S, not in SF (Fig. 7). The profile of the stroke

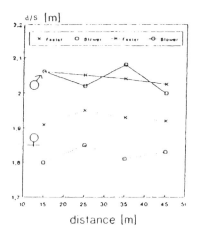

Fig. 6. Distance per stroke profile of faster and slower groups of
50 m freestyle.

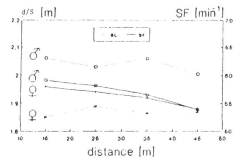

Fig. 7. Distance per stroke and stroke frequency profile of the 50 m
freestyle.

frequency was similar for all groups: after the highest frequency in
the start section the values decreased continuously. This reduction
of frequency caused the loss of velocity throughout the distance for
all swimmers.

(iv) The groups of faster swimmers were distinguished by a
constant profile of d/S, while the faster women achieved longer pulls
than their slower counterparts. The faster men gained their
advantage of velocity by a significantly smaller decrease of SF
compared to the slower athletes.

(v) The SF differed systematically among men whereas d/S differed
in women. Therefore SF could be classified as the determinant
kinematic factor in 50 m freestyle performance for males. For
females that factor is the d/S.
Nevertheless we must be conscious of one fact. Both d/S and SF vary
more than their product, the velocity.

8 References

Ballreich, R. (1979) Modell zur Bestimmung biomechanischer Einflussgrössen sportmotorischer Leistungen und zur Schätzung ihrer Einflusshöhen. Leistungssport, 9, 1.

Büsken, P. (1986) Zur Geschwindigkeitsgestaltung im Schwimmen. University Examen Thesis, Bielefeld.

Christensen, C.L. and Smith, G.W. (1987) Relationship of maximum sprint speed and maximal stroking force in swimming. **J. Swimming Res.**, 2, 18-20.

Clarys, J.P., (1988) Muscular specificity and intensity in swimming against a mechanical resistance surface EMG in MAD and free-swimming, in **Swimming V** (eds B. Ungerechts, K. Wilke and K. Reischle), Human Kinetics, Champaign, Ill., pp. 191-199.

Clarys, J.P. and Olbrecht, J. (1983) Peripheral control of complex swimming movements using telemetric and conventional electromyo-graphy, in **Motorik- und bewegungsforschung** (eds H. Rieder, K. Bös, H. Mechling and K. Reischle), Schorndorf, pp. 111-116.

Costill, D.L. (1978) Adaptation and skeletal muscle during training for sprint and endurance swimming, in **Swimming Medicine IV** (eds B. Erikson and B. Furberg), University Park Press, Baltimore, pp. 233-248.

Costill, D.L., Sharp, R. and Troup, J.P. (1980) Muscle strength: contributions to sprint swimming. **Swimming World**, 21, 29-34.

Counsilman, J.E. (1976) The importance of speed in exercise. **Athletic Journal**, 56, 72-75.

East, D. (1971) Stroke frequency, length and performance. **Swimming Technique,** 8, 68-73.

Grimston, S.K. and Hay, J.G. (1986) Relationship among anthropometric and stroking characteristics of college swimmers. **Med. Sci. Sports Exerc.**, 1, 60-68.

Hopper, R.T. (1983) Measurements of power delivered to an external weight, in **Biomechanics and Medicine in Swimming** (eds P.A. Hollander, A.P. Huijing and G. de Groot), Human Kinetics, Champaign, Ill., pp. 112-119.

Hultman, E. and Sjöholm, H. (1986) Biochemical causes of fatigue, in **Human Muscle Power** (eds N. Jones, N. McCartney and A. McComas), Human Kinetics, Champaign, Ill., pp. 215-238.

Maglischo, E.W. (1982) **Swimming Faster.** Mayfield, Palo Alto, CA.

Maglischo, E.W. (1988) **Sprint Training. Report.** Stichtung Congress, Swim 2000, Venlo.

Monpetit, R.R. and Smith, H. (1988) Build for speed. **Swimming Technique,** 24, 30-33.

Newes, R.E. and Brown, P.T. (1977) Sprint swimming and voluntary hyperventilation. **Swimming Technique,** 12, 86-93.

Patton, R.W. (1979) The effect of hypoxic training upon sprint freestyle swimming performance. **Swimming Technique,** 16, 89-92.

Petzer, V. (1990) **Zugfrequenz und Zugläge als Leistungsparameter im Kraulsprint. Ein Vergleich zwischen österreichischen und internationalen Spitzenschwimmern.** Diplome Thesis, University of Innsbruck.

Pfeifer, H. (1988) **The Extent and Intensity of the Training for a Sprinter. Report** Stichtung Congress: SWIMM 2000, Venlo.

Rasulbekov, R.A. (1986) Explosive strength in pulling. **Swimming Technique,** 23, 30-32.

Reischle, K. (1988). **Biomechanik des Schwimmens.** Bockenem.

Ryan, W. (1980) Sprinttraining und Langstreckentraining nach dem Overload - Prinzip. **Schwimmagazin,** 1, 1-3.

Sharp, R.L. (1986) Muscle strength and power as related to competitive swimming. **J. Swimming Res.,** 2, 5-10.

Sharp, R.L., Troup, J.P. and Costill, D.L. (1982) Relationship between power and sprint freestyle swimming. **Med. Sci. Sports Exerc.,** 14, 53-56.

Smith, L. (1978) Anthropometric measurements, and arm on speed performance of male and female swimmers as predictors of swim speed. **J. Sports Phys. Fit.,** 18, 153-167.

Strass, D. and Haberer, K. (1987) Der Einfluss von Maximalkrafttraining auf die Sprintleistung des Wettkampfschwimmers. **Leistungssport,** 23, 49-53.

Stroup, F., Harris, A. and McCormick, J. (1967) Anthropometric measurement and swimming performance. **Swimming Technique,** 3, 13-15.

Takahashi, G., Yoshida, A. and Tsubakimoto, S. (1983) Propulsive force generated by swimmers during a turning motion, in **Biomechanics and Medicine in Swimming** (eds P.A. Hollander, A.P. Huijing and G. de Groot), Human Kinetics Publishers, Champaign, Ill., pp. 192-199.

Thayer, A.L. and Hay, J.G. (1984) Motivating start and turn improvement. **Swimming Technique,** 20, 17-20.

Torma, Z.D. and Szekely, G. (1978) Parameters of acid-base equilibrium at various swimming intensities and distance. **Swimming Medicine IV,** University Park Press, Baltimore, pp. 274-281.

Toussaint, H.M. and Vervoorn, K. (1990) Effects of specific high resistance training in the water on competitive swimmers. **Int. J. Sports Med.,** 11, 228-233.

Watkins, J. and Gordon, T.W. (1983) The effects of leg action on performance in sprint front crawl stroke, in **Biomechanics and Medicine in Swimming** (eds P.A. Hollander, P.A. Huijing and G. de Groot), Human Kinetics Publishers, Champaign, Ill., pp. 310-314.

Zaciorskij, V.M. and Safarjan, J.G. (1972) Untersuchung von Faktoren zur Bestimmung der maximalen Geschwindigkeit im Freistilswimmen. **Theorie und Praxis der Körperkultur,** 21, 695-709.

PART TWO

BIOMECHANICS

INTENSITY AND PERFORMANCE RELATED DIFFERENCES IN PROPELLING AND
MECHANICAL EFFICIENCIES

J.M. CAPPAERT, M. BONE and J.P. TROUP
U.S. Swimming, International Centre for Aquatic Research, Colorado
Springs, CO, USA

Abstract
The purpose of the study was to determine propelling (PE) and
mechanical efficiency (ME) of freestyle swimming under two
conditions: (i) at velocities having high aerobic or anaerobic demand
and (ii) during swims specific to sprint, middle distance and
distance competitors. The results suggest that PE decreases as the
anaerobic energy sources increase. Mechanical efficiency does not
seem to be affected by the predominant energy source used.
Keywords: Propelling Efficiency, Mechanical Efficiency, Power Output,
Power Input, Three-dimensional Cinematography.

1 Introduction

The freestyle events contain a wide range of competitive distances.
Swimming events of 100 m and below have been shown to require a
predominant anaerobic energy contribution. Races of 200 m and
longer, in contrast, have been shown to rely more heavily on the
aerobic system (Troup et al., 1989). Previous studies have shown
that anaerobic metabolism is less efficient than aerobic metabolism
(Åstrand and Rodahl, 1977; di Prampero et al., 1974) which may affect
the overall efficiency of work possible by athletes. Whether or not
propelling and mechanical efficiencies change as the relative contributions of energy sources change is not known. The purpose of the
study therefore, was to determine propelling (PE) and mechanical
efficiencies (ME) of freestyle swimming (i) at velocities having
either a high aerobic demand or anaerobic demand and (ii) during
swims specific to sprint, middle distance and distance competitors.

2 Methods

2.1 Data collection
Seventeen highly trained competitive swimmers (16 $\pm$ 1.5 years)
performed a pre-test, five point economy (four submaximal swims and a
maximal swim). All subjects were tested at a submaximal aerobic pace
(67% of $\dot{V}O_2$max) in a swimming treadmill. Accumulated O_2 uptake (1)
was measured during the test and expressed in 10 s increments. The
values were converted into watts and used to measure the power input
per pull. During the entire swim, subjects were videotaped with two
underwater video cameras (60 Hz).

Next the subjects were tested at a highly anaerobic pace (corresponding to 134% of VO_2max). The total O_2 demand (1) of the swim was extrapolated from the economy curve for each subject and multiplied by the time swum. This energy cost was converted into watts and expressed as power input per pull. Subjects were also videotaped with two underwater cameras during the swim.

The subjects were divided into the following groups based on their competitive speciality, (1) sprinter (50-100 m) (n = 5), (2) middle distance (200-500 m) (n = 7) and (3) distance (800-1500 m) (n = 5). The swimmers performed a third test in which they swam at their individual race pace based on the speciality event. This was a highly anaerobic, maximal swim. During this swim, subjects were videotaped. Total O_2 demand (1) of the swim was found by taking products of the extrapolated O_2 (l/min) value at 134% of VO_2max from the economy curve and the time swum. This value was then converted to watts for power input and expressed as power per pull.

2.2 Analysis of data

One arm in the two camera views was digitized for the aerobic, anaerobic and race specific swims. Using the DLT method, three-dimensional coordinates of the arm were calculated followed by the calculation of arm kinematic data. Instantaneous resultant hand forces were calculated (Schleihauf, 1984). The resultant force was projected onto the forward direction and defined as effective force. Average propelling efficiency for the whole stroke was calculated using the theory described by Toussaint (1986)

$$PE = \frac{P_d}{\text{Power output}} = \frac{P_d}{P_d + P_k} \tag{1}$$

where PE is propelling efficiency, P_d is the power to overcome drag and P_k is the power used to give water kinetic energy. Using this theory, and assuming that most of the propulsion in freestyle swimming is generated from the upper body rather than the legs (Hollander et al., 1988), the hand forces were used to calculate power output in the theoretical equation:

$$PE = \frac{RE*V_{body}}{((RE*V_{body}) + ((R - RE)*HV)} \tag{2}$$

where RE is the effective component of the resultant force, V_{body} is the velocity of the body or swim, R is the resultant force and HV is the hand velocity (for more detail see Cappaert et al., 1990).

Average mechanical efficiency for the whole stroke was also calculated during the same three swims from Toussaint's (1986) theory.

$$ME = \frac{\text{Power output}}{\text{Power input}} = \frac{P_d + P_k}{\text{Power input}} \tag{3}$$

The power input values in watts were calculated as described earlier. Again, the hand force data were used to calculate the power output:

$$ME = \frac{((RE*V_{body}) + ((R - RE)*HV))}{\text{Power input}} \qquad (4)$$

where ME is the mechanical efficiency, RE is the effective component
of the resultant force, V_{body} is the velocity of the body of swim, R
is the resultant force and HV is the hand velocity.
  Both PE and ME were calculated for the aerobic (67% of VO_2max)
swim, anaerobic (134% of $\dot{V}O_2$max) swim, and the race specific swims.

3 Results

The results show a significant difference ($P < 0.01$) in PE between
the groups while they were swimming their race specific paces. No
significant difference was found in ME between these swims.

Table 1. Propelling and mechanical efficiencies between the groups
          at race specific paces

Group	PE (%)	ME (%)
Sprint	47.8 ± 7.1	5.1 ± 1.5
Middle distance	55.9 ± 10.1	4.0 ± 1.1
Distance	61.5 ± 10.2	4.8 ± 1.5

  Power input and input values for the race specific swims are
presented in Table 2.

Table 2. Power output (PO) and power input (PI) for the race
          specific swims

Group	PO (watts)	PI (watts)
Sprint	86.2 ± 30.2	1906.5 ± 551.8
Middle distance	64.5 ± 20.3	1659.1 ± 305.7
Distance	58.1 ± 15.3	1218.9 ± 230.6

  There was also a significant difference ($P < 0.05$) in PE between
the aerobic swims. Mechanical efficiency (ME) was not different
between the two swims (Table 3).

Table 3. Propelling and mechanical efficiencies of aerobic and
          anaerobic swims

Group	PE (%)	ME (%)
Aerobic	43.5 ± 4.8	6.2 ± 1.1
Anaerobic	33.4 ± 3.9	4.4 ± 1.6

4 Discussion

In examining the race specific data (Table 1), there was an increase in PE as the contribution of aerobic energy systems increased. Since 50 m and 100 m races are considered more anaerobic events than aerobic, the results suggest that propelling efficiency decreases as anaerobic energy contributions increase. This was again reflected in comparing the anaerobic and aerobic swims of the group as a whole (Table 3). This suggests that anaerobic energy sources are less efficient than aerobic and agrees with Åstrand and Rodahl (1977) and di Prampero (1974) discussed earlier. It was interesting to note however, that PE did not increase further with the lower intensity, possibly more aerobic, swim (67% $\dot{V}O_2$max). This may suggest that while PE increases, there may be an optimal amount of work that must be performed to optimize PE.

Mechanical efficiency does not seem to be affected by the predominant energy system used. Both power output and input showed a general trend of decreasing as the intensity decreased (sprint to distance, Table 2) and thus do not have an overall effect on mechanical efficiency. Therefore, even though the more aerobic, less intense swims seem more efficient requiring less power output and input, this is not reflected in the mechanical efficiency data.

5 References

Åstrand, P. and Rodahl, K. (1977) **Textbook of Work Physiology.** McGraw-Hill Book Company, New York, NY.

Cappaert, J.M., Franciosi, P.Q., Langhans, G.W., Troup, J.P. (1990) Indirect calculation of mechanical and propelling efficiency. **VIth International Symposium on Biomechanics and Medicine in Swimming, Liverpool.**

de Groot, G. and van Ingen Schenau, G.J. (1988) Fundamental mechanics applied to swimming: Technique and propelling efficiency, in **Swimming Science V** (eds B.E. Ungerechts, K. Wilke and K. Reischle), Human Kinetics Books, Champaign, IL., pp. 39–44.

di Prampero, P.E., Pendergast, D.R., Wilson, D.W. and Rennie, D.W. (1974) Energetics of swimming in man. **J. Applied Physiol.,** 37, 1–5.

Hollander, A.P., de Groot, G., van Ingen Schenau, G.J., Kahman, R. and Toussaint, H.M. (1988) Contribution of the legs to propulsion in front crawl swimming, in **Swimming Science V** (eds B.E. Ungerechts, K. Wilke and K. Reischle), Human Kinetics Books, Champaign, IL, pp. 39–44.

Schleihauf, R.E. (1979) A hydrodynamic analysis of swimming propulsion, in **Swimming Science III** (eds J. Terauds and W. Bedingfield), University Park Press, Baltimore, pp. 70–109.

Toussaint, H.M. (1988) **Mechanics and Energetics of Swimming.** Rodopi, Amsterdam.

Troup, J.P. (1989) Swimming economy. **Communication to Eighth FINA World Congress on Aquatic Sports,** London, England.

INDIRECT CALCULATION OF MECHANICAL AND PROPELLING EFFICIENCY DURING FREESTYLE SWIMMING

J.M. CAPPAERT, P.Q. FRANCIOSI, G.W. LANGHANS and J.P. TROUP
U.S. Swimming, International Center for Aquatic Research, Colorado
Springs, CO, USA

Abstract
Mechanical and propelling efficiencies during swimming have been
defined and calculated using the direct method of modified underwater force pads (MAD-system, Toussaint, 1988). The limitation of
this approach is that the whole stroke cycle is not taken into
consideration in the calculations of propelling and mechanical
efficiencies. The purpose of this study was to calculate propelling
and mechanical efficiencies by phases of the stroke using three-
dimensional cinematography. The results indicate that by taking the
whole stroke into consideration, propelling efficiencies might be
less than previously reported data.
Keywords: Biomechanical Analysis, Propelling Efficiency, Mechanical
Efficiency, Three-dimensional Cinematography.

1 Introduction

1.1 Mechanical efficiency
As related to the freestyle stroke and creating propulsion, power
output can be considered the sum of the forces made by the limbs
(Toussaint, 1988):

$$P_o = F_{feet}*V_{feet} + F_{hand}*V_{hand} \qquad (1)$$

where F_{feet} is the force made by the feet, V_{feet} is the velocity of
the feet, F_{hand} is the force made by the hands and V_{hand} is the
velocity of the hands.

Hollander et al. (1988) estimated the contribution by the feet as
minimal during freestyle swimming and that the addition of the legs
did not affect the power output from the arms. Additionally they
suggest that the addition of the legs in distance events might
actually hinder performance. Therefore, it can be assumed that the
power output by the feet is zero.

Concentrating on the arms for propulsion, mechanical efficiency
for freestyle has been measured during a submaximal swim by Toussaint
(1988) and others using the following theoretical equation (2):

$$ME = \frac{\text{Power output}}{\text{Power input}} = \frac{P_d + P_k}{\text{Power input}} \qquad (2)$$

53

where power input is the steady state oxygen value from a submaximal swim converted into watts, P_d is the power used to overcome drag and P_k is the power used to give water kinetic energy.

Using three-dimensional cinematography and a hydrodynamic analysis method of Schleihauf (1979), the resultant or total force produced by the hand can be calculated during swimming. This total force is calculated based on the velocity and orientation of the hand. The projection of the resultant force onto the forward direction, called effective force, is used to determine the propulsive component of the resultant force. Hand force data calculated from film analysis can be used to calculate the power output making the following assumptions:

(a) P_d is equal to the effective forces of the hand (RE) multiplied by the velocity of the swim.

(b) P_k is "wasted" energy and is the difference between the total force and the effective force from the hands (R-RE).

Using these assumptions, we can calculate ME using the hand force data described above and presented in equation (3).

$$ME = \frac{((RE*V_{body}) + ((R - RE)*HV)}{Physiological\ power\ input} \tag{3}$$

where ME is the mechanical efficiency, RE is the effective component of the resultant force, V_{body} is the velocity of the body or swim, R is the resultant force, HV is the hand velocity and physiological power input is an on-line steady state oxygen uptake value from a sub-maximal swim converted into watts.

1.2 Propelling efficiency
Propelling efficiency can be defined as in equation (4):

$$PE = \frac{P_d}{P_o} = \frac{P_d}{P_d + P_k} \tag{4}$$

where PE is propelling efficiency, P_o is power output, P_d is the power used to overcome drag and P_k is the power used to give water kinetic energy. Using the above assumptions for mechanical efficiency, calculated hand forces can be used to calculate propelling efficiency (equation (5)):

$$PE = \frac{RE*V_{body}}{((RE*V_{body}) + ((R - RE)*HV))} \tag{5}$$

The availability of high resolution cameras along with the computer capabilities that provide the opportunity to examine underwater technique make it possible to determine overall stroke efficiency. Of greater significance is the ability to analyze each phase of the stroke. This is an advantage since the freestyle swimming pull involves sweeping actions that can be divided into the catch, insweep and outsweep/finish. While the outsweep/finish segment is known to be the more propulsive phase (Schleihauf et al., 1983), all phases will affect the efficiency of the stroke. The purpose of the study therefore, was to determine propelling and mechanical efficiencies of the whole stroke as well as for each stroke phase.

2 Method

2.1 Physiological data collection
Six female college swimmers participated in this study. Each subject swam at a constant velocity (1.3 m/s) in a swimming treadmill for 5 min. Expired air samples were collected during the swim and accumulated O_2 uptake values expressed at 10 s increments. The values recorded at steady state (i.e. 5 min) were used to describe the energy demand of the workout. These energy demand values (1) were converted into watts and used as the power input value for the mechanical efficiency. For purposes of estimating mechanical efficiency per stroke phase, it was assumed that at steady state oxygen consumption, no difference existed at each stroke phase. Therefore, power input was expressed based on the time for each segment of the pull.

2.2 Biomechanical data collection
During the last minute of the test swimmers were filmed using two underwater video cameras (60 Hz). One arm cycle was chosen for analysis. Both views of the arm cycle were digitized and three-dimensional coordinates of one arm were calculated using the direct linear transformation method (Abdel-Aziz and Karara, 1971). Resultant hand forces were calculated instantaneously (Schleihauf, 1979). The resultant hand force was projected onto the forward direction and defined as effective or propulsive force.

Propelling and mechanical efficiencies were calculated as described above (equations (3) and (5)) using the instantaneous hand forces, instantaneous hand velocities and the velocity of the swim.

3 Results

The results of propelling and mechanical efficiencies of the stroke and its phases are presented in Table 1.

Table 1. Propelling and mechanical efficiencies during the free-style stroke

	PE (%)	ME (%)
Whole stroke	25.1 ± 12.4	4.5 ± 1.8
Catch	-9.7 ± 6.4	3.3 ± 1.3
Insweep	57.2 ± 7.3	4.3 ± 2.0
Finish	58.9 ± 27.3	8.7 ± 4.6

4 Discussion

Previous studies reported propelling efficiency from 46-77% and mechanical efficiency 8-12% (Toussaint, 1988) using the MAD-system. By virtue of the MAD-system's design, the forces generated appear to correspond to the insweep and outsweep phases denoted in this study. These data show similar propelling and mechanical efficiencies when examining the insweep and outsweep.

Total efficiency for the whole stroke, the product of PE and ME ranged from 1.1-2.7%. These values were lower than the range of 5-8% reported by Toussaint (1988). They were in closer agreement to Pendergast et al. (1974) who reported total efficiency values 2.7-9.4%.

The resultant vector from the hand during the catch is usually pointed towards the swimmer's head as the hand enters the water. This causes the effective force during the catch phase of freestyle to be negative. Therefore, when the catch is taken into consideration our propelling and mechanical efficiencies measured for the whole stroke are approximately 50% less than those calculated using the MAD-system.

This study shows that propelling and mechanical efficiencies might actually be lower and power output might be greater than previously thought. It also emphasizes the importance of examining the whole stroke cycle.

5 References

Abdel-Aziz, Y.I. and Karara, H.M. (1971) Direct linear transformation: from comparator coordinates into object coordinates in close-range photogrammetry. **Proceedings ASPUI Symposium on Close-Range Photogrammetry**, American Society of Photogrammetry, Church Falls, Va., pp. 1-19.

Hollander, A.P., de Groot, G. van Ingen Schenau, G.J., Kahman,. R. and Toussaint, H.M. (1988) Contribuition of the legs to propulsion in front crawl swimming, in **Swimming Science V** (eds B.E. Ungerechts, K. Wilke and R. Reischle), Human Kinetics Books, Champaign, Ill., pp. 39-44.

Pendergast, D.R., di Prampero, P.E., Craig, A.B., Wilson, D.R. and Rennie, D.W. (1974) Quantitative analysis of the front crawl in men and women. **J. Appl. Physiol.**, 475-479.

Schleihauf, R.E. (1979) A hydrodynamic analysis of swimming propulsion, in **Swimming III** (eds J. Terauds and W. Bedingfield), University Park Press, Baltimore, pp. 70-109.

Schleihauf, R.E., Gray, L. and DeRose, J. (1983) Three-dimensional analysis of hand propulsion in the sprint freestyle front crawl stroke, in **Biomechanics and Medicine and Swimming** (eds A.P. Hollander, P.A. Huijing and G. de Groot), Human Kinetics Publishers Inc., Champaign, Ill., pp. 173-183.

Toussaint, H.M. (1988) **Mechanics and Energetics of Swimming**. Rodopi, Amsterdam.

EFFECTS OF TWO TYPES OF BIOMECHANICAL BIO-FEEDBACK ON CRAWL PERFORMANCE

D. CHOLLET[*], M. MADANI[*] and J.P. MICALLEF[+]
[*]Centre D'Etude et d'Optimisation de la Performance Motrice, UFRSTAPS, Montpellier, France; [+]Unité 103 "Appareil moteur et Handicap", INSERM, Montpellier, France

Abstract
This study aims at perfecting and evaluating experimental equipment which responds to the bio-feedback principle. The equipment is composed of two systems which can be used separately or simultaneously by the swimmer. The first is composed of stroke information paddles allowing the swimmer to be informed about the hydrodynamic pressure in his hand during the stroke, whilst the second is composed of a swimmer's speed variation measuring device which transforms the data into auditory information. In order to evaluate the use of the bio-feedback in crawl, a study was performed using four groups of swimmers. Three groups were equipped with the informative equipment and the fourth was the control group (neutral equipment). The results obtained after 5 and 15 days demonstrated that a swimmer informed on the speed variations parameter first and then simultaneously receiving the pressure and speed information, can significantly improve swimming performance.
Keywords: Bio-feedback, Biomechanics Parameters, Stroke Technique, Crawl.

1 Introduction

In order to improve performance, the swimmer must receive information about the efficiency of his technique, the kinetic and kinematic parameters being essential as information feedback in the acquisition of propulsive skill (Newell and Walter, 1981). The information given at the end of the session may not be precise as it is subjective. When some technique evaluation systems are used, both precision and objectivity of information can be improved although feedback only occurs after the task has been completed.

On the contrary, the bio-feedback techniques consist of changing in real time internal processes of biological origin associated with auditory or visual information (Gauthier, 1985). The use of those techniques has already been studied in swimming (Svec, 1982; Van Tilborgh and Persyn, 1984). In our first experiment (Chollet et al., 1988) parameters of distance per cycle were improved, although the experimental group (manual hydrodynamic pressure bio-feedback) did not change the timing performance in a significant way. The purposes of this research are to improve the experimental group's performance at short and average term (after 5 and 15 days) due to the use of two types of biomechanical bio-feedback, and to evaluate the effects of the equipment according to the methods used.

2 Methods

2.1 Experimental equipment
The conception of the equipment involved several conditions: firstly to supply the swimmer with objective information in real time on the biomechanical parameters, secondly to be individually adaptable and simple in order not to worry the swimmer in action, and finally, to understand the nature of crawl swimming.

This experimental installation is composed of two systems which can be used either separately or simultaneously by the swimmer:

(i) a system which picks up the hand propulsive hydrodynamic pressure or the stroke informative paddles (P);

(ii) a system which picks up the instantaneous speed variations of the swimmer in motion (S).

2.2 Stroke informative paddles
These have already been described (Chollet et al., 1988) and are composed of swimming paddles fixed on the swimmer's hand and equipped with a pressure sensor, sound generator and an electrical source of energy. The information given by the sensors is transmitted to the acoustic transmitter fixed in the bathing cap.

2.3 System capturing the instantaneous speed variations of the swimmer's movement
This system is composed of the following components:

(a) a pressure sensor composed of a potentiometer provided with a spring;

(b) an electronic part including a multivibrator and an electrical source of energy, this part being linked to the sensor by a wire;

(c) an acoustic transmitter linked to the electronic part by a wire; this transmitter is placed in the ear of the swimmer during the learning sessions;

(d) a round moss lump connected to the sensor by a linking cable (2 m). This block is placed at the back of the swimmer and lies as a floating anchor so as to allow a resistance outside the turbulence areas;

(e) a belt around the swimmer's waist on which are fixed the speed sensor and the electronic part.

To ensure the system remain watertight, the speed sensor is placed in a waterproof enclosure, while the electronic part is kept within an airtight box. On the latter, a slewing plastic beam containing a magnet is stuck so as to close the circuit. The system for measuring the speed variations is driven by the rubbing strengths caused by the moving moss which forms a resistance located at the back of the swimmer, proportionately varying according to the speed of the swimmer's motion. The variations of the resistance trail (the accelerations) are registered by the sensor and then sent to the multivibrator (electronic part) which transforms them into electrical variations of frequencies proportional to the resistance variations created by the motion of the moss. They are then transformed into auditory signals of equal amplitude by the acoustic transmitter.

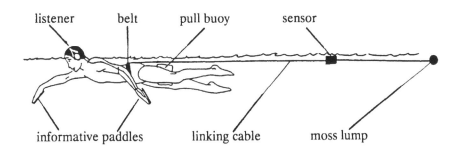

informative paddles   linking cable   moss lump

Fig. 1.   The swimmer is equipped with the experimental bio-
feedback equipment.   At the front (hands), are informative swimming paddles (pressure), at the back, a
system of instantaneous speed analysis.

Consequently, the higher the speed the higher is the pitch.   The
swimmer receives the information in a sustained way during swimming.
The sound stops for only a short moment because the moss becomes
stationary during the turn.   The total charge for both types of
experimental system (Figure 1) is quite insignificant and represents
a slight constraint in the swimming action.

2.4 Subjects
Fifty-eight Moroccan male swimmers (aged from 14 to 18 years) of
regional level took part in the experimental study.   The subjects
formed a homogeneous swimming population in terms of swim times.
Their training level allowed them to easilly perform the sessions
proposed in this experiment.

2.5 Experimental procedures
Three maximal front crawl 'test' swims over 100 m and four training
sessions made up the experimental procedure.   The training sessions
involved a 4 × 50 m front crawl swim at 80% of the first 'test' speed
followed by a 100 m swim, followed by 2 × 50 m front crawl swims at
95% of the first 'test' speed.   The procedures were performed within
15 days and took place as follows:
    Day 1: standardised warm-up (200 m crawl, 100 m arms only, 100 m
two strokes) followed by first 'test' (T0) followed by the first
training session.
    Days 2 to 4: second, third and fourth training sessions.
    Day 5: second 100 m 'test' (T5) after standardised warm-up.
    Day 15: third 100 m 'test' (T15) after standardised warm-up.
    During the testing sessions the equipment used was the same for
all subjects and consisted of:
    (a) Swim paddles, of approximate hand size, fixed by two
adjustable elastic supports.
    (b) Pull buoy placed between the thighs which was composed of two
floating cylinders joined by elastic, thus enabling the swimmer to
work the arms specifically whilst maintaining leg flotation.
    Based on the times achieved for T0, the 58 subjects were divided
into four matched groups:
    (a) A control group (C) performed all the tasks and training
sessions without any bio-feedback equipment.

(b) Experimental group 1 (E1) performed the first two training sessions with the stroke informative paddles (P) and the speed variations system (S) and P during the last two sessions.

(c) Experimental group 2 (E2) performed the first two training sessions with S equipment and the last two sessions with S and P equipment.

(d) Experimental group 3 (E3) performed the first training session with S, the second with P, and the final two sessions with S and P.

The three 100 m front crawl tests (T0, T5, T15) represented the performance criteria relating to the specified training sessions, and as such necessitated that the subjects in each of the four groups were matched for swimming speed. There were no significant differences in swim speed betwen the four groups for T0.

3 Results

Tables 1 and 2 show the results from analysis of the 100 m swim times using the Student-Fisher test and Mann-Witney U test. The data analysis was performed on the mean of the 100 m time differences i.e. T5-T0 and T15-T0. Such a methodology would allow for an examination of the optimal training periods necessary to show any improvements using the bio-feedback devices. Furthermore, the experimental groups were compared to the control in order to evaluate the effectiveness (or otherwise) of the devices.

Table 1. Comparison of the time criteria performances of each experimental group compared with those of the control group at short (T5-T0 gaps) and at an average term (T15-T0 gaps)

Comparison of the groups two by two	(T5-T0)		(T15-T0)	
C/E1	t = 1.00	NS	t = 2.42	P < 0.02
C/E2	t = 2.27	P < 0.05	t = 2.27	P < 0.03
C/E3	t = 0.70	NS	t = 2.88	P < 0.001

Table 2. Comparison of the time criteria performances of each group compared to themselves at short (T5-T0 gaps) and at an average term (T15-T0 gaps)

Groups	(T5-T0)		(T15-T0)	
C	t = 0.18	NS	t = 1.48	NS
E1	t = 1.28	NS	t = 1.86	NS
E2	t - 3.17	P < 0.005	t = 2.19	P < 0.05
E3	t = 0.85	NS	t = 2.42	P < 0.05

4 Discussion

When we consider the values and mean differences obtained for the control group, there were no significance differences after 5 and 15 days. It is unlikely that the time taken for the training (four days) would be sufficient to develop the energy capacities of the swimmers and so lead to a timing improvement. The performances in time express a stability between the three tests.

The averages of the timing performances obtained by the E1 group were significantly different from those of the control group after 15 days ($P < 0.05$). The results did not show a significant improvement after 5 days. At the beginning of the learning (first two sessions), the informative paddles enabled the swimmers to evaluate the hydro-dynamic pressure of the hand. During this period, the subjects received complete information or no information at all (the auditory signal being launched when the chosen strength limit is overtaken) concerning the action of the hand. In this case, we can suppose that the propulsive distance of the arm has been optimized because the subject can judge the nature of the responses to be corrected early (no pause between the propulsive distance of the hand auditory sound or none). The speed equipment which was used at the end of learning (last two sessions) provided global information. In fact, the speed is the result of all the actions included in the stroke. This information, characterized by a progressive sound, constantly varies according to the swimmer's speed. Because of its specification this information was more complex for evaluation by the swimmer. The latter, having two feedback informations would attempt to link them to begin correction of the mistakes pointed out by the systems.

In the case of Experimental group E2 who used the first two learning sessions with the speed variation measuring equipment, followed by the two systems of pressure and speed variation, we noted the appearance of a number of important results. In time the average performance differences showed a significant improvement in the stroke after 5 and 15 days compared with that of the control group ($P < 0.05$) and also between the three tests ($P < 0.005$, $P < 0.05$). It would appear that the subjects in E2 managed to realise a global correction of their action (S), and then during a second phase, assimilating the information given by the informative paddles (P), to carry out a finer correction of propulsive distance of the hand, thus leading to an improvement in their swimming.

Experimental group E3, who used S first then P and finally S and P, showed a significant improvement after 15 days compared to the performance of the control group ($P < 0.01$). A significant progression of the stroke performance between T0 and T15 tests ($P < 0.05$) was also found. It would appear that E3 needed to assimilate the information from the two separate devices initially and then put that information in the final two training sessions in order to show swimming improvements. Hence the findings were significant only after 15 days.

5 Conclusion

Two conclusions were drawn from this study:

(i) All the swimmers benefited from bio-feedback learning and improved in their performances when compared to those of the control group.

(ii) The best results were successively registered by E2, then E3, and finally the E1 group.

In our study, the use of the bio-feedback technique appears as a self-control means using the stroke and leading to improvement in performance.

8 References

Chollet, D., Micallef, J.P. and Rabischong, P. (1988) Biomechanical signals for external biofeedback to improve swimming techniques, in **Swimming Science V** (eds B.E. Ungerechts, K. Wilke and K. Reichle), Human Kinetics Books, Champaign, Il., pp. 389-396.

Gauthier, G.M. (1985) Visually and acoustically augmented performance feedback as an aid in motor skill acquisition. **J. Sports Sci.**, 3, 3-26.

Newell, K.M. and Walter, C.B. (1981) Kinematic and kinetic parameters as information feedback in motor skill acquisition. **J. Human Mov't Stud.**, 7, 235-254.

Svec, O.J. (1982) Biofeedback for pulling efficiency. **Swimming Technique**, 19, 1, 38-44.

Van Tilborgh, L. and Persyn, U. (1984) Sensorimoter and visual feedback for swimming technique. **Project for the Leuven Evaluation Center for Swimmers in collaboration with Heidelberg Swimming Research.** Katholicke Universitein Leuven, Leuven.

BIOMECHANICAL ASPECTS OF PADDLE SWIMMING AT DIFFERENT SPEEDS

K.M. MONTEIL and A.H. ROUARD
Centre de Recherche et d'Innovation sur le Sport, UFRAPS, Université
Lyon I, France

Abstract
The influence of speed on biomechanical parameters of swimming with
paddles has rarely been studied. Seven skilled long and sprint
distance swimmers were examined. Each subject performed 25 m front
crawl swims with the same paddles (arena paddle - 264 cm^2 cross-
sectional area) at three different speeds. Electromyographic (EMG)
parameters were recorded with a telemetric system for five muscles of
the upper limb. Lateral subaquatic views were obtained simultaneously during all the tests. Results showed that there was a close
relationship between the increase in speed and the decrease of the
total time of the stroke. Electromyographic results indicated a non-
linear relationship between muscular activity and swimming speed.
The greatest muscular activity was not obtained for the highest
speed.
Keywords: Electromyography, Kinematic, Paddles, Swimming.

1 Introduction

Since 1970, several authors have investigated the influence of speed
on biomechanical swimming parameters. For example, Lewillie (1971)
showed that the electrical activity of the M. triceps brachii did not
increase linearly with increasing speed. In addition, Craig et al.
(1985) indicated that there was a strong relationship among different
kinematic parameters (velocity/frequency/distance per stroke). These
results were confirmed by Rouard (1987) who found no linear relationship between the amount of muscle activity and swimming speed. These
investigations were followed by a study of the influence of paddle
size on the front crawl stroke (Monteil and Rouard, 1990). The
temporal parameters of the stroke seemed to be increased, and muscular recruitment was modified by the use and size of the paddles. In
addition, competitive sprint swimmers seemed to be more disturbed by
the use and size of the paddles than long distance swimmers.
    The objective of this study was to further investigate the
influence of speed on kinematic and electromyographic parameters in
the front crawl stroke with paddles.

2 Methods

2.1 Subjects
Seven skilled sprinters and long distance swimmers were tested.
Subjects' ages ranged from 15 to 17 years. General subject
characteristics are summarized in Table 1.

Table 1. General characteristics of the subjects

	Age (years)	Height (cm)	Weright (kg)
Men (n = 4)			
Mean	16.7	180.8	65.8
SD	0.4	4.3	8.7
Range	16-17	176-187	56-80
Women (n = 3)			
Mean	15.6	164.6	49.5
SD	0.4	7.4	4.2
Range	15-16	158-175	46-55

2.2 Tests
Each subject performed six 25 m front crawl swims with the same
paddles (arena paddle - 264 cm^2 cross-sectional area) at different
speeds.

Three different speeds were studied (slow, medium and fast) in a
random order. These speeds were expressed as a percentage (65, 80
and 100% respectively) of their maximal speed in the 100 m front
crawl stroke with these paddles. The legs were fixed to a pull-buoy
to eliminate their actions. To minimize fatigue, a rest of 3 min was
allowed between each repetition.

Lateral subaquatic views were captured with a JVC Gx N7S video
camera (25 Hz) fixed in a moving box. Kinematic data were derived
from the video. Electromyographic parameters were recorded during
all swims.

Muscular activity was recorded with a multichannel telemetric
system (Rouard, 1987). Activity was monitored for the following
muscles: the M. pectoralis major, the M. deltoidus pars anterior, the
M. biceps brachii, the M. triceps brachii caput medialis, and the M.
flexor carpi ulnaris. After skin preparation, 11 mm Beckman
electrode pre-amplifier units were affixed to the belly of each
muscle and connected to a box on the swimmer's back. The sensors
were waterproof. Signals were encoded with a subcarrier frequency
and summed. It was then transmitted to a receiving device located at
the side of the pool. The demodulated signals were recorded on an
audio-tape.

2.3 Data treatment
For kinematic data a frame by frame analysis was undertaken to
calculate the total time of the stroke (T) (from the entry to the
next entry of the same hand), and the hip displacement per stroke
(DH) to evaluate the efficiency of the swimmer.

For electromyographic data, raw EMG signals were rectified to obtain the full wave rectified signal. The integration of the rectified EMG was calculated, per unit of time for each stroke. To normalize the results, each integrated part of the signal per unit of time of each muscle was expressed as a percent of the maximal value recorded during the whole test (dynamic reference). Each muscle was used as its own reference for each subject.

For each variable, the mean (M), and the standard deviation (SD) values were calculated. For some of the selected variables, correlation coefficients (r) and analyses of variance were computed.

3 Results and discussion

Kinematic results (Fig. 1) indicated that for all subjects, the total time of the stroke decreased (2.25 s for 65%, 1.70 s for 80% and 1.52 s for 100%) when the speed increased (P < 0.05). This increase in the stroke frequency confirmed findings of Craig et al. (1985). Standard deviation values were similar for the three paces (0.13 for 65%, 0.10 for the 80% and 0.08 for 100%) and indicated no difference within the subject sample.

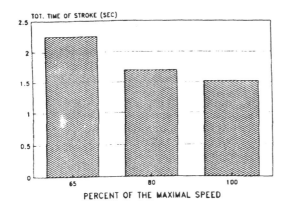

TOT. TIME OF STROKE (SEC)

PERCENT OF THE MAXIMAL SPEED

Fig. 1. Influence of the speed on the total time of the stroke.

Additionally, the hip displacement per stroke (Fig. 2) decreased when the speed increased (2.33 m for 65%, 2.12 m for 80%, and 2.10 m for 100%). There was a strong trend, and perhaps if the sample size were larger, a statistically significant difference may have been found. There was a 10% difference for the hip displacement per stroke between the slow and fast speeds; however, this was not significant (P = 0.10). Standard deviation values were also similar for the three paces (0.21 for 65%, 0.26 for 80%, and 0.27 for 100%).

From these results, it was concluded that a speed increase was associated with a total time of the stroke and hip displacement per stroke decrease. These results were observed for all subjects.

Electromyographic results showed that all muscles had a higher activity for the medium speed (80%) except for the M. biceps brachii, which had its greatest activity for the maximal speed. It was also

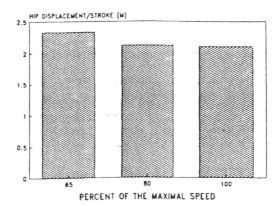

HIP DISPLACEMENT/STROKE (M)

PERCENT OF THE MAXIMAL SPEED

Fig. 2. Influence of speed on the hip displacement per stroke.

noted that the smallest electrical activity (38.0%) was recorded for
all muscles during the slow speed condition. These results seemed to
indicate that there was no linear relationship (r = 0.59) between
swimming speed and muscular activity, as observed in a previous study
without paddles (Rouard, 1987).

The hierarchy of muscular activity (from the highest to the
lowest) did not display large variations through all the speeds
studied. The M. triceps brachii had the highest activity (51.43%)
with the muscle flexors of the upper limb, except for the M. biceps
brachii which had the lowest activity (28.92%) as found in previous
studies (Clarys, Jiskoot and Lewillie, 1973; Rouard, 1987). The
order of the muscles from the highest to the lowest was:
M. triceps brachii > M. flexor carpi ulnaris > M. brachioradialis >
M. pectoralis major > M. biceps brachii.

The comparison between sprint and long distance swimmers showed
higher muscular activity for the long distance swimmers than for the
sprinters, for all the muscles and paces studied. These results
could be explained by the greater use of the upper limb rather than
the lower limb for the long distance swimmers. The standard
deviation values were larger for the sprint swimmers than for the
long distance swimmers. The sprinters demonstrated larger variations
in their crawl stroke technique. They used more kicking in free
swimming than the long distance swimmers. This greater use of
kicking could explain that when they swim with a pull-buoy (fixation
of the legs), no pattern in their muscular recruitment with the
increase of the speed is observed.

4 Conclusion

The study of the biomechanical aspects of paddle swimming at
different speeds showed that there was a close relationship between
increase in speed, decrease of total time (r = -0.98) which was
significant at P < 0.10, and hip displacement per stroke (r = -0.95).

Electromyographic results showed a non-linear relationship between
muscular activity and swimming intensity. The greatest activity

recorded was not obtained during the fastest pace, but was observed for the medium speed. Higher activities were recorded for the M. triceps brachii and some flexors of the upper limb.

Additionally, sprint swimmers seemed to be more sensitive to an increase in swimming speed. These observations could lead to multiple uses of paddles in training. In a longitudinal study, it might be interesting to observe changes in muscular patterns in paddle swimming.

5 References

Clarys, J.P., Jiskoot, J. and Lewillie, L. (1973) A kinematographical, electromyographical, and resistance study of water-polo and competition front crawl. **Medicine and Sport**, 8: Biomechanics III, Karger, Basel, pp. 446-452.

Craig, A.B. Jr., Skehan, P.L., Pawelczyk, J.A. and Boomer, W.L. (1985) Velocity, stroke rate, and distance per stroke during elite swimming competition. **Med. Sci. Sports Exerc.**, 17, 6, 625-634.

Lewillie, L. (1971) Quantitative comparison of the electromyogram of the swimmer, in **Swimming I** (eds L. Lewillie and J.P. Clarys), Vrije Universiteit Brussel, Brussels, pp. 53-57.

Monteil, K.M. and Rouard, A.H. (1990) Influence de la taille des plaquettes sur les paramètres biomécanique du crawl. **STAPS** (accepté à cette revue, publication pour février 1992).

Rouard, A.H. (1987) Étude biomécanique du crawl: évolution des paramètres cinématiques et électromyographiques avec la vitesse. Thèse présentée pour obtenir le grade de docteur, Université Grenoble 1.

THE INTERRELATION OF HYDRODYNAMIC FORCES AND SWIMMING SPEED IN BREASTSTROKE

B.E. UNGERECHTS
Olympic Training Center, Hanover, Germany

Abstract
In swimming the hydrodynamic forces of arms and legs in motion propel the swimmer resulting in a certain swimming speed. This paper examines whether the intracyclic velocity of a swimmer's body can be explained by a 3-dimensional kinematic analysis of the movements of the hands - based on the present knowledge in biomechanics of swimming. Calculating both the fluid forces of the hands in motion and the forces necessary to reach a certain swimming speed (thrust forces) respectively, the degree of coincidence of both forces can be checked. Ninety-nine pairs of forces, calculated for the propulsive part of the armstroke of eight breaststrokers, were compared statistically. The results reveal that 80% of all pairs of forces were statistically equal, indicating close covariation.

Moreover, the comparison of the absolute values of the different force terms demonstrated that the fluid forces produced by the hands account for only about half of the entire thrust forces. This in turn requires the consideration of the fluid forces provided by the arms which account for the second half.

It is concluded that the biomechanical approach chosen here, supplemented with some adjustments, might be a valuable method for diagnosis and prognosis of elite swimmers' technique and efficiency.
Keywords: Flow Forces, Hand Motion, Thrust Forces, Hip Motion, Breaststroke, Hydrodynamics, Laws of Motion.

1 Introduction

In swimming the limbs in motion interact with the surrounding water and in reaction to that the body is propelled forward. The moving limbs can be considered as obstacles disturbing the resting water in the vicinity. Since the water cannot penetrate the limbs, it is set in motion, resulting in a flow. Due to the properties of the water some **flow forces** are created. These flow forces can be separated into **lift** and **drag forces** resulting in the **fluid force**. The fluid force is the origin of the propulsive action which is transferred via the limbs of the body itself, and which in reaction is pushed ahead. The swimming speed is determined by the fluid force interacting with the resistance of the body.

For practical use the knowledge to understand how the limbs should be moved in order to create as much thrust as possible "under the condition of a human being" is obvious. Biomechanical studies in swimming therefore serve at least two purposes. Firstly these studies reveal an insight into the correct relation of origin and effect - the basic or determining factors - and secondly the studies influence the reflections of the strokes resulting in appropriate learning strategies.

It was Counsilman in 1971 who prepared the water-related view of swimming strokes, introducing the sweeping motion; Schleihauf et al. (1979, 1983) introduced the appropriate fluid laws; Ungerechts (1979) demonstrated that the sweeping motions will match with the anatomical properties of human limbs, and van Tilborgh et al. (1988) demonstrated the effect on the body's motion.

In the past we thus had two approaches, one considering the strokes' effect on the water and the other the resulting swimming speed. The purpose of this study is to check if the calculated fluid forces created by the limbs explain the intracyclic swimming speed of the body, based on the Laws of Motion.

2 Methods

2.1 Subjects
Twenty-two breaststrokers of the FRG Swimming Team took part in the investigation; they were aged from 14.5 to 20.5 years and the best times per 100 m ranged from 1:12.9 to 1:17.3 for the women (n = 9) and from 1:03.4 to 1:13.4 for men (n = 13). The breaststroke was selected due to the unique situation of the synchronisation of the propulsive parts of arms and legs which are more or less separated.

The swimmers were filmed by two underwater cameras, each operating at 40 Hz. The kinematic analysis of the films provided three-dimensional coordinates of the movement of the left hand and two-dimensional coordinates of the hip's motion in the swimming direction.

2.2 Measurements
The calculation of the hydrodynamic parameters for example: relative flow velocity v(hd), angle of attack, and sweepback angle were calculated using to the algorithms introduced by Schleihauf et al. (1983). The calculation of the temporal distribution of the fluid force; the resultant of the lift and drag, was well executed according to the algorithms of Schleihauf et al. (1983). The calculation of the intracyclic swimming speed u of the hip was obtained by a method introduced by van Tilborgh et al. (1987). If the velocity-time relation of a swimmer is known the necessary thrust force Fs can be calculated based on the laws of motion.

$$Fs = 2Fx$$
$$2Fx = m.u/t + D.u^2 \tag{1}$$

Equation (1) implies that theoretically the propulsive force (2Fx) equal the resistance force ($D.u^2$) plus a term, the inertial term, dependent of the acceleration of the body (m.u/t).

In this study the question was whether the theoretical ideal could be justified biomechanically. For eight swimmers some 99 pairs of force-data (2Fx(t)/Fs(t)) regarding the propulsive part of the armstroke were checked statistically to answer the following questions:

1. How large is the deviation factor k between Fx(t) and Fs(t)?
2. Is there a systematic covariation between the forces?
   and
3. What are the regression equations?

3 Results

In order to calculate equation (1) the individual body mass m was taken; the coefficient of resistance D for women was D_w = 29.2 kg/m, for men D_m = 27.4 kg/m. The acceleration u/t was calculated by differentiation of u(t) for each time sequence (t) considered.

Table 1.   Results of some parameters concentrated on statistical terms; mean and standard deviation, for eight swimmers regarding the propulsive part of the armstroke in breast-stroke

	I (N)	II (N)	III –	IV –	V –
1	66.7 +54.3	147.2 +75.5	4.9 +6.5	0.69 n = 13	6.55 + 0.49x
2	57.2 +32.7	118.4 +34.0	3.3 +3.0	0.47 n = 11	0.01 + 0.45x
3	55.3 +26.9	126.9 +30.9	3.2 +2.5	0.52 n = 13	-2.0 + 0.45x
4	45.0 +20.8	113.0 +18.0	3.2 +1.8	0.64 n = 13	-38.60 + 0.73x
5	47.0 +18.5	125.8 +17.9	2.8 +1.6	0.70 n = 14	24.26 + 0.18x
6	57.6 +37.9	193.1 +150.6	5.1 +5.7	0.59 n = 14	28.64 + 0.15x
7	94.9 +34.9	138.9 +27.9	2.1 +2.2	0.74 n = 10	-34.12 + 0.92x
8	36.3 +19.1	185.3 +93.8	10.9 +17.2	0.66 n = 11	11.24 + 0.13x

I: Fluid force 2Fx in swimming direction for both hands, (means),
II: Thrust force Fs, depending on the velocity of the hip, (means),
III: Factor of deviation, (means),
IV: Correlation coefficient r (Fx/Fs),
V: Regression equation.

Some details not included in Table 1 should be emphasized
additionally:
- peak acceleration occurred 70-50 ms earlier than peak velocity.
- the maximal calculated body drag was $(D.u^2)$ = 106 N, the maximum
  calculated inertial force was 466 N, 4.4 times higher than the body
  drag; in total peak forces were 572 N which were only opposed by
  maximal hand forces of 136 N.
- in seven of 99 force pairs the deviation k was exaggerated; in
  overwhelming cases k was between 2-3, indicating close covariation
  for about 80% of pairs of forces.
- the coefficient of correlation when considering the cases of eight
  swimmers separately are placed in the range of 0.47-0.74. The
  critical value is r(0.058) = 0.6. On this basis in five out of
  eight cases (62.5%) the correlation is significant, which means
  there is a reasonable trend that the experimental data fulfil the
  laws of motion.
- if 2Fx should be assessed on the basis of the forces Fs calculated
  for the hip's motion the regression equations can be referred to.
  If the regression coefficient b is for example b = 0.44 it implies
  that if Fs = 10 N, then 2Fx = 4.4 N. This indicates that for a
  given time unit the fluid force produced in the vicinity of the
  hands are too small to match with the forces related to the actual
  swimming velocity.

4 Conclusion

The assumption that the interrelationship of the hydrodynamic forces
and the swimming velocity can be based on the fluid force of the
hands exclusively is questionable. It is concluded that fluid forces
of the arms - which are about the same value as the drag forces of
the hands (Löhr and Ungerechts, 1976) - should be considered as well.
   The covariation of fluid and thrust forces showed large deviations
in some cases. Close scrutiny revealed an accumulation during the
phase when the hands change direction, from outwards to inwards.
This may be attributed to an insufficient theory, when using the
hydrodynamics of foils. In conjunction with changes in direction of
propelling body parts, Ungerechts (1981, 1988) demonstrated that the
flow behaviour is better explained by the "vortex theory".
   The examination of the interrelationship of forces and swimming
speed revealed the variability of propulsive and resistive force
resulting in intracyclic velocity distributions. It is questionable
if these intracyclic velocity structures can be optimized to lower
the resistance of the body by emphasizing the undulation of the total
body.

5 References

Counsilman, J.E. (1971) The application of Bernoulli's principle to
   human propulsion in water, in **Biomechanics in Swimming** (eds
   J.P. Clarys and L. Lewillie), Université Libre de Bruxelles,
   Brussels, pp. 59-71.
Löhr, R. and Ungerechts, B. (1976) Experimental estimation of the
   optimal finger position in front of crawl. **Leistungssport**, 4,

312-314.

Schleihauf, R.E. (1979) A hydrodynamic analysis of swimming propulsion, in **Swimming III** (eds J. Terauds and E.W. Bedingfield), University Park Press, Baltimore, pp. 70-109.

Schleihauf, R.E., Gray, L. and De Rose, J. (1983) Three dimensional analysis of hand propulsion in sprint front crawl stroke, in **Biomechanics and Medicine of Swimming** (eds A.P. Hollander, P.A. Huijing and G. de Groot), Human Kinetics Publishers, Champaign, Ill., pp. 173-183.

Ungerechts, B.E. (1979) Optimizing propulsion in swimming by rotation of the hands, in **Swimming III** (eds J. Terauds and E.W. Bedingfield), University Park Press, Baltimore, pp. 55-61.

Ungerechts, B.E. (1981) Propulsive principle of fast swimming vertebrates analysed by flow-visualising technique, in **Abstracts VIIIth International Congress of Biomechanics**, Nagoya, p. 165.

Ungerechts, B.E. (1988) The relation of peak body acceleration to phases of movements in swimming, in **Swimming Science V** (eds B.E. Ungerechts, K. Wilke and K. Reischle), Human Kinetics Books, Champaign, Ill., pp. 779-784.

Van Tilborgh, L.M., Stijnen, V.V. and Persyn, U.J. (1987) Using velocity fluctuations for estimating resistance and propulsive forces in breaststroke swimming in **Biomechanics X-B** (ed B. Jonsson), Human Kinetics Publishers, Champaign, Ill., pp. 779-784.

Van Tilborgh, L.M., Willems, E.J. and Persyn, U.J. (1988) Estimation of breaststroke propulsion and resistance-resultant impulses from film analysis, in **Swimming Science V** (eds B.E. Ungerechts, K. Wilke and K. Reischle), Human Kinetics Books, Champaign, Ill., pp. 67-72.

MOVEMENT ANALYSIS OF THE FLAT AND THE UNDULATING BREASTSTROKE PATTERN

U. PERSYN, V. COLMAN and L. VAN TILBORGH
Instituut voor Lichamelijke Opleiding, K.U. Leuven, Leuven, Belgium

Abstract
A new video-analysis system was used to derive hypotheses regarding advantages of an extremely undulating breaststroke pattern. To obtain supporting evidence on the effectiveness of undulation, relationships between several specific body segment positions (or angles) in the stroke and resultant impulses per phase (difference between propulsion and drag) were specified (Tau-B coefficients, significant at the 5% level).

In the stroke cycle of the undulating pattern of an 'experimental' swimmer, higher peaks and less decrease in velocity of the centre of gravity are seen. Apparently, this is obtained due to a vertical propeller-like propulsion of the hands and feet, and up- and downhill movements of the entire body.

The following correlations were found between impulse and respectively the amount of upward spreading of the arms (0.44), the amount of keeping the hands in front of the vertical under the shoulders (0.38), the depth of closing the legs (0.47), the more vertical foot position (0.41), the amount of the most downhill (0.59) and uphill trunk position (0.37).

Although this uphill, hydroplaning position takes place in the recovery phases, the symmetry in the undulation of the body is not significantly disturbed and the vertical displacements of the centre of gravity are small.
Keywords: Breaststroke Swimming, Movement Analysis, Flat and Undulating Pattern.

1 Introduction

The study of the new breaststroke patterns and of the evolution of one international female swimmer, from a flat to an undulating and faster pattern, influenced to some extent the FINA rule change, which allows the head to dive under the water (Persyn et al., 1988; Van Tilborgh et al., 1988). This rule change made even extreme undulation possible, and this has resulted in one swimmer exhibiting a still faster pattern. For a follow-up of this swimmer, a new video-analysis system was used to derive hypotheses regarding advantages of this extremely undulating pattern. In addition, to obtain supporting evidence on the effectiveness of undulation, relationships between several specific body segment positions (or angles) in the stroke and resultant impulses per phase (difference between propulsion and drag) were specified. To calculate these impulses, a method was developed to estimate the body centre of gravity for swimmers, using a personalized computer model of the human body (Hanavan, 1964; Stijnen et al., 1980; Van Tilborgh, 1987). These relations were checked on a group of 18 West German national and international breaststroke swimmers.

2 Methods

Swimming movements are normally recorded with a fixed camera. Since the swimmer must remain on screen for at least one complete stroke cycle, the field of view is wide and the swimmer appears small and poorly visible. To obtain a larger image of the swimmer, he must be filmed in close-up and, consequently, the camera must be rotated. Because the swimmer is moving under water and in the air, a periscope was constructed dividing a single video field into two parts.

Due to the different refractions of light in water and in air, body segments above the water surface appear much smaller than those under water, and not in the correct position. In addition, the zone at the water level, separating the two views, is distorted so that no direct digitizing is possible in this area. To solve these problems, a manual digitizing system was developed providing specific procedures for the reconstruction of the image (Colman and Persyn, 1989).

After digitizing 18 body markers on 12 specific frames (delimiting the phases in one cycle), diverse movement variables were calculated (angles, paths and velocities of body segments). Simultaneously the necessary corrections were made for the rotating camera. Furthermore, the exact position of the body's centre of gravity was determined in each frame.

In Fig. 1A space and time aspects of the flat (I) and undulating (II) patterns are visualized:

- In Aa the digitized frames are presented in stick figures. The displacement per phase is specified by the horizontal distance between the position of the body's centre of gravity in the successive stick figures (indicated by a circle approximately at the level of the navel). The duration of the phases is indicated by the vertical distance between each water level (the dotted lines).
- In Ab this timing is drawn vertically (successively for the propulsive kick and pull phase and for the recovery).
- In Ac the mean velocity of the centre of gravity of the swimmer is given for each phase.

More details of the movement can be seen in Fig. 1B-F:

- In B-E, the displacement of the body segments, in relation to a fixed background are visualised: in B for the entire body, hip and centre of gravity, in C for trunk and thigh only (the drag surface) and in D-E for the foot and hand (the propulsion paths). In E,II the trunk inclination is also indicated.
- In F, the amplitudes of the leg and arm movements, in relation to the hip and shoulder, artificially fixed at the same horizontal level are visualized (there is neither displacement nor rotation of the trunk).

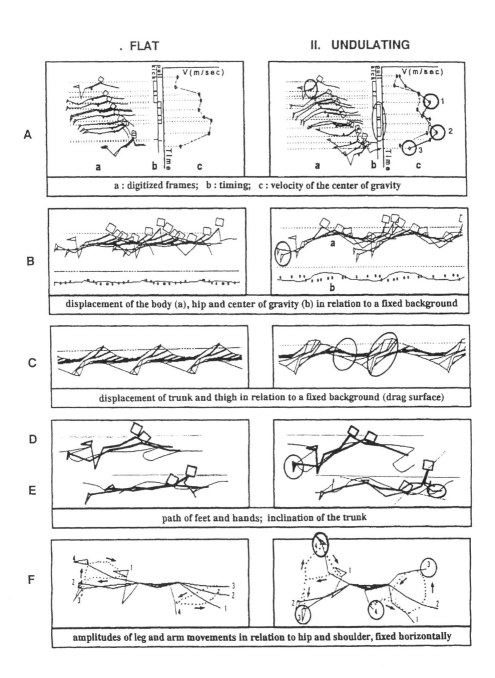

Fig. 1.   Some space and time aspects of the flat (I) and the undulating (II) breaststroke pattern used by one international swimmer, visualized by video-analysis.

3 Results and discussion

From these visualizations, hypotheses were derived with regard to advantages of undulation. To support this, correlations (Tau-B coefficients, significant at the 5% level) between resultant impulses per phase and specific movement variables (positions or angles) are presented.

In Fig. 1,II Ac higher peaks (1,2) and decrease in velocity (3) are seen for the undulating pattern. Apparently, this is obtained because of a vertical propeller-like propulsion of the feet and hands, and up- and downwards movements of the entire body (Fig. 2).

3.1 Vertical propeller-like propulsion of the hands and the feet

The more vertical and less backward slipping paths of hands and feet in the undulating pattern indicate that more lift (propeller) than drag (paddle) propulsion is applied (Fig. 1,D-E).

During this propeller-like movement the **hands** come close to the surface twice (Fig. 2): first, during the spreading of the arms (1) and, next, during the recovery (2). Approaching this second moment, the hands (positioned horizontally) can lift the body upwards (Fig. 1,II,E).

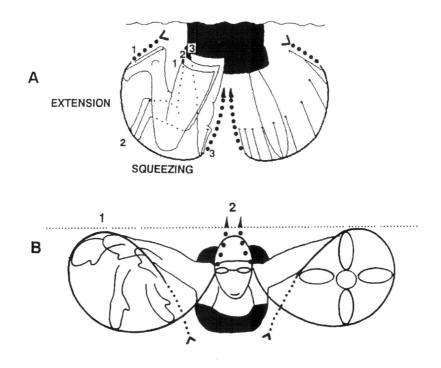

Fig. 2. Front view of the paths of the propeller-like propulsion of the feet and hands

In this up-, down- and upward arm action the propulsion will probably act through the centre of gravity, only slightly upwards (Fig. 1,II,Bb). Furthermore, this propeller-like arm action lasts longer (Fig. 1,Ab), probably generating a greater impulse. The correlation between the amount of upward spreading of the arms and impulse is 0.44 and between the time spent keeping the hands in front of the vertical under the shoulders and impulse is 0.38.

In the undulating pattern it is easier to keep the soles of the feet vertical (the position of a propeller blade) during the closing of the legs (Fig. 1,II,B and D). Even when the ankles are slightly extended, this vertical position can be maintained due to the bottomward kick. (It is interesting to note that with slight ankle extension, greater supination is possible as well.) The correlation between the depth of closing the legs and impulse is 0.47, and between a more vertical foot position and impulse is 0.41.

When the paths of the **hands** and **feet** are drawn in relation to the hip and the shoulder, artificially fixed at the horizontal level, it can be seen that in the undulating pattern both movement amplitudes are approximately double that of the flat pattern (Fig. 1,F). One can expect that greater flexibility in the hips, trunk and shoulders and more strength in the M. pectoralis are required to obtain these amplitudes.

3.1 Upward and downward movements of the body

Because of the vertical pull and kick the trunk moves considerably up and down (respectively 44° and -10°) (Fig. 1,II,E). The correlation between the angle of the greatest upward trunk position and impulse is 0.37, and of the lowest downward trunk position and impulse is 0.59. Paradoxically, these impulses occur in phases without arm and leg propulsion. Additional propulsion can thus only be generated by the surrounding water.

In the lowest downward position the body is S-shaped (Fig. 1,II,E). This body position can be obtained by holding the hips flexed while spreading the arms upwards and trying to camber in the lumbar region. Following this, the entire body undulates through an S-shaped path to the greatest upward and cambered body position. This is obtained during a quick and large bottom- and upward arm action and upward leg action (Fig. 1,II,F,3-4).

This undulation could decrease the drag surface to a minimum (Fig. 1,II,C) and/or generate additional propulsion by moving a mass of water, a wave along the body, from shoulders to feet: indeed, in the stroke cycle a curve in the body moves from the shoulders to the lumbar region, the hips, the knees and the feet.

Regarding the greatest upward, hydroplaning position (during the recovery) the hypothesis was formed that an (added) mass of water, being displaced behind the trunk during the preceding pull, could push against the back (Fig. 1,II,E). This could be compared to a cyclist wearing a backpack, who is thrown forward over the handlebars when braking suddenly.

This hydroplaning position can be maintained by cambering the trunk and keeping the hips sufficiently extended during the recovery (Fig. 1,II,Aa). Apparently, due to the upward body position in the following spreading of the legs (Figs. 1,II,D) the symmetry in undulation of the body is not significantly disturbed by the recovery (Fig. 1,B-C). In addition, the vertical displacements of the centre of gravity are small (Fig. 1,Bb).

4 Conclusions

The correlations between impulse and specific movement variables in
the undulating pattern provide some evidence of advantages of this
pattern. However, interpretations from video-analysis of one international swimmer does not allow one to provide each individual with
advice regarding the best pattern. Therefore, the movement patterns
as well as the corresponding physical characteristics of a large
group of international swimmers must first be investigated.

An important prerequisite to undulate could be specific flexibility (Fig. 1,II,F). This may mainly be necessary during the most S-
shaped and cambered body positions (shoulder inward rotation, upward
extension and abduction, lumbar camber and hip and knee hyperexten-
sion), as well as during the kick (ankle flexion, outward rotation
and supination and hip in- and outward rotation).

5 Acknowledgements

The evaluation of the swimmers investigated was done with the help of
D. Daly, D. Verhetsel and F. Van Oost.

6 References

Colman, V. and Persyn, U. (1989) PC-seminars on sport technique and
    training, in **Schwimmen lernen und optimieren Band 2 DSV** (ed
    W. Freitag), Mainz, pp. 69-110.
Hanavan, E. (1964) **A Mathematical Model of the Human Body** (Technical
    report AMRL-TDR-64-102) Wright-Patterson Air Force Base, OJ:
    Wright Air Development Center.
Persyn, U., Van Tilborgh, L., Daly, D., Colman, V., Vijfvinkel, D.
    and Verhetsel, D. (1988) Computerized evaluation and advice in
    swimming, in **Swimming Sciences V** (eds B. Ungerechts, K. Wilke and
    K. Reischle) Human Kinetics Books, Champaign, Ill., pp. 341-349.
Stijnen, V., Spaepen, A. and Willems, E. (1980) Models and methods
    for the determination of the center of gravity of the human body
    from film, in **Biomechanics VII-A** (eds A. Morecki, K. Fidelus, K.
    Kedzior and A. De Wit), University Park Press, Baltimore, pp.
    558-564.
Van Tilborgh, L. (1987) **Stuw- en rembrachten bij schoolslagzwemmers:
    berekening uit filmanalyse (Propulsion and drag forces in breast-
    stroke swimmers: calculation from film analysis)**, Unpublished
    doctoral dissertation in Physical Education, K.U. Leuven, Leuven.
Van Tilborgh, L., Willems, E. and Persyn, U. (1988) Estimation of
    breaststroke propulsion and resistance resultant impulses from
    film analysis, in **Swimming Sciences V** (eds B. Ungerechts, K. Wilke
    and K. Reischle), Human Kinetics Books, Champaign, Ill., pp.
    66-72.

PROPULSION IN THE BUFFERFLY STROKE

B.R. MASON, Z. TONG and R.J. RICHARDS
Australian Institute of Sport, Canberra, Australia

Abstract
This study examined the intra-stroke velocity and acceleration of the
centre of gravity (CG) of elite bufferfly swimmers. The purpose of
the research was to understand more about the propulsive nature of
the stroke and identify if the velocity and acceleration profiles of
the swimmers' hip would adequately reflect the corresponding CG
profiles. An analysis of the results (n = 11) revealed that the hip
parameters could not reliably be substituted for those of the
swimmers' CG. The profiles of the swimmers' hips were found to
fluctuate with greater magnitude and were out of phase with the
velocity and acceleration profiles of the CG. The CG acceleration
profiles illustrated that there were five distinct propulsive phases
in the stroke. If hand entry was considered as the start of the
stroke, the acceleration peaks occurred at the kick (1.9 m/s^{-2}),
outsweep of arms (1.4 m/s^{-2}), insweep of arms (4.2 m/s^{-2}), concurrent
kick with upsweep of arms (2.3 m/s^{-2}) and finally catching the wave
(0.0 m s^{-2}). The last propulsive phase did not correspond to any
particular movement of the arms or legs and on observation was
associated with the swimmers' actions of riding the wave produced by
the swimming action itself.
Keywords: Swimming, Biomechanics, Butterfly, Propulsion,
Acceleration.

1 Introduction

The intra-stroke acceleration profile of a swimmer indicates where
the swimmer utilises effective propulsive actions to propel himself
forward and where effective streamlining is used to reduce drag. The
intra-stroke velocity profile indicates the effect of propulsion on
the swimmer's motion. The relationship between the intra-stroke
velocity profile of a swimmer and efficiency in swimming was reported
in the literature (Kornecki and Bober, 1978).

It is important that the centre of gravity (CG) of the swimmer is
used to compute the velocity and acceleration profiles. The movement
pattern of the CG reflects the true movement of the whole swimmer.
It is the most accurate method presently used to diagnose the propulsive efficiency of competitive swimmers (Maglischo et al., 1987). It
is almost impossible to obtain accurate velocity and acceleration
information about the CG of the body directly from a transducer as
this method only measures the movement occurring at one point on the

body. Large changes in body position occur in butterfly and this
affects the location of the CG. In order to obtain accurate measurements of velocity changes which occur during a stroke cycle, these
shifts in the location of the CG need to be considered. Movement
parameters of the CG can be obtained by digitising specific anatomical landmarks from film and computing the location of the CG a frame
at a time. The velocity and acceleration parameters can then be
calculated. Previous research has examined the velocity and acceleration profiles of swimmers. In many cases such studies only
investigated the hip motion.

The major aim of this project was to obtain accurate intra-stroke
velocity and acceleration profiles of elite butterfly swimmers. This
would result in an improved understanding of the mechanics of propulsion in the stroke. The research also investigated the velocity and
acceleration profiles associated with the hip movement to evaluate
whether they could reliably be substituted for the CG profiles, such
that information about hip movement would be sufficient for the
evaluation of stroke mechanics.

2 Methods

2.1 Subjects
Eleven elite Australian butterfly swimmers, two females and nine
males, were filmed at the Australian Institute of Sport. All
swimmers were instructed to swim their regular competitive distance
at competition pace and the filming was done as they completed the
last two laps, in a 25 metre pool.

2.2 Filming procedures
A 16 mm high speed Photosonics camera, operating at 100 Hz, was used
to film each swimmer. The camera was positioned three lanes distant
from the swimmer just beneath water level, at right angles to the
swimmer's movement plane. The camera was behind the viewing window
(1.3 m × 1.2 m), which extended above and below the water level. The
camera was panned to obtain a large image size of the swimmer over
approximately three strokes. A periscope attachment on the camera
permitted a split image which provided pictures of the swimmer's body
above and below the water on each frame of the film. Reference
markers were located both above and below the water level to enable
the digitised information to be adjusted. This was necessary due to
the complex filming procedures. Adjustments had to be made because
of the differences in the size and displacement of those parts of the
swimmer's body which were out of the water as opposed to those parts
which were under water, caused by the different refractive indices of
light in air and water. The markers also enabled adjustments to be
made to the varying displacement measurements which arose because of
the changing camera angles to the plane of motion that resulted from
using a panned camera.

2.3 Data processing
The start of the stroke was considered to be hand entry. For each
swimmer, 22 body segmented endpoints represented the swimmer's body,
and four reference markers were digitised in every frame over an
entire stroke length. An additional 20 frames before and after the

stroke were digitised to provide the information to permit accurate data smoothing over the entire stroke. The reference markers were digitised so the computer could scale and correct the displacement of the body's segmental endpoints for the information obtained in each film frame during the digitising process.

2.4 Calculated parameters
The adjusted two dimensional data, representing the location of the swimmer's body landmarks, were smoothed using a digital filtering technique. The data were then adjusted to account for the phase shift which occurred during the digital smoothing process. The displacement of the swimmer's CG in the horizontal plane was computed for each frame digitised. The velocity and acceleration of each swimmer was computed as the first and second derivative respectively of the CG's horizontal displacement with respect to time. Digital filtering techniques were applied after each derivative computation. This extra smoothing resulted in the profiles being a representative but conservative measure of the intra-stroke velocity and acceleration patterns for the individual swimmers. To investigate whether hip movement could be accurately substituted for CG movement, similar computations were performed on the horizontal displacement of the hip. Average data from both the left and right hips were used to compute velocity and acceleration parameters of the hip.

2.5 Data presentation
The velocity and acceleration profiles for each swimmer were plotted and displayed simultaneously with animated stick figures drawn from the smoothed digitised data on a computer terminal. The animated stick figures produced a simulation of the swimmer's stroke. Pointers moved along the velocity and acceleration profiles to show exactly which part of the profile corresponded to the stick figure.

2.6 Analysis

The analysis consisted firstly of observing the velocity and acceleration profiles of the CG of each swimmer in conjunction with the animated stick figure which represented the action of that swimmer's stroke. Here the various phases of the stroke for each swimmer were identified. The values for the timing and peak acceleration of the events representing each propulsive phase were ascertained for all swimmers tested. Similar values for the timing and maximum deceleration were obtained for the troughs between each propulsive phase. This averaged information provided the data to compute a composite graph which represented a general acceleration parameter for all the swimmers tested. The integral of this curve was computed and adjusted for the integration constant to represent the composite parameter for velocity.

To evaluate whether the velocity and acceleration profiles associated with hip movement could reliably represent CG movement, the following analysis was performed. The velocity and acceleration profiles obtained for the hip were plotted together with the corresponding profiles obtained for the CG. Separate graphs for acceleration and velocity were produced for each swimmer. This enabled a visual inspection and comparison of the hip and CG profiles to be made. A correlation coefficient was calculated to determine the degree of relationship between the hip and CG profiles for each swimmer tested. The Pearson product moment correlation coefficient was computed using the paired values on each curve representing the velocity or acceleration values at corresponding points in time. The number of pairs of values used in the correlation calculation corresponded with the number of film frames from which the information for each swimmer's stroke was derived.

3 Results

The composite acceleration parameter developed from the eleven butterfly swimmers identified that five major propulsive phases occurred during the butterfly stroke. The duration of the entire stroke was 1.29 s. The first event was the kick immediately following hand entry (0.007 s, 1.9 m s^{-2}). This was followed by the outsweep;/downsweep (0.35 s, 1.4 m s^{-2}), the insweep (0.57 s, 4.2 m s^{-2}), the kick and upsweep (0.79 s, 2.3 m s^{-2}) and lastly the catch wave (1.06 s, 0.0 m s^{-2}). See Figure 1 for the composite acceleration and velocity parameter. Ten of the eleven swimmers demonstrated the catch wave phase. The hand catch was noticeable as a slight bump in the acceleration profiles of four of the swimmers and occurred in the composite acceleration parameter 0.22 s after hand entry. A comparison of hip versus CG profiles revealed that velocity and acceleration of the hip could not reliably be substituted for that of a swimmer's CG. The profiles of the swimmers' hips were found to fluctuate with greater magnitude and were out of phase with the acceleration and velocity profiles of the CG. The researchers believe that for the hip profiles to be considered as representative of the CG, the correlation coefficient representing the relationship between the time based paired points on the CG and hip profiles should be as high as 0.95. The results of this research indicated a mean correlation coefficient computed over all subjects of 0.84 for velocity and 0.75 for acceleration using a mean of 129 paired points on the curves.

4 Discussion

The analysis revealed that five distinct propulsive stages occur in butterfly swimming. On the basis of magnitude in the composite acceleration parameter, the most propulsive to the least propulsive were as follows: insweep of hands, upsweep of hands and second kick, the first kick, the outsweep and downsweep of the hands and lastly the catch wave phase. Previous research (Barthels and Adrian, 1975) also reported large body accelerations during the insweep which were produced by lift forces on the hand. Research conducted at the USOC reported that the largest forces in butterfly usually occurred during the insweep (USOC Biomechanics Report, 1989). The propulsive stage associated with the catch wave phase was not associated with any obvious propulsive action of the swimmer. The researchers hypothesised that this acceleration peak was associated with the swimmer catching the wave produced by the swimming action itself. During the arm pull propulsion phases of the stroke the swimmer moves a large volume of water forward with the trunk. The main cause of this

MEAN BUTTERFLY INTRASTROKE PROFILE

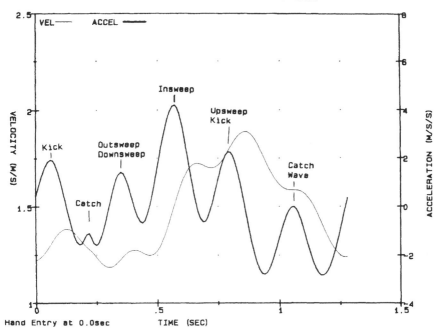

Fig. 1. Composite graph of intra-stroke velocity and acceleration
         parameter computed from individual profiles of 11 butter-
         fly swimmers.

phenomenon is the relatively large surface area of the trunk moving
forward against a still, incompressible volume of water. The resulting moving wall of water is sometimes referred to as an accelerated
mass. When the swimmer decelerates after the completion of the arm
pull, a volume of water or wave tends to surge forward past the
swimmer and may be used as a source of propulsion. This may be
explained in terms of a transfer of momentum from the swimmer to the
water, during the arm pull phases, and then some of the momentum is
transferred back to the swimmer, during the catch wave phase. A
similar phenomenon is experienced in a moving motor boat when the
motor is switched off. Shortly after being switched off a wave
catches up to the boat and causes it to surge forward as it rides the
wave.

   The CG acceleration profiles were very informative and disclosed
the degree to which each propulsive action in the stroke was successful in achieving its aim. Both the magnitude and duration of the
effective propulsive forces were displayed. The value of the velocity profiles became apparent at this point as they enabled an
assessment to be made of the combined effect of both the magnitude,
shape and duration of the acceleration peaks and troughs which
reflected each propulsive and resistive event.

   Although the correlation coefficients for the relationship between the hip and CG acceleration profiles were reasonably high for most swimmers tested in the present study, this was to be expected because the movement of the hip was related to the movement of the entire body. However, no consistent relationship could be identified between the hip and CG movement for all swimmers. It would therefore be invalid to evaluate stroke technique based on the acceleration profile obtained for only the hip, or for any other single point on the body. The shift in phase of the velocity and acceleration curves produced for the hip, from the true movement pattern of the entire body, considerably limits the value of the hip parameters. The shift was found to be inconsistent from one swimmer to the next which further reduces the reliability of a modified hip movement profile for stroke correction purposes.

5 References

Barthels, K. and Adrian, M.J. (1975) Three-dimensional spatial hand positions of skilled butterfly swimmers, in **Conference Proceedings - International Symposium on Biomechanics in Swimming** (eds J. Clarys and L. Lewillie), University Park Press, Baltimore, pp. 154-160.

Kornecki, S. and Bober, T. (1978) Extreme velocities of a swimming cycle as a technique criterion, in **Swimming Medicine IV** (eds B. Eriksson and B. Furberg), University Park Press, Baltimore, pp. 402-407.

Maglischo, C.W., Maglischo, E.W. and Santos, T.R. (1987) The relationship between the forward velocity of the centre of gravity and the forward velocity of the hip in the four competitive strokes. **J. Swimming Res,** 3(2), 11-17.

USOC (1989) Report by United States Swimming - Sports Medicine and Science Biomechanics Summary: Analysis of Competitive Races. USOC, Colorado Springs.

A BIOMECHANICAL ANALYSIS OF THE NOVICE SWIMMER USING THE BUTTERFLY STROKE

T. TOGASHI and T. NOMURA*
Faculty of General Education, Ibaraki University, Mito, Japan
*Institute of Sport Science, University of Tsukuba, Tsukuba, Japan

Abstract
The purpose of this study was to clarify the technical characteristics of novice swimmers using the butterfly stroke. Twenty-five novice swimmers swam two 25 m maximal trials which were filmed by an underwater VTR camera. The velocity and angle of joints and segments were calculated by the Direct Linear Transformation (DLT) method using a microcomputer. Significant correlations were found between (1) elbow angle at catch point and average swimming velocity, (2) appearance time of high elbow and average swimming velocity, (3) fluctuations in horizontal velocity and average swimming velocity, (4) horizontal distance from entry point to release point and average swimming velocity. In conclusion, the high elbow technique and early appearance of high elbow at the catch point were considered very important for the correct butterfly stroke in novice swimmers.
Keywords: Evaluation, Biomechanical Analysis, Butterfly Stroke, Novice Swimmer.

1 Introduction

The butterfly stroke is perceived by most coaches and national swimming associations to be the most difficult to learn and possibly the most tiring. A consequence of this fact is that it is the last of the four strokes to be taught by coaches. This study analysed the biomechanics of the butterfly stroke, as performed by novice swimmers, in order to determine the difficulties associated with it, and with a view to providing useful information to coaches and teachers.

2 Methods

Twenty-five novice butterfly swimmers were filmed. They swam two 25 m trials at their maximal effort, during which an underwater VTR camera filmed several locations of their body parts which had been marked with black vinyl tape, i.e. wrist joint, elbow joint, shoulder joint, top of the head, knee and ankle joint.

The camera was fixed 50 cm underwater by a tripod to record side views. The VTR film was digitized using a personal computer with superimposed board and using a VTR deck. The digitized data were calculated by the same computer, and two dimensional data of the body parts were calculated using a DLT program (Walton, 1979). The following parameters were calculated:

1. angle of upper arm;
2. angle of elbow joint;
3. angle of trunk joint;
4. angle of knee joint;
5. the angle of elbow joint at high elbow appearance;
6. horizontal velocity of trunk joint;
7. average horizontal velocity of trunk joint;
8. first and second kick phase in whole stroke;
9. appearance of high elbow phase in whole stroke;
10. appearance of maximal velocity phase in whole stroke;
11. the standard deviation of horizontal velocity of trunk joint;
12. the standard deviation of angle of trunk joint in whole stroke;
13. the distance from entry point to release point of wrist joint.

In order to evaluate the swimming technique of the swimmers, the relationship between averaged horizontal velocity, and (a) angle of elbow joint at catch point, (b) pull and kick phase in whole stroke, and (c) horizontal distance from entry to release point of wrist joint were examined.

3 Results and discussion

3.1 Evaluation of high elbow at catch point
The angle of the elbow joint at the catch point ranged from 128.0° to 240.6° ($\bar{x}$ = 187.9°, SD $\pm$ 2.8°). Fig. 1 shows the relationship between the mean horizontal velocity and angle of the elbow joint at the catch point, where a significant correlation was found (r = -0.606, $P < 0.005$). This result suggests that the swimmer who has a higher average swimming velocity tends to have a smaller angle of elbow joint at the catch point. Many coaches consider the dropped elbow position a weak propulsive element (Counsilman, 1977; Maglischo, 1988).
A significant correlation (r = -0.570, $P < 0.025$) was also found between mean horizontal velocity and the appearance phase of high elbow (Fig. 2). This result can be explained, in that the early appearance of a high elbow makes a longer downsweep, insweep and upsweep possible. Therefore, the early appearance of a high elbow results in a greater horizontal velocity.

3.2 The fluctuation of horizontal velocity
The fluctuation of horizontal velocities ranged from 19.0 to 43.3 cm/s ($\bar{x}$ 32.8 cm/s). Fig. 3 shows the relationship between mean horizontal velocity and fluctuation of horizontal velocity. A significant correlation was exhibited (r = 0.509, $P < 0.025$). A large fluctuation in horizontal velocity causes a swimmer to use a greater amount of energy for propulsion and is therefore inefficient.

3.3 Horizontal distance from entry to release point of wrist joint
Fig. 4 shows a highly significant correlation (r = -0.777, $P < 0.005$) between horizontal distance from entry to release point of the wrist joint. The horizontal distance assesses the slip of the fore-arm in

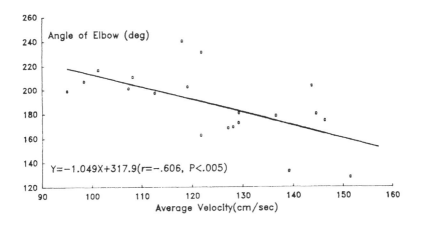

Fig. 1.   Relationship between angle of elbow and average velocity.

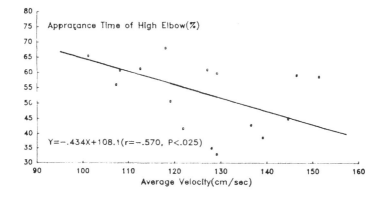

Fig. 2.   Relationship between appearance time of high elbow and
average velocity.

the underwater stroke.   Therefore, it is clear that novice swimmers
cannot swim faster because they are unable to perform a propeller-
like vertical and lateral arm stroke thus incorporating lift forces.

4 Conclusion

A smaller angle of elbow at the catch point and the earlier
appearance of a high elbow results in a higher average swim velocity.
Therefore for the novice swimmer using the butterfly stroke, it is
clear that a high elbow is of prime importance for increases in
average velocities.   Novice swimmers who have lower horizontal
velocities also have a lower horizontal distance from entry to the

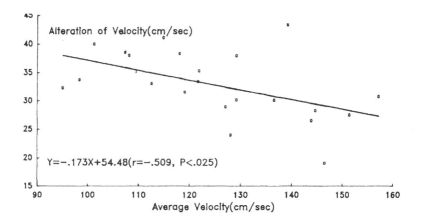

Fig. 3. Relationship between fluctuation of velocity and average
        velocity.

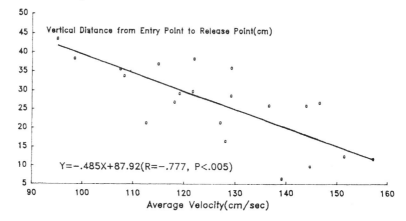

Fig. 4. Relationship between horizontal distance from entry to
        release point and average velocity.

release point of the wrist joint resulting in a slip of the fore-arm
during the underwater stroke.

5 References

Counsilman, J.E. (1977) **Competitive Swimming Manual for Coaches and
    Swimmers.** Prentice-Hall, New York.
Maglischo, E.W. (1988) A biomechanical analysis of the 1984 US
    Olympic freestyle distance swimmers, in **Swimming Science V** (eds
    B.O. Ungerechts, K. Wilke and K. Reischle), Human Kinetics Books,
    Champaign, Ill., pp. 351-360.
Walton, J.S. (1979) Close-range cine-photogrammetry: Another approach
    to motion analysis, in **Science in Biomechanics. Cinematography**
    (ed J. Terauds), Academic Publishers, Del Mar., pp. 69-91.

PART THREE

ELECTROMYOGRAPHY

EFFECTS OF SPEED ON EMG AND KINEMATIC PARAMETERS IN FREESTYLE

A.H. ROUARD*, G. QUEZEL** and R.P. BILLAT**
*CRIS, Université Lyon, Lyon, France; **LIME, Grenoble, France

Abstract
The purpose of this study was to investigate the evolution of
kinematic and electromyographic parameters with increasing speed in
freestyle. Fifty subjects (30 males, 20 females) with average age of
over 18.1 years were tested. The subjects performed 2 × 25 m at 4
different speeds: 75%, 85%, 95% and 100% of their best performance
over 100 m. Side-underwater video views were obtained and
simultaneously EMGs of 6 muscles of the upper limb were recorded with
a telemetric system. The EMGs, normalised to the highest values
found throughout the test, were related to hip displacement and the
total time of the stroke using principal component analysis. Results
indicated that swimmers increased their speed by decreasing the total
time of the stroke and by sustaining their hip displacements. A
linear relationship between speed and muscular activity was not
observed. The six muscles studied had their higher activities for
the lowest and highest speed and their lower recruitments for the
intermediate paces. The greater activities of the legs, associated
with a higher position of the body on the water, could explain the
lower muscular activities of the upper limb for the intermediate
speeds.
Keywords: Freestyle, Speed, Electromyographic, Kinematic, Sex.

1 Introduction

The application of the electromyography (EMG) in swimming research
started in 1964 with Ikai's studies. Since that time, many authors
(e.g. Clarys, 1983; Nuber et al., 1986) have been using surface or
fine wire electrodes to evaluate the roles of different muscles in
the front crawl stroke. In other ways, kinematic data were obtained
to determine the swimming skill (Craig et al., 1985; Schleihauf et
al., 1986). However, little information was available on the
relationships between kinematic variables and EMG activity in
swimming. The purpose of this study was to investigate the change in
kinematic and EMG parameters with increasing speed in front crawl.

2 Methods

2.1 Subjects
Fifty subjects (30 males, 20 females) participated in this study.

They had an average age of 18.1 (SD ± 2.7) years. Subjects'
characteristics (Table 1) were in the same range as observed in
previous studies (Hebbelinck et al., 1975; Grimston and Hay, 1986).

Table 1. Subjects' characteristics

Characteristics	Males	Females
Height (cm)	181.5	167.4
Weight (kg)	70.4	54.8

2.2 Testing procedure
The test distance was 25 m to minimize the influence of fatigue on
the EMG and to obtain higher swim speeds. Each subject performed
2 × 25 m swims at four different speeds in a random order. The given
paces were 75%, 85%, 95% and more than 100% of the swimmer's best
performance over 100 m. A rest of 3 min was observed between each
repetition.

2.3 Recordings
Using a telemetric system (Rouard et al., 1988), surface EMGs were
obtained from the following muscles: M. deltoidus pars anterior and
medialis, M. biceps brachii, M. triceps brachii, M. brachioradialis
and M. flexor carpi ulnaris. Beckman type electrodes (11 mm
diameter) were fixed on the belly of each muscle after cleaning the
skin. The differential amplifier was on the site of the electrodes
to minimize artefacts. Each amplified signal was coded with a subcarrier frequency and summed together before being transmitted to a
receiving device located on the side of the pool.
Side underwater video views were synchronised with EMG recordings
during all tests. A video camera (25 Hz) was fixed in a waterproof
case and moved alongside the pool in pace with the swimmer.

2.4 Data analysis
Raw EMGs were rectified to obtain the full wave rectified signals.
The integration of the rectified EMG was calculated per unit of time
for each stroke and its phases. To normalize the results, each
integrated part of the signal per unit of time was expressed as a per
cent of the maximal value found during the whole test. Each muscle
of each subject was used as its own reference.
Video recordings were analysed view by view to obtain kinematic
data. The longitudinal displacement of the hip from the hand entry
to the next same hand's entry was calculated, together with the total
time of the stroke.
A principal component analysis was used for each speed studied to
treat the relationships between speed, normalized EMG and kinematic
data. The results were represented by the correlation circle. Each
axis of the circle was defined by the combination of different parameters. The most important parameters are those which are projected,
on the axis, nearest to the periphery of the circle.

3 Results and discussion

Results (Fig. 1) indicated that, whatever the circle, the speed
(No. 2) was in close proximity to the hip displacement during the
stroke (No. 3) and to the subject's height (No. 1). It was opposite
to the muscles' activity (Nos. 6 to 11) and to the total time of the
stroke (No. 4).

These positions showed that the hip displacement was dependent on
the height of the subjects. These two parameters were determinants
of the swimming speed i.e. the taller the subject, the greater was
his hip displacement and the higher his swim speed. The results
confirmed previous studies (Sprague, 1976; Smith, 1978; Pai et al.,
1984; Craig et al., 1985). The situation of the muscles' activities
and the total time of the stroke was opposite to the mean speed,
indicating that they were not determinant parameters for the swim
speed. The best swimmers were not those who had higher muscular
requirements. Similar results were observed in other activities
(Kamon, 1968; Basmajian, 1978).

The change in kinematic parameters indicated that the swimmers
decreased the total time of the stroke and sustained their hip
displacement to increase their swimming speed. The comparison of the
four circles indicated differences in the relative position of the
six muscles studied. For the lower speed (75%) and the highest speed
(more than 100%), muscles were grouped together near the periphery of
the circle. This position showed that all the muscles had high
activities for these two speeds. For the intermediate paces (85% and
95%), muscles were more dispersed and nearer the centre of the
circle, indicating their lower recruitments compared to extreme
speeds (75% and more than 100%). The relationships between speed and
muscular activities of the upper limb were not linear; muscular
recruitments were greater for lower and higher speeds and moderate
for the intermediate speeds.

These results could be explained by the most important activity of
the legs during the intermediate paces. As the subject swam faster,
the activity of his legs increased. As a result, the lift force
exerted on the body increased, and the swimmer had a higher position
on the water and offered lower frontal drag. The decrease of the
frontal drag could be associated with less muscular activity of the
upper limb to propel the body through the water.

4 Conclusion

The change in kinematic and electromyographic parameters with
increasing speed indicated an increase in the stroke rate and a
stable hip displacement which seemed to be non-linearly dependent on
the muscular activity of the upper limb. Muscular recruitments were
maximum at lowest and highest speeds. During intermediate speeds,
muscles were used less. This moderated activity could be a
consequence of the decrease of the frontal body drag resulting from
an increase of the lift force of the body due to the greater activity
of the legs.

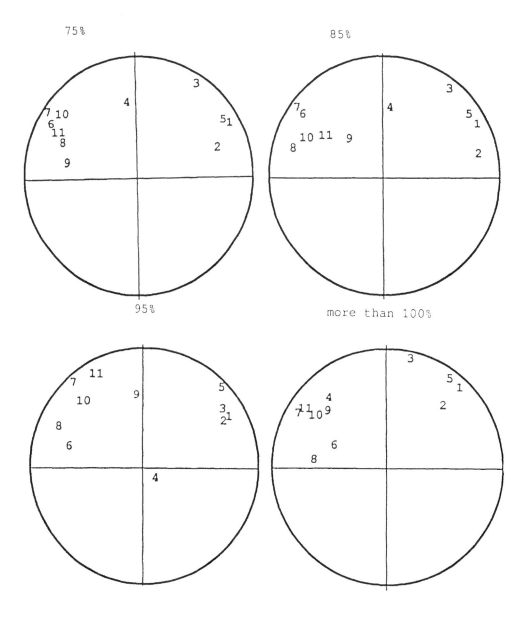

Fig. 1. Correlation circles of the different speeds (percentage
         values refer to percent of the fastest speed achieved
         over 100 metres).

No. 1: height, No. 2: displacement of the hip, No. 3: mean speed,
No. 4: time of the total stroke, No. 5: index of performance, Nos. 6
to 11: normalised activities of the M. triceps brachii (6), biceps
brachii (7), deltoidus pars anterior (8) and medialis (11), brachioradialis (9), flexor carpi ulnaris (10).

5 References

Basmajian, J.V. (1978) **Muscles Alive. Their Functions Revealed by Electromyography.** 4th Ed. Williams & Wilkins Co., Baltimore.

Clarys, J.P. (1983) A review of EMG in swimming, in **Biomechanics and Medicine in Swimming** (eds A.P. Hollander and P.A. de Groot), University Park Press, Baltimore, pp. 123-125.

Craig, A.B., Skehan, P.L., Pawelczyk, J.A. and Boomer, W.L. (1985) Velocity, stroke rate and distance per stroke during elite swimming competition. **Med. Sci. Sports Exerc.**, 17, 625-634.

Grimston, S.K. and Hay, J.G. (1986) Relationships among anthropometric and stroking characteristics of college swimmers. **Med. Sci. Sports Exerc.**, 18, 60-68.

Hebbelinck, M., Carter, L. and de Garay, A. (1975) Body build and somatotype of Olympic swimmers, divers and water polo players, in **Swimming II** (eds J.P. Clarys and L. Lewillie), University Park Press, Baltimore, pp. 285-305.

Ikai, M., Ishii, K. and Miyashita, M. (1964) An electromyographic study of swimming. **Res. J. Phys. Educ.**, 7, 3, 47-54.

Kamon, E. and Gormley, J. (1968) Muscular activity pattern for skilled performance and during learning of horizontal bar exercise. **Ergonomics**, 11, 4, 345-357.

Nuber, G.W., Jobe, F.W. and Perry, J. (1986) Fine wire electromyography analysis of muscles of the shoulder during swimming. **Am. J. Sports Med.**, 14, 1, 7-11.

Pai, Y.C., Hay, J.G. and Wilson, B.D. (1984) Stroking techniques of elite swimmers. **J. Sports Sci.**, 2, 225-239.

Rouard, A.H., Quezel, G. and Billat, R.P. (1988) A telemetric system for the analysis of six muscles activities in swimming, in **Swimming Science V** (eds B.E. Ungerechts, K. Wilke and K. Reischle), Human Kinetics Books, Champaign, Ill., pp. 201-205.

Schleihauf, R.E., Higgins, R. and Hinricks, R. (1986) Models of aquatic skill in sprint front crawl stoke. **New Zealand J. Sport Med.**, March, 6-12.

Smith, L.E. (1978) Anthropometry related to speed. **J. Sport Med. Phys. Fit.**, 18, 153-168.

Sprague, H.A. (1976) Relationship of certain physical measurements to swimming speed. **Res. Quart.**, 47, 810-814.

INFLUENCE OF THE SIZE OF THE PADDLES IN FRONT CRAWL STROKE

K.M. MONTEIL and A.H. ROUARD
Centre de Recherche et d'Innovation sur le Sport, UFRAPS, Université
Lyon I, France

Abstract
Many coaches use paddles in the training programme of their swimmers.
The purpose of the research was to study the influence of the size of
these paddles on biomechanical parameters (total time of the stroke,
hip displacement per stroke, phases of the stroke) in front crawl
swimming. Seven long (n = 4) and short (n = 3) distance swimmers
were examined. Each subject performed 25 m swims with and without
three different paddles. Electrical activity of five muscles of the
upper limb were recorded with a multichannel telemetric system.
Underwater sideviews were captured simultaneously. Results showed
that the use and size of the paddles did not change the temporal
partitioning of the phases and the hip distance covered per stroke.
Electromyographic results indicated similar recruitment patterns
through the different tests. The M. biceps brachii had the lowest
firing, but the use of paddles increased its activity during the pull
phase. There was no linear increase in muscle activity with the
increase of size of the paddles. The short distance swimmers seemed
to be the more disturbed by the use and size of the paddles.
Keywords: Electromyographic, Front Crawl, Kinematic, Paddles.

1 Introduction

In swimming, development of muscular strength seems to be regarded as
an important factor in performance (Birrer and Levine, 1987). The
same observations could be found in other sports such as the javelin
throw (Fuchs, 1987; Kovacs, 1987), shot putt (Poprawski, 1988),
sprint running (Mero and Komi, 1986; Farrar and Thorland, 1987), long
jump (Ramey, 1973), tennis (Plagenhoef, 1973), gymnastics
(Plagenhoef, 1973; Dyhre-Poulsen, 1987), skiing (Hauser and Schaff,
1987) and speed-skating (Boer et al., Cabri, 1987) among others.
In swimming, one principle of the specificity of exercise includes
designing strength training exercises to imitate the skill of the
activity (Costill et al., 1980).
  Maglischo (1987) has shown the importance of increasing specific
strength in training; this improvement would generate a greater power
which would increase swimming speed. From past research, it was
found that improving this specific strength can be considered an
important link in the swimmer's training programme. For example,
these exercises could be used in dry-land exercises (weight-lifting,
elastics, pulleys, swim bench and so on) or wet exercises (swimming

against a resistance, paddles, pull-buoy and others) (Maglischo, 1987). Few authors have investigated these relationships. Clarys (1983) conducted an electromyographic study of the paddle swimming front crawl. Other findings of Rouard (1987) underlined the importance of muscular dissociation and economy in highly skilled swimmers. The purpose of the study was to quantify the kinematic and muscular modifications due to the size of paddles.

2 Methods

2.1 Subjects
Seven skilled swimmers were tested. The general characteristics are given in Table 1.

Table 1. General characteristics of the subject

	Age (years)	Height (cm)	Weight (kg)
Men (n = 4)			
Mean	16.7	180.8	65.8
SD	0.4	4.3	8.7
Range	16–17	176–187	56.80
Women (n = 3)			
Mean	15.6	164.6	49.5
SD	0.4	7.4	4.2
Range	15–16	158–175	46–55

2.2 Tests
Subjects performed ten 25 metre front crawl swims at 80% of their maximal speed in the 100 m paddle front crawl. All tests were carried out with paddles. The reason for choosing the short swimming distance was to minimize the degradation of the muscular activity due to eventual fatigue. Between each repetition, three minutes of active rest (25 m back), and passive rest (subjects stayed in the pool without moving for 2 min 30 s) were allowed.

The 25 m tests were performed in a randomized experimental protocol:
- small paddles: 8 cm × 12 cm (area: 96 cm^2)
- medium paddles (arena paddle) used during training: 12 cm × 22 cm (area: 224 cm^2)
- large paddles: 11 cm × 34 cm (area: 374 cm^2)

All these paddles were bigger than the hand surface area which was 70 cm^2 for the men and 55 cm^2 for the women.

During the test, subjects pulled a pull-buoy, fixed at the middle of the thigh.

Electromyographic data were recorded from five muscles of the upper limb (M. pectoralis major, M. brachioradialis, M. biceps brachii, M. triceps brachii caput medialis, and M. flexor carpi ulnaris) using a multichannel telemetric system (Rouard, 1987) and surface electrodes. Sensors were 11 mm Beckman electrodes, in Ag/AgCl. The amplifiers were in the same box as the sensors. Gains were set at 1000 V/V.

Lateral views were obtained using a video camera JVC Gx N7S
(25 Hz) fixed in a moving box.

2.3 Data treatment
A frame by frame kinematic analysis was completed to calculate:
- the total time of the stroke (T): from the hand entry to the next
  entry of the same hand;
- the hip displacement covered per stroke (DH) to evaluate the
  efficiency of the swimmer.

The aquatic part of the stroke was divided into four phases from
the angle arm-trunk (Hay, 1985; Rouard, 1987):
- phase 1: entry of hand into the water-angle arm-trunk 45° = catch
- phase 2: angle arm-trunk 45° to 90° = pull phase;
- phase 3: angle arm-trunk 90° to 135° = push phase;
- phase 4: angle arm-trunk 135° to exit of the hand out of the water
  = finish.

For each phase, the time (t) was expressed as a percentage of the
total time (T) of the stroke, to normalize the results.

Raw EMG data were rectified to obtain the full wave rectified
signals. The integration of the rectified EMG was calculated per
unit of time, for each stroke. To normalize the results, each
integrated part of the signal per unit of time of each muscle was
expressed as a percentage of the maximal value found throughout all
the test (dynamic reference).

For each variable, mean ($\bar{X}$) and standard deviation (SD) values
were calculated. Analyses of variance and coefficients of
correlation were computed.

3 Results and discussion

3.1 Kinematics results
The total time of the stroke was greater for the swimming paddle
condition than for the free swimming. The statistical difference was
non-significant ($p = 0.09$), but with a larger subject sample a
significant difference might be found. For all the subjects, the
total time increased from 1.59 s ($\pm$ 0.11) without paddles to 1.72 s
($\pm$ 0.14) with paddles. This result could be explained by the
increase in the resistance exerted by the hand on the water with the
paddles. The standard deviation values were rather small (SD = 0.11
without paddles and SD = 0.14 with paddles) and indicated that the
subjects were homogeneous. The second standard deviation value
(SD = 0.14) indicated that there was no temporal difference between
strokes swum with various sizes of paddles.

The temporal division seemed to be stable for all the repetitions
of the test (Fig. 1); the standard deviation values were small (from
0.065 for the recovery phase to 1.185 for the catch). The temporal
division did not seem to be a pertinent variable for comparing
swimming with and without paddles. The values obtained for the
aquatic phase 74.71%) and the recovery phase (25.29%) without paddles
were slightly different from the values given by Vaday and Nemessuri
(1975). They found 68.9% for the aquatic phase and 31.1% for the
recovery phase.

The comparison of the hip displacement covered per stroke did not
indicate any significant differences ($p = 0.57$) when the subjects

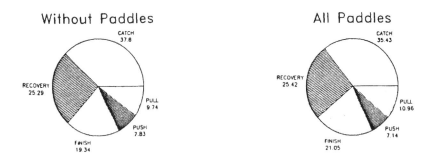

Figs. 1 and 2.   Temporal division of the phase of the stroke.

swam with or without paddles ($\overline{X}$ = 1.990 m without paddles and $\overline{X}$ = 2.062 m with paddles). However, for the sprinters, this parameter was variable and dependent on the size of the paddles. Sprinters seemed to be more influenced by the size of paddles than long distance swimmers.

3.2 Electromyographic results
The muscular activity was unchanged during the different repetitions. For all subjects, standard deviation values were very small: 3.14 for the M. biceps brachii ($\overline{X}$ = 32.10%), 2.41 for the M. pectoralis major ($\overline{X}$ = 49.64%), 3.83 for the M. triceps brachii ($\overline{X}$ = 63.36%), 4.69 for the M. flexor carpi ulnaris ($\overline{X}$ = 52.03%) and 3.96 for the M. brachioradialis ($\overline{X}$ = 49.54%) (Table 2).

Table 2.   Influence of the different conditions on the normalized muscular activity (percentage of the maximal dynamic contraction)

Tests/Muscles		M1	M2	M3	M4	M5
T1	M	28.33	52.93	59.95	52.54	46.64
	S	1.61	8.34	5.36	4.20	7.98
T2	M	29.88	51.46	63.91	50.26	45.68
	S	0.36	9.43	9.47	6.38	16.14
T3	M	36.51	49.99	61.31	49.40	51.85
	S	12.46	4.59	9.21	10.64	6.40
T4	M	30.71	46.67	61.06	47.18	56.25
	S	6.34	3.75	9.62	13.08	11.98
T5	M	35.10	47.16	70.59	60.77	47.30
	S	11.17	11.66	11.91	15.95	7.60

Legend: T1: 25 m – without paddles; T2: 25 m – medium paddles;
        T3: 25 m – small paddles: T4 25 m – large paddles;
        T5: 25 m – without paddles.
        M1: M. biceps brachii; M2: M. pectoralis major;
        M3: M. triceps brachii; M4: M. flexor carpi ulnaris
        M5: M. brachioradialis

There was no significant (p = 0.05) linear increase between the size of the paddles and the electrical activity of the muscles. The greatest muscular activity was not obtained with the large paddles (T4), but with the medium paddles (T2) or small ones (T3). Important standard deviation values for each test indicated that the swimmers did not have the same muscular recruitment. As already observed for the hip displacement per stroke, sprinters seemed to be more disturbed by the size of paddles. This result could be explained by an important use of kicking during free swimming. Swimming with a pull-buoy could modify their muscular recruitment.

Since the use of paddles did not involve an increase in muscular activity, it seemed interesting to observe if the subjects could improve the specific role of the muscles for a specific phase. According to the findings of Clarys et al. (1973) and Rouard (1987), the M. biceps brachii displayed the best correlation with the swimming speed. The measure of the demand of the biceps during phase 2 (pull-phase: flexion of the forearm on the arm) was obtained in calculating a coefficient without dimension - coefficient of dissociation:

$$Cd = \frac{\text{area phase 2}}{\text{total area}}$$

If the demand of the M. biceps brachii during phase 2 is important, the coefficient of dissociation Cd will be larger.

The results indicated that the use of paddles was favourable to muscular recruitment of the M. biceps brachii during phase 2. During the pull-phase, individual variations were observed, but for most subjects, the greatest electrical activity of the M. biceps brachii was recorded with the medium paddles. This highest electrical activity could be explained by the habit of these subjects to swim with this size of paddles.

4 Conclusion

The study of the swimming paddle in front crawl pointed out that the use of the paddles involved an increase of the total time of the stroke. However, the size of the paddles did not influence this parameter. The temporal division of phases of the stroke was not modified by the use and size of paddles. The hip displacement covered per stroke was not significantly altered when the subject used paddles.

There was no linear increase in muscular activity with an increasing size of paddles. The M. biceps brachii had the lowest activity, but its demand seemed to be greater during phase 2 with the use of paddles (especially with the medium and small ones).

The sprint swimmers seemed to be more influenced by the variations of the different sizes of paddles.

5 References

Birrer, R.B. and Levine, R. (1987) Performance parameters in children and adolescent athletes. **Sports Med.**, 1, 211-227.

Boer, R.W. de, Cabri, J. , Vaes, W., Clarys, J.P., Hollander, A.P., Groot, G. de, and Ingen Schenau, G.J. van (1987) Moments of force, power and muscle coordination in speed-skating. **Int. J. Sports Med.**, 8, 371-378.

Clarys, J.P. (1983) A review of EMG in swimming: explanation of facts and/or feedback information. **Biomechanics and Medicine in Swimming, International Series on Sports Sciences,** 14, 123-135.

Clarys, J.P. (1985) Hydrodynamics and electromyography: ergonomics aspects in aquatics. **Appl. Ergonomics,** 16, 1, 11-24.

Clarys, J.P., Jiskoot, J. and Lewille, L. (1973) A kinematographical, electromyographical and resistance study of water-polo and competition front crawl. **Medicine and Sport,** 8, Biomechanics III, 446-452.

Costill, D., Sharp, R. and Troup, J. (1980) Muscle strength: contributions to sprint swimming. **Swimming World,** 21, 2, 29-34.

Dhyre-Poulsen, P. (1987) Analysis of split leaps and gymnastics skill by physiological recordings. **Eur. J. Appl. Physiol.,** 56, 390-397.

Farrer, M. and Thorland, W. (1987) Relationship between isokinetic strength and sprint times in college-age men. **J. Sports Med. Phys. Fit.,** 27, 368-372.

Fuchs, R. (1987) Strength training for women javelin throwers. **Modern Athlete and Coach,** 25, 3, 11-13.

Hauser, W. and Schaff, P. (1987) Ski boots: biomechanical issues regarding skiing safety and performance. **Int. J. Sport Biomech.,** 3, 326-344.

Hay, J.G. (1985) Swimming. **Biomechanics of Sports Techniques, Starting, Stroking and Turning,** 1-52.

Kovacs, E. (1987) Complex development of strength, velocity and technique of young javelin throwers. **New Studies in Athletics,** 1, 43-45.

Maglischo, E.W. (1987) **Swimming Faster.** Coll. Metiers de L'Eau.

Mero, A. and Komi, P.V. (1986) Force, EMG, and elasticity-velocity relationships at submaximal, maximal, and supramaximal running speeds in sprinters. **Eur. J. Appl. Physiol.,** 55, 553-561.

Plagenhoef, S. (1973) The joint force and moment analysis of all body segments when performing a nonsymmetrical, three-dimensional motion. **Medicine and Sport,** 8, Biomechanics III, 165-171.

Poprawski, B. (1988) Aspects of strength, power and speed in shot putt training. **New Studies in Athletics,** 1, 89-93.

Ramey, M.R. (1973) Use of force plates for long-jump studies. **Medicine and Sport,** 8, Biomechanics III, 370-380.

Rouard, A.H. (1987) Étude biomécanique du crawl: évolution des paramètres cinématiques et électromyographiques avec la vitesse. **Thèse présentée pour obtenir le grade de docteur, Université Grenoble 1.**

Vaday, M. and Nemessuri, M. (1971) Motor pattern of freestyle swimming. **Biomechanics and Medicine in Swimming,** 173-187.

AN ERGONOMIC ELECTROMYOGRAPHIC STUDY OF DIFFERENT SWIMMING FINS

J. CABRI, V. SLACHMUYLDERS and J.P. CLARYS
Department of Experimental Anatomy, Vrije Universiteit Brussel,
Belgium

Abstract
The purpose of this study was to investigate leg muscle activity
during fin-swimming (two-legged) using kinesiological electromyography (EMG) techniques. Six differently shaped commercial flippers
were tested by nine male recreational divers during a 15 m maximal
leg propulsion swim at a depth of 1.5 m. For all muscles
investigated results showed a cyclic activation pattern, as could be
expected from prior front crawl swimming studies. Averaged
integrated EMG (iEMG) of M. rectus femoris was significantly higher
when compared to the M. biceps femoris, as was the case for the M.
gastrocnemius in comparison to the M. tibialis anterior. No
significant differences in iEMG of the muscles investigated were
found when the different types of flippers were taken into
consideration. Because of its significant performance improvement,
without any alteration in EMG activity, it was concluded that the
Nordic fin can be preferred over the other fins tested.
Keywords: Kinesiology, EMG, Fin Swimming, Scuba Diving.

1 Introduction

The tremendous popularity of scuba diving has resulted in an
increasing interest of companies to invest in the design of the
equipment. An example of this is the marketing of the 'super-fins',
where the knowledge of hydrodynamic principles was applied to develop
fins which are larger in surface area than conventional fins, and
which contain such sophisticated designs as venturis, louvers, or
ridges to direct the water flow (McMurray, 1977).

Scuba divers rely only on their lower limbs for propulsion; they
use swim fins to increase kicking forces and to help resolve the
sideways motion into thrust that is directed parallel to the diver's
body (Lewis and Lorch, 1979). Therefore, a lot of attention has been
given to the design of fins in producing a better (or more efficient)
underwater movement. Efficiency, in this case, was defined as the
ratio between forward movement in the water and the energy needed to
generate movement.

The purpose of this study was to investigate the muscle activity
during fin-swimming with six commercially available differently
shaped flippers:
the Nasa Carboflex (New Advanced Swimming Apparatus; NC):

- the Nasa Yellow (NY),
- the Compro Fin (CO)
- the Nordic Fin (NO)
- the Sea Wing (SW), and
- the Squid Fin (SQ).

2 Methods

Nine male recreational divers (aged 24 to 40 years; with an average
diving experience of 8 years) were asked to perform a 15 m maximal
leg propulsion swim in apnoea at a depth of 1.5 m. The time of the
last 4 m was recorded as a measure of all-out performance. The tests
were repeated for all the fins (i.e. NC, NY, CO, NO,, SW and SQ), in
a randomized way. Physical characteristics of the fins are given in
Table 1.

Table 1. Characteristics of the fins used in the experiment

	Max.length (cm)	Max.width (cm)	Surface (cm^2)
Nasa Carboflex	57.3	24.0	978
Nasa Yellow	57.3	24.0	978
Compro Fin	53.7	23.2	688
Sea Wing	58.5	22.7	1056
Nordic Fin	50.7	26.0	1068
Squid Fin	58.2	24.3	1097

Electromyography (EMG) of the (right) M. rectus femoris, M. biceps
femoris, M. tibialis anterior, and M. gastrocnemius (caput laterale)
was registered during the last four propulsion cycles, using active
bipolar surface electrodes (gain: 10; CMRR: 90 db) and additional
amplifiers (gain: 100; CMRR: 85 dB). The EMG was recorded on-line by
means of an FM-tape recorder (Clarys and Publie, 1985; Clarys, 1988:
Clarys and Cabri, 1988). The skin was thoroughly prepared (shaved,
rubbed and cleaned), and the electrodes were fixed using adhesive
tape and plastic film.
After the experiments at the swimming pool, analysis of the EMG
signals was carried out in the laboratory, using the Electromyography
Signal Processing and Analysis System (ESPAS; Cabri, 1989). The
signals were low-pass filtered (cut-off frequency 500 Hz), analogue-
to-digital converted (sample frequency 2 KHz), full-wave rectified
and averaged (time constant 10 ms).
Analysis included integrated values of the EMG (iEMG) and maximal
amplitudes (maxEMG) during the last four propulsions. The EMGs were
normalised for time and for the highest dynamic peak (i.e. maxEMG).
Furthermore, for the qualitative analysis of the data, the IDANCO
system (Clarys and Cabri, 1988) was used to identify specificity of
the EMG patterns.
The statistical analysis of both iEMG and maxEMG included
Kologmorov-Smirnov tests (for normal spreading of the data), one-way
analysis of variance (df 5,48), a-posteriori protected Fisher-test,
and simple correlation analysis. The level of significance was

chosen at P < 0.05.

3   Results

The qualitative analysis of the EMG patterns demonstrated a cyclic
activation pattern for all muscles investigated, as could be expected
from prior front crawl swimming studies (Clarys, 1988).   The linear
envelopes during the scuba test are exemplified in Fig. 1.   Five
percent of all patterns proved to be identical, 25% were analogue,
and 48.2% were considered to be conform.   Thus, 78% of the linear
envelopes showed a form of cyclic reproducibility, and only 21.7%
could not be reproduced.   Most of the differing patterns were found
in the M. biceps femoris (46%).

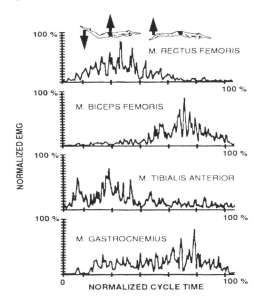

Fig. 1.   Normalized linear envelopes (mean rectified EMG) of the
          muscles investigated while scuba diving with the Nordic
          fin.

Averaged iEMG of M. biceps femoris was significantly higher when
compared to the M. rectus femoris, as was the case for the M.
gastrocnemius in comparison to the M. tibialis anterior.   No
significant differences in iEMG of the muscles investigated were
found when the different types of fins were taken into consideration
(P > 0.05).
The analysis of variance of the maxEMG showed significant
differences in the M. rectus femoris, M. biceps femoris and M.
tibialis anterior (P < 0.05; Table 2).   The a-posteriori protected
Fisher-tests showed a significantly higher mean value for the SW fin
in comparison to the NC, NY and SQ fins for the M. rectus femoris.
In the M. biceps femoris significantly higher values were found for
SQ in comparison to NC, CO, and NO, whereas in the M. tibialis

anterior swimming with NC provoked significantly higher activities in comparison to NY, CO, SW, NO and SQ (P < 0.05).

Table 2. One-way analysis of variance (dF 5,48) of the maxEMG (condition: NC,NY,CO,SW,NO,SQ); *P < 0.05.

Muscle investigated	F	P
M. rectus femoris	2.2781	0.028*
M. biceps femoris	2.79	0.027*
M. gastrocnemius	0.195	0.093
M. tibialis anterior	3.945	0.005*

Significant correlations were found between the synchronized time and both maximal width and surface area of the fin (r = 0, P < 0.001 and r = 0.61, P < 0.001, respectively). The performance measurements showed a significantly better performance time in both NO, SQ, and SW fins. However, no significant correlations were found between the EMG results (iEMG and maxEMG) and the performance time nor with any of the physical characteristics of the find (P > 0.05).

Table 3. Mean values (± SD) of the time of all-out performance (time to swim the last 4 m of the scuba test)

Fin type	Time (s)	SD
Nasa Carboflex	3.28	0.25
Nasa Yellow	3.25	0.31
Compro Fin	3.27	0.39
Sea Wing	3.12	0.30
Nordic Fin	2.99	0.29
Squid Fin	2.96	0.37

Table 4 represents the averaged iEMG and maxEMG values. It is a quantification of the total mean muscular activity for all muscles investigated, during the scuba dive tests. In these cases, no significant differences were found when comparing the different fin types (P > 0.05), both in iEMG as well as in maxEMG.

Table 4. Values of integrated EMG (iEMG) and maximal EMG amplitudes (maxEMG) for all muscles investigated during the scuba test. Values are means (± SD)

Fin Type	iEMG (%)	SD	maxEMG (µV)	SD
Nasa Carboflex	20.3	7.9	229.7	29.4
Nasa Yellow	20.1	6.4	229.8	29.3
Compro Fin	18.2	3.5	214.3	20.1
Sea Wing	18.7	5.0	227.3	28.6
Nordic Fin	18.8	5.2	213.9	26.1
Squid Fin	21.2	6.8	220.6	19.7

4 Discussion

The M. rectus femoris and M. tibialis anterior are both activated during the extension phase, whereas the M. biceps femoris and M. gastrocnemius are simultaneously active during the extension phase. The M. rectus rectus femoris becomes silent when the activity of the M. biceps femoris becomes increasingly important. However, the M. gastrocnemius seems to have a longer period of activity than the M. tibialis anterior, and peaks at full flexion movement (together with the M. biceps femoris). These findings are in concordance with previous reports (Clarys, 1983; Olbrecht and Clarys, 1983; Clarys, 1988).

The muscular activity of the M. biceps femoris is on average higher than for the M. rectus femoris, indicating that the effort is more strenuous for the knee flexors and hip extensors. On the other hand, iEMG was also significantly higher in the M. gastrocnemius in comparison to the M. tibialis anterior. This finding suggests that the movement investigated required more activity from the flexor apparatus, rather than from the extensors probably because of the higher resistance (drag) during evacuation of the water after the extension phase.

This study could not conclusively test the hypothesis that the form of the fin used significantly influences the muscular activity (both intensity and pattern). However, muscular efficiency (defined as the muscular activity required to perform a given task) proved to be influenced by the surface area and the maximal width: the performance time using the Nordic fins was significantly reduced in comparison to the other fins, without changing the EMG. This could mean that when swimming with the Nordic fin (in maximal effort conditions), the diver will swim significantly faster without having to increase the muscular activity. Picken and Crowe (1974) came to the conclusion that the efficiency depends more on other parameters (forward speed, kicking rate) than construction aspects (length, width). However, performance was positively influenced by the flexibility of the fin.

The positive correlations found in our investigation between maximal width (span) and surface area of the fin on the one hand, and the performance time on the other, indicated that a greater span resulted in a better propulsion, and thus a better performance. This finding was regarded elsewhere by Lewis and Lorch (1979). In an older study (Fisher, 1957), oxygen consumption was found to be reduced by 15% using a fin with a large, well stiffened blade in comparison to others. McMurray (1977) found a significant correlation between oxygen consumption and surface area ($r = -0.90$), and noted a direct relationship between flexibility and the maximal speed that could be attained ($r = 0.90$). He concluded that a large surface area contributes to a better efficiency of the fin. In our study, the Nordic fin had a surface area which was, except for the Squid fin, the largest; the latter statement can thus be corroborated.

As muscle intensity (expressed as iEMG) was not altered significantly by the choice of the flipper, with an improvement of the all-out performance test using the NC, it was concluded that the Nordic fin can be preferred over the other flippers.

5 References

Cabri, J. (1989) The influences of different doses alprazolam on muscle activity. Ph.D. Thesis, Vrije Universiteit Brussel, p. 196.

Clarys, J.P. (1983) A review of EMG in swimming: explanation of facts and/or feedback information, in **Biomechanics and Medicine in Swimming** (eds A.P. Hollander, P.A. Huijing and G. de Groot), Human Kinetics Publishers, Champaign, Ill., pp. 123-135.

Clarys, J.P. (1988) The Brussels EMG project, in **Swimming Science V** (eds B. Ungerechts, K. Wilke and K. Reischle), Human Kinetics Books, Champaign, Ill., pp. 152-172.

Clarys, J.P. and J. Cabri (1988) EMG of repetitive and rhythmic (sport) movements. **IEEE Proceedings**, 10, 58-59.

Clarys, J.P. and Publie, J. (1985) A portable EMG data acquisition system with active surface electrodes for monitoring kinesiological research, in **Biomechanics X-A** (ed B. Jonsson), Human Kinetics Publishers, Champaign, Ill., pp. 233-240.

Fisher, W.G. (1957) Comparative evaluation of swim fins, Evaluation Report 18-57, Naval Experimental Diving Unit, Washington, p. 32.

Lewis, E.R. and Lorch, D. (1979) Swim fin design utilizing principles of marine animal locomotion, in **Swimming III** (eds J. Terauds and E.W. Bedingfield), University Park Press, Baltimore, pp. 289-297.

McMurray, R.G. (1977) Comparative efficiencies of conventional and super-swimfin designs. **Hum. Fact.**, 19, 495-501.

Olbrecht, J. and Clarys, J.P. (1983) EMG of specific strength training exercises for the front crawl, in **Biomechanics and Medicine in Swimming** (eds A.P. Hollander, P.A. Huijing and G. de Groot), Human Kinetics Publishers, Champaign, Ill., pp. 136-141.

Picken, J. and Crowe, C.T. (1974) Performance efficiency of swim fins, **Ocean Engng.**, 2, 251-258.

AN ELECTROMYOGRAPHIC AMD IMPACT FORCE STUDY OF THE OVERHAND WATER POLO THROW

J.P. CLARYS, J. CABRI and P. TEIRLINCK
Experimental Anatomy, Vrije Universiteit, Brussels, Belgium

Abstract
Ten elite water polo players were monitored during the performance of
the overhand throw from 4 m and 8 m distance to a force platform
target using surface EMG of arm, trunk and lower limb muscles. The
impact force of the ball was simultaneously registered with the raw
EMG. The linear envelope was used for pattern and throwing
synchronisation detection, the iEMG was used as a reference value for
muscular intensity and the force plate target gave an approximation
of throwing precision. Good throwing synchronisation was initiated
by the co-contraction of the M. biceps femoris and the M. rectus
femoris followed by an important activity of the M. pectoralis major.
The actual swing phase showed an important co-contraction of the M.
triceps brachii with the M. biceps brachii. The impact forces ranged
from 598 N to 981 N (4 m) and 402 N to 961 N (8 m). The impact force
profile of the subjects was not reflected in the precision scores.
Keywords: EMG, Impact Force, Precision, Co-ordination.

1 Introduction

In many countries, waterpolo is a popular team sport and is linked
with swimming through the aquatic environment. Apart from some
similarities in the swimming drills there is little further
comparison possible, even on the research level. The great amount of
literature on swimming contains little objective information on
drills and skills of water polo. The existing research into water
polo can easily be summarized completely. It comprises: morphological aspects of water polo players (Kolraush, 1929; Medved and
Friedrich, 1966; Leek, 1968; Clarys and Borms, 1971; Szögy and Rosca,
1973; Hebbelinck et al., 1975; Medved and Medved, 1976; Vertommen et
al., 1979; Clarys, 1983), drag measurements of water polo front crawl
drills with a ball (Clarys et al., 1973), pressure registrations of
the interior malleoli of the egg-beater kick during upward and
forward propulsion of players during training and water polo games
(Goodwin and Cumming, 1966; Lilley, 1982; Cazorla et al., 1987;
Pinnington et al., 1987, 1988). Only five studies have analysed the
biomechanics of throwing techniques (Clarys, 1970, 1971; Clarys and
Lewillie, 1971; Davis and Blanksby, 1977; Whiting et al., 1985 and
Elliot and Armour, 1988). At this point it is known that the
overhand throw accounts for up to 90% of all passes and shots during
a water polo game (Lambert and Gaughran, 1969). It results in

67.3% of scoring chances from a 4 m distance (penalty throw) and
26.5% of scoring chances from a 8 m distance (average N = 30; Clarys,
1970). The overhand throw allows for ball release velocities ranging
from 14.5 to 25.8 m/s with peak elbow angular velocities averaging
19.8 rad/s (Whiting et al., 1985) with a ball velocity recorded
immediately following the release averaging 19.1 m s^{-1} (Elliot and
Armour, 1988). The average elbow angle at release was 155° in the
study of Whiting et al. (1985) of the United States Men's water polo
team and ranged from 122 to 158° as reported by Davis and Blanksby
(1977) who studied Australian waterpolo players. In addition it has
been reported that during practices comprising shooting at goal and
passing the ball with overhand technique, the mean rate attains
respectively 173 $\pm$ 2 and 168 $\pm$ 1 heart beats/min with an estimated
$\dot{V}O_2$ of 86.8 $\pm$ 1.6% and 79.9 $\pm$ 1.3% $\dot{V}O_2$max (Pinnington et al., 1988).
   The purposes of this study were: (i) to determine the muscular
activity – patterns, intensity and coordination – of selected arm,
truck and leg muscles associated with the overhand throw and (ii) to
record simultaneously the ball impact force and precision, shooting
from 4 m and 8 m distances.

2 Methods

Ten members of the Belgian 1st and 2nd National Division participated
in the study. The EMG and force data were acquired in the University
swimming pool. All subjects were prepared for the measurements
(shaving and cleaning of the skin – electrode fixation) before a 10
min warm-up with ball handling, including shooting at the target
(force platform) of the test set-up. The active electrodes were
fixed on the midpoint of the M. rectus femoris, the M. biceps
femoris, the M. rectus abdominis, the M. pectoralis major, the biceps
brachii and the triceps brachii; the reference electrode was on the
manubrium sterni. All electrodes were covered with plastic varnish
(Nobecutane).
   The hardware for the electromyography system was designed for
multidisciplinary purposes. The subject (waterpolo player) was not
to be disturbed during the throwing movement (total freedom of
movement), the system should have a certain freedom of action
(continuous measurement over several minutes), several muscles as
well as synchronization signals were to be monitored simultaneously.
Simplicity of operation was to be a predominant characteristic,
influences of complex skin resistance phenomena were to be eliminated
(by means of high input impedance amplifiers), and user-friendly
analysis was to be installed.
   The analog raw EMG is recorded on-line on a 7-channel FM data
recording system (IEAC HR30) with preamplified "active" bipolar
surface electrodes supplied with a precision instrumentational
amplifier (AD 524, Analog Devices, Norwood, USA). With the
Electromyographic Signal Processing and Analysis System (ESPAS,
Cabri, 1989) the raw signal is full-wave rectified and enveloped
using a moving average principle. This linear envelope is normalized
according the highest peak amplitude procedure per subject and is
integrated in order to obtain a reference value of throwing
intensity.
   The impact force of the ball is measured with a vertically fixed

force platform mounted on four strain gauge sensors with a combined resonance frequency of 152 HZ. The ball contact time averaged 0.009 s, resulting in a significant inferior frequency of 55.5 Hz, avoiding the influence of the self-resonance of the platform. Data are registered in volts and transformed to N or kg.

The dimensions of the force plate were 62.0 cm wide and 32.5 cm high. Its fixation against a starting block of the swimming pool gave the effect of a target and a reference for precision. The subjects were allowed 5 shots from both 4 and 8 m distance with the explicit task to throw as hard as they could manage. The EMG and impact force were registered simultaneously if the target was touched. Given the fact that not all subjects or shots touched the target, the precision could be approximated.

The force plate-target was fixed at a "natural" throwing height; consequently the subjects were allowed to shoot with their proper skill mechanics. Prior to the series of shots the force plate was calibrated statically (in horizontal position) with weights of 10 and 20 kg followed by a dynamic (plate in vertical position) calibration using a slinger of 185 cm with a metal bullet of 5 kg which was released at 40, 60 and 80 cm from the target. This way the impact force could be calculated and compared with the measured impact value.

From the frequency of the force input ($\frac{1}{2}T$ = 0.008 s) f = 1/T = 1/0.01 s = 62.5 Hz, it appears that we are far below the natural frequency of the platform which was 152 Hz. The contact time of the water polo ball averaged 0.009 s ($\pm$ 0.001): it has a frequency of 55.5 Hz and remains below the platform's own frequency also, so avoiding spurious data.

3 Results and discussion

The qualitative analyses of the averaged muscle patterns indicated similar activity for the shots from both 4 and 8 m and confirm the mechanics of the overhand waterpolo shot. Since each subject was instructed to make normal throws similar to a penalty throw motion and since subjects were encouraged to throw with maximum velocity at the force plate target, no pattern differences were observed between the subjects.

It was noted that the upward propulsion of the body at the start of the throw is initiated by the M. rectus femoris, the upward position and the activity of the M. rectus femoris is maintained and supported by the co-contraction of the M. biceps femoris within the egg-beater kick. The forward motion of the arm and shoulder girdle becomes clear through the activity of the M. pectoralis major and the M. biceps brachii with the latter very active half way through the swing movement and ending with a dynamic contraction of the M. triceps brachii prior to the release of the ball and beyond. In other words the M. triceps continues its activity to a full extension of the arm and beyond the elbow angle at release as stated by Davis and Blanksby (1977). All muscles investigated indicated a continuous static activity level over the full range of the movement.

However, the comparison of the iEMG values of all muscles between the 4 m and 8 m distances confirm that the subject's muscular activity adapts itself to the distance. With a decrease of precision

of almost 30%, a decrease of ball impact force averaging 0.064 V
(± 0.006) or 157 N was found. The decrease of the impact force can
certainly be attributed partly to drag phenomena, although not
measured, but is mainly the result of the neuromuscular adaptation to
the distance of the throw. These adaptations are necessary to limit
the decrease of precision.

For the 4 m overhand throw the impact forces ranged from 598 N to
981 N and for the 8 m throw the impacts ranged from 402 N to 961 N.
Experienced waterpolo players and coaches recognise that velocity and
force of the overhand throw are high but the authors never assumed
them to be that high. However, they seem to be comparable with the
high angular and release velocities found by Whiting et al. (1985)
and Elliot and Armour (1988). The impact force profile was not
reflected in the precision scores where 6 out of 10 players threw
with a 100% precision from the 4 m and where the 8 m throw resulted
in a variable precision range of 37.5% to 75%.

If the muscular intensity (iEMG) of each muscle is correlated
separately with both impact force and precision the same tendencies
are found (Table 1). From this it can be deduced that not all
muscles correlate significantly with impact and precision and if they
do reversed correlations are often noted. This suggests, for
example, that the high activity of the M. rectus abdominis and lower
limb muscles might decrease precision, ball velocity and impact,
contrary to the beliefs of coaches and players.

Table 1. Muscle intensity (iEMG) correlations (P < 0.05 level) with
          impact force and precision scores (N = 10)

Muscle	Impact force		Precision	
	4 m	8 m	4 m	8 m
M. rectus femoris	N.S.	−0.56	−0.89	N.S.
M. biceps femoris	N.S.	N.S.	0.94	N.S.
M. rectus abdominis	−0.99	−0.96	−0.99	−0.99
M. pectoris major	N.S.	0.87	N.S.	0.67
M. biceps brachii	0.76	0.73	N.S.	0.58
M. triceps brachii	0.58	N.S.	0.71	0.63

4 Conclusions

These data suggest that the lower limbs and abdominal wall activity
is dominant in both the upward propulsion of the body and during the
forward throwing motion mechanics. The precision and ball impact
decrease with increasing distance, but the EMG patterns remain
similar.

It becomes obvious that the waterpolo goalkeeper's shoulder, elbow
and wrist joints are submitted to very high impacts.

5 Acknowledgements

The expertise of the electronic engineers Simon Sleutel and the help

of Jan Publie of the Technical University of Mechelen (Belgium) in
the development of the force-plate and Mr. Louis Van Lierde for
design of the plate-target in the swimming pool are gratefully
acknowledged.

6 References

Beatty, G.W. (1973) **Prospectus of a biomechanical analysis of the
egg-beater kick in waterpolo.** Personal communication and partial
fulfilment of the degree of Masters of Arts, University of Western
Ontario, Canada.

Cabri, J.M.H. (1989) **The influences of different doses of alprazolam
on muscle activity, in function and cardiovascular responses to
concentric and eccentric efforts in isokinetic movement
conditions.** Doctoral thesis for the fulfilment of the degree of
doctor in Physiotherapy. Vrije Universiteit Brussel.

Cazorla, C., Montpetit, R. and Chatard, J.C. (1987) Metabolic and
cardiac responses of swimmers, modern pentathletes and waterpolo
players during free swimming up maximum, in **Biomechanics and
Medicine in Swimming** (eds B. Ungerechts, K. Wilke, K. Reischle),
Human Kinetics Publishers, Champaign, Ill., pp. 251-258.

Clarys, J.P. (1970) Informatieveen praktische wenken in het precisie
domein van de waterpolo (Information and practice of the precision
domain of waterpolo). **Sport,** 13, 54-58.

Clarys, J.P. (1971) Emploi des traces lumineuses lors d'une analyse
de trajet au cours de plusieurs shots de waterpolo.
Kinanthropologie, 3, 27-42.

Clarys, J.P. (1975) Analysis of the egg-beater and breaststroke kick
in waterpolo, in **Swimming II** (eds J.P. Clarys and L. Lewillie),
University Park Press, Baltimore, pp. 241-246.

Clarys, J.P. (1983) Biomechanical and morphological aspects of
waterpolo, in **Collected Papers on Sports Biomechanics** (ed G.A.
Wood), University of Western Australia Press, Perth, pp. 192-222.

Clarys, J.P. and Borms, J. (1971) Typologishe studie van waterpolo
spelers in gymnasten (typological study of waterpolo players ands
gymnasts). **Geneeskunde en Sport,** 4, 2-8.

Clarys, J.P. and Lewillie, L. (1971) The description of wrist and
shoulder motion of different waterpolo shots using a simple light-
trace technique, in **First International Symposium on Biomechanics
in Swimming, Waterpolo and Diving, Proceedings,** Press
Universitaires de Bruxelles, Bruxelles, pp. 249-256.

Clarys, J.P., Jiskoot, J. and Lewillie, L. (1973) A kinematographic,
electromyographic and resistance study of waterpolo and
competition frontcrawl, in **Biomechanics III** (eds S. Cerguillini,
A. Verenando and J. Wartenweiler), S. Karger Verlag, Basel, pp.
446-452.

Davis, T. and Blanksby, B.A. (1977) Cinematographic analysis of the
overhand waterpolo throw. **J. Sports Med. Phys. Fit.,** 17, 5-16.

Elliot, B.C. and Armour, J. (1988) The penalty throw in waterpolo: a
cinematographic analysis. **J. Sports Sci.,** 6, 103-114.

Goodwin, A.B., Cummings, G.R. (1966) Radio telemetry of the
electrocardiogram fitness tests, and oxygen uptake of waterpolo
players. **Can. Med. Ass. J.,** 95, 402-406.

Hebbelinck, M., Carter, J.E.L. and de Garay, A.L. (1975) Body build and somatotype of Olympic swimmers, divers and waterpolo players, in **Swimming** II (eds J.P. Clarys and L. Lewillie), University Park Press, Baltimore, pp. 285-305.

Kolraush, W. (1929) Zusammenhange von Korperform und Leistung. **Arbeitsfysiologie,** 1877-2204.

Lambert, A.F. and Gaughran, R. (1969) **The Technique of Water Polo.** Swimming World, North Hollywood, CA,

Leek, G.M. (1968) The physique of New Zealand waterpolo players. **New Zealand J. Phys. Educ.,** 1, 39-47.

Lilley, G. (1982) A basis for the conditioning of state level waterpolo players. PELOPS: Studies in Physical Education, Leisure Organisation. **Play and Sport,** 25-29.

Medved, R.V. and Friedrich, V. (1966) Oarsmen and waterpolo players, sportsmen with the largest hearts. **Proceedings World Congress for Sports Medicine,** Hanover.

Medved, R.J. and Medved, V.I. (1976) To which limit values has the athlete's heart enlarged? **J. Sports Med. Phys. Fit.,** 16, 138-143.

Pinnignton, H.C., Dawson, B., Blanksby, B.A. (1987) Cardiorespiratory responses of waterpolo players performing the head-in-the-water and head-out-of-the-water front crawl swimming techniques. **Austr. J. Sci. Med. Sport,** 19, 15-19.

Pinnington, H.C., Dawson, B. and Blanksby, B.A. (1988) Heart rate responses and the estimated energy requirements of playing waterpolo. **J. Human Movt. Stud.,** 15, 101-118.

Szögy, A. and Rosca, E. (1973) Einige spiroergometrische Befunde und Hertzvolumenbestimmungen bei Wasserballspielern. **Sportartz und Sportmedicin,** 253-258.

Vertommen, L., Clarys, J.P. and Welch, W. (1979) Body measurements and heart morphology of waterpolo players, in **Swimming III,** International Series on Sport Science, Vol. 8 (eds J. Terauds and E.W. Bedingfield), University Park Press, Baltimore, pp. 307-319.

Whiting, W.C., Puffer, J.C., Finerman, G.A., Gregor, R.J. and Maletis, G.B. (1985) Three-dimensional cinematographic analysis of water polo throwing in elite performers. **Am. J. Sports Med.** 13, 95-98.

SYNCHRO-SWIMMING: AN EMG-STUDY OF THE ARM MUSCLES DURING THE SCULL MOVEMENT IN THE "SINGLE BALLET LEG ALTERNATE"

E. ZINZEN, J. ANTONIS, J. CABRI, P. SERNEELS and J.P. CLARYS
Experimental Anatomy, Vrije Universiteit Brussel, Brussels, Belgium

Abstract
Electromyography of five arm muscles was measured on-line from the scull movement in the Single Ballet Leg Alternate. The patterns of the arm EMG were compared using the IDANCO system for co-contraction and specificity. The iEMG was used as a reference for muscular intensity. Normalization of data was made according to the highest peak principle.

On analysing relations between synergist, agonist and antagonist muscles, significant differences were found ($P < 0.05$) in integrated EMG during the lifting of the leg (iEMG of M. brachioradialis = 40%, iEMG of M. flexor carpi ulnaris = 60% of the normalized highest peak contraction). A comparison of the movement phases with leg lifted versus the "Back Layout" phases, found significant differences in iEMG for the M. pectoralis major. During the "Ballet Leg" phase the iEMG-level was lower (45%) than during the "Back Layout" phase.
Keywords: MREMG, iEMG, Sculling, Synchro-swimming.

1 Introduction

Synchronised swimming has evolved from a "Show case" in the 1930's into an Olympic sport in the 1990's. It requires a high degree of sophisticated and graceful artistic movements and is related to both ballet and swimming. Its routine events comprise music and a lot of floating. Since it gained Olympic status it combines the artistic characteristics with dynamic and powerful movement mechanics. At the same time synchro-swimming has aroused a first, albeit limited, scientific interest (Takamoto et al., 1988) primarily in the U.S.A., Japan and Canada.

The existing research can be summarized as follows:
- Body composition of synchro-swimmers (Atwater et al., 1988; Kirkendall et al., 1982; Moffat et al., 1980; Ross et al.,1977)
- Physiological assessment (including heart rate studies) of synchro-swimming (Erickson and Wells, 1987; Jamnik et al., 1987; Poole et al., 1980; Roby et al., 1983; Lakamoto et al., 1987; 1988).
- Medical problems affecting synchro-swimmers (Davies, 1987); Daniel, 1978; Mutoh et al., 1988; Tucker, 1979; Weinberg, 1986).
This short review might not be complete, but to our knowledge there are no biomechanical nor electrophysiological studies of synchro-swimmers. Therefore the main purpose of this investigation was to

enlarge the little insight in the muscular movement patterns of the arm muscles during the "sculling skill" in basic synchro figures (e.g. the Single Ballet Leg Alternate).

2 Methods

The EMG-signals of five arm muscles were measured using active surface electrodes. Subjects were the best 10 out of 73 participants at the Belgian Championship 1989 (N = 10, age: 19.6 ± 3.3 yrs). The EMG signals were synchronised on 11 parts of the movement (from "Back Layout" over "Ballet Leg" to "Back Layout" exerted with the right leg, and the same skill repeated with the left leg).

An overall view of the electromyographic data acquisition is given in Fig. 1. The EMGs of the five arm muscles – the M. brachioradialis, the M. flexor carpi ulnaris, the M. biceps brachii, the M. triceps brachii and the M. pectoralis major – were measured on the right arm.

The raw EMG and subsequently the presentation of the linear envelope, the MREMG and the iEMG, the normalization and the analyses of data were done using the Electromyographic Signal Processing and Analyses System - ESPAS (Cabri, 1989).

The muscular activity patterns of the sculling movements were compared between right and left leg (the pattern being obtained as each leg executed the requisite skills), using the IDANCO-system. The term IDANCO stands for IDentical, ANalogue and COnform muscular patterns. These three criteria indicate three different levels of muscular specificity. The IDANCO-system is a quantitative way of

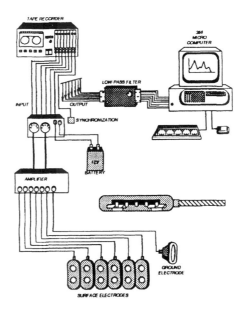

Fig. 1. The electromyographic data acquisition set up.

118

comparing the quality of muscular activity patterns (Clarys et al., 1988, Fig. 2). This comparison is based on the full-wave rectified and normalised in time and amplitude) linear envelope of the raw EMG-signal.

3 Results and discussion

During 3/5 of the movement executions of the different phases of the Single Ballet Leg (Fig. 3), one leg and part of the head and trunk were observed to be above the water surface. This assumes an increase in the gravitation influence and thus on the upward drag or propulsion to be created by the sculling of the arms. For this reason the EMG data were analysed separately for the "Back Layout" (1), "Bent Knee" (2)' "Ballet Leg" (3) "Bent Knee" (4) and again the "Back Layout" (5) and for both right and left leg. On analysis of the mechanics of the scull movement in combination with the muscular activity patterns, a high level of dynamic activity was found for all muscles, especially during sideward scull movement and during the

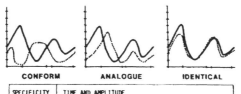

SPECIFICITY CRITERION	TIME AND AMPLITUDE CRITERION
IDENTICAL	No difference in time and amplitude
IDENTICAL	Difference in time and/or amplitude (0 - 10%)
ANALOGUE	Difference in time and/or amplitude (11 - 20%)
CONFORM	Difference in time and/or amplitude (21 - 30%)
CONFORM	Equal numbers of peaks with total time shift
DIFFERENT	Unequal number of peaks and/or total disproportion of dynamic and static contraction

Fig.2.   The IDANCO system for "specificity" of control of EMG patterns.

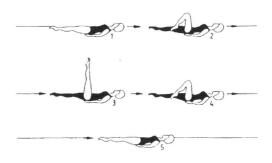

Fig. 3.   The Single Ballet Leg.

119

rotation of the hand at the level of the wrist. These parts of the skill increased their intensity during the "Bent Knee - Ballet Leg - Bent Knee" phases. However, looking at the overall muscular intensity (iEMG - Fig. 4) in the 11 left-right movement phases, it is seen that each of the five muscles react differently ranging from ±35% to ±65% of the highest peak maximum.

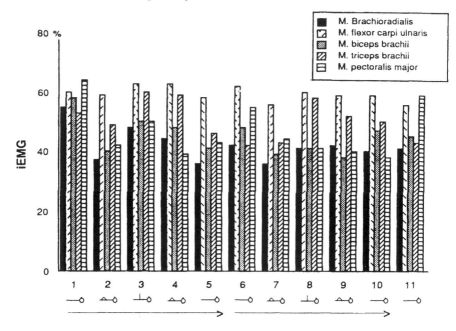

Fig. 4.   Percentage of muscular intensity (iEMG - all subjects) per muscle during the 11 phases of the Single Ballet Leg alternate.

For all subjects, muscles and numbers of movement executions it was found that 85% of the patterns were ANalogue or COnform (40% ANalogue, 45% COnform); 15% were different patterns. This suggests that the sculling movements during "Single Ballet Leg Alternate" are symmetrical, although there were small differences in time shift and amplitude level. The qualitative analysis of the data failed to provide evidence of co-contractions.

For synergist, agonist and antagonist muscles (e.g. M. brachio-radialis versus M. flexor carpi ulnaris; M. brachioradialis versus M. biceps brachii, M. triceps brachii versus M. pectoralis major and M. triceps brachii versus M. biceps brachii), significant differences were found ($P < 0.05$) in integrated EMG during the lifting of the leg (iEMG of M. brachioradialis = 40%, iEMG of M. flexor carpi ulnaris = 60% of the normalized highest peak contraction). Comparing the movement phases with leg lifted versus the "Back Layout" phases, significant differences in iEMG for the M. pectoralis major were seen; during the "Ballet Leg" phase the iEMG was lower (45%) than during the "Back Layout" phase (both in the left and right execution).

4 Conclusions

These data suggest that due to the absence of co-contractions, the scull movement has no stabilisation function. It is a fully dynamic motion, solely for the support of the trunk position and a slowly executed "Single Ballet Leg Alternate".

The level of the integrated EMG as a reference for muscle intensity was lower than expected, and showed intensities similar to other sports movements in submaximal efforts. This suggests that an increase of muscular activity might increase precision in executing the "Single Ballet Leg Alternate".

It can also be concluded that the M. flexor carpi ulnaris has a stabilisation function for the wrist and hand in comparison with the forearm. The M. brachioradialis and M. biceps brachii are as expected the flexors of the elbow and the M. triceps brachii is the extensor with an obviously different muscular activity. The M. pectoralis major is mostly working during the "Back Layout" and less while lifting the leg. It can be concluded that the sculling propulsion effect is initiated by the elbow and not by the shoulder as assumed by coaches and athletes.

5 References

Atwater, A., Puhl, J. and Roby, F. (1988) Sport science and medicine committee: body composition. **Synchro,** 26, 37-38.

Cabri, J. (1989) **The influences of different doses of alprazolam on muscle activity, in function and cardiovascular responses to concentric and eccentric efforts in isokinetic movement conditions.** PhD thesis, Vrije Universiteit Brussel.

Clarys, J.P., Cabri, J., De Witte, B. and Toussaint, H. (1988) Electromyography applied to sport ergonomics. **Ergonomics,** 31, 1605-1620.

Daniel, L. (1978) Physical evaluation. **Synchro Info.,** 16, 26.

Davies, T. (1987) Shoulder problems. **Synchro,** 25, 28-30.

Erickson, G.K. and Wells, C.L. (1987) Heart rates of elite synchronized swimmers. **Phys. Sportsmed.,** 15, 99-107.

Jamnik, V., Gledhiull, N., Hunter, I. and Murray, P. (1987) Physiological assessment of synchronized swimming and elite synchronized swimmers. **Med. Sci. Sports Exerc.,** 19, 305.

Kirkendall, D.T., Delio, D.J., Hagerman, G.R. and Fox, E.T. (1982) Body composition of elite and intermediate class synchronized swimmers. **Synchro,** 20, 10-11.

Moffat, R., Katch, V.L., Freedson, P. and Lindeman, J. (1980) Body composition of synchronized swimmers. **Canad. J. Appl. Sport Sci.,** 5, 153-155.

Mutoh, Y., Takamoto, M. and Miyashita, M. (1988) Chronic injuries of elite competitive swimmers, divers, waterpolo players and synchronized swimmers, in **Swimming Science V** (eds B.E. Ungerechts, K. Wilke and E. Reischle), Human Kinetics Books, Champaign, Ill., pp. 333-338.

Poole, G.W., Crepin, B.J. and Sevigny, M. (1980) Physiological characteristics of elite synchronized swimmers. **Canad. J. Appl. Sport Sci.,** 5, 156-160.

Roby, F.B., Buono, M.J., Constable, S.H., Lowdon, B.J. and Taso, W.Y.

(1983) Physiological characteristics of champion synchronized swimmers. **Phys. Sportsmed.**, 11, 136–139; 142–144; 147.

Ross, W.D., Corlett, J., Drinkwater, D., Faulkner, R. and Vajda, A. (1977) Anthropometry of synchronized swimmers (abstract). **Canad. J. Appl. Sport Sci.**, 2, 227.

Takamoto, M., Mutoh, Y. and Myashita, M. (1987) Heart rate response to routine performance in synchronized swimming, in **VIIth World FINA Medical Congress**, USOC (Red.), Orlando, FL, p. 71.

Takamoto, M., Nakamura, Y., Motoyoshi, M., Mutoh, Y. and Miyashita, M. (1988) Physiological characteristics of Japanese elite synchronized swimmers, in **Swimming Science V** (eds B.E. Ungerechts, K. Wilke and K. Reischle), Human Kinetics Books, Champaign, Ill., pp. 121–128.

Tucker, M. (1979) Common orthopaedic problems affecting synchronized swimmers. **Synchro Info.**, 17, 18–20.

Weinberg, S.K. (1986) Medical aspects of synchronized swimming. **Clin. Sports Med.**, 5, 159–167.

PART FOUR

SWIM TECHNIQUE

CONSEQUENCES OF ALTERING STROKE PARAMETERS IN FRONT CRAWL SWIMMING AND ITS SIMULATION

D. McARDLE and T. REILLY
Centre for Sports and Exercise Sciences, Liverpool Polytechnic, Byrom Street, Liverpool L3 3AF, England.

Abstract
The aim of the study was to examine the effect of altering the normal stroke parameters in front crawl swimming. Seven club swimmers completed a series of 366 m free style trials at five different stroking rates ranging from very slow to very fast. A clear 'inverted U' pattern was observed between stroke frequency and swim velocity; the optimum stroke rate (S_{opt}) freely chosen by the subject producing the highest swim velocity. Each subject then simulated the front crawl arm action on a swim bench using the five stroke frequencies determined during the pool tests. These were conducted at three different levels of exercise intensity. Oxygen uptake ($\dot{V}O_2$), $\dot{V}E$ and heart rate were affected by changes in stroke rate at all intensities. Mean power per stroke varied according to an inverted U curve; the correlation between mean power at S_{opt} and maximum swimming velocity was 0.88 ($P < 0.01$) at the highest level of exercise. Total power output at S_{opt} was also related to swimming performance ($r = 0.85$; $P < 0.01$). Maximum swimming velocity was not significantly related to $\dot{V}O_2$ peak measured either on the swim bench or during arm cycling. Results suggest that analysis of responses to varying stroke parameters, particularly power output, may have more relevance for the swimmer than $\dot{V}O_2$ peak measured in a dry-land test.
Keywords: Heart rate, Stroke frequency, Swim bench, Ventilation, $\dot{V}O_2$.

1 Introduction

The swimmer's horizontal velocity in water is a product of the stroke frequency (SF) and the distance travelled per stroke (d/S). Maximum velocity is attained at a unique combination of these stroke parameters. The combination seems to differ between individuals, with competitive distance and with swimming competence. Elite swimmers have a greater d/S than less successful counterparts (Craig et al., 1985). They increase their own swim velocity by an increase in SF which more than compensates for a fall in d/S (Swaine and Reilly, 1983). Within a single competitive event the speed of the stroking action rather than the actual SF decreases as the event progresses.

Previous work has shown that altering the preferred SF results in impaired swimming performance (Swaine and Reilly, 1983). The optimal stroke frequency (SF_{opt}) coincided with the highest $\dot{V}O_2$ peak

and the highest V̇E peak (r = 0.98) when SF was experimentally
manipulated on a swim-simulator. It was concluded that the
combination of SF and d/S employed spontaneously by competitive
swimmers has a significant influence in maximising swimming velocity
and $\dot{V}O_2$ in all-out efforts. It was not possible to establish whether
power output was maximised at SF_{opt}, since no measurement of power
output on the swim bench was made.

This study aimed to further examine factors affecting front-crawl
swim performance, specifically to:-
i)   establish the consequences of altering stroke parameters on
front crawl swimming and on physiological responses to sub-maximal
and all-out performance on a swim-simulator;
ii)   examine the relation between swim performance, peak
physiological responses and power output on the simulator;
iii)   determine the relationship between physiological responses on
swim-specific ergometry and swimming performance.

2 Methods

Seven male swimmers from the City of Liverpool squad - mean ($\pm$ SD)
age 15.8 $\pm$ 1.2 years, height 174 $\pm$ 6 cm, body mass 64.7 $\pm$ 7.4 kg -
acted as subjects. They were tested in the pre-competitive season
and at the time were swimming about 6.3 km each day in training.
They first swam a series of 366 m all-out front crawl trials to
determine five different SF rates, ranging from their slowest
possible to the fastest, their preferred SF being intermediate. This
was done at the same time of day (18:15 hours) but over different
days in a 30.5 m pool. Subjects were requested to maintain maximum
d/S and the same leg-kick and breathing patterns over the five
trials. Prior to any testing all subjects did a standard warm up
(1260 m). Mean SF and mean velocity were calculated for each swim
from the total number of complete arm cycles and the time taken for
the full distance. The SF_{opt} and maximum velocity were identified
for each swimmer when decreases in SF brought no further increase in
velocity.

Each subject then simulated the front-crawl arm action on a
Biokinetic Swim Bench (Isokinetics Inc., Albany, CA) using the five
stroke frequencies determined during the pool tests. These were
conducted at three different levels of subjective exercise intensity,
corresponding to low, moderate and the highest tolerable. The stroke
frequencies corresponded to very fast, fast, optimum, slow and very
slow. Each SF condition was administered on a separate occasion, the
order of administration being randomised and each trial lasting 4
min. For each SF the subject started at the low intensity,
progressing to the moderate and then maximal levels, subjects being
fully rested between the 4 min trials. During performance the power
output was monitored using the display on the swim-bench which was
pre-calibrated according to Sharp et al. (1982). Throughout exercise
metabolic responses ($\dot{V}O_2$ and $\dot{V}E$) were monitored continuously using an
automated system (P.K. Morgan, Rainham) and heart rate recorded using
short-range radio telemetry (Sport-Tester). The highest value over
60 s for $\dot{V}O_2$ and $\dot{V}E$ at the most strenuous exercise intensity was
taken as the peak value. At the end of each subjectively-determined
exercise level, the perception of effort was rated according to Borg

(1982).

Peak values for physiological responses on the swim-bench were compared to those obtained using standard arm-cycling ergometry (Monark AB) and using a progressive continuous test to voluntary exhaustion on the swim-bench. The work-rate was increased every 2 min until the subject was unable to continue. During the test $\dot{V}O_2$, $\dot{V}E$ and heart rate were measured continuously using the same procedures as previously described.

Effects of varying the SF on performance and physiological variables were analysed using ANOVA. Tukey's honestly significant difference (HSD) test was used to localise specific differences.

3 Results

3.1 Water tests

A clear 'inverted U' pattern was observed, relating SF to swim velocity. The optimum SF freely-chosen by subjects was that which produced the best swim performances. The SF (mean $\pm$SD) values from slowest to fastest were 34 ($\pm$ 3.4), 38 ($\pm$3.8), 45($\pm$2.4), 48 ($\pm$1.9) and 53 ($\pm$1.6) S min^{-1}. The corresponding swim velocities were 1.34 ($\pm$ 0.04), 1.38 ($\pm$0.04), 1.45 ($\pm$0.05), 1.38 ($\pm$0.07) and 1.24 ($\pm$0.06) m s^{-1}. These compared with the best competitive performances of the subjects at 400 m freestyle of 4 min 30 s ($\pm$ 13 s), the mean corresponding to 1.48 m s^{-1}. The distance per stroke (d/S) was inversely related to SF ($r = -0.995$). The correlation coefficient between maximum swimming velocity and optimum d/S was $r = 0.764$ ($P < 0.05$).

3.2 Experimental alterations of stroke parameters on the swim-bench

The three levels of exercise were significantly separated according to the Borg ratings. Mean values were 10.7, 12.3 and 16.7, corresponding to fairly light, somewhat hard and very hard, respectively.

A linear relationship was noted between SF and $\dot{V}O_2$ at the lowest ($r = 0.903$) and moderate exercise ($r = 0.930$) intensities. At the highest exercise intensity the $\dot{V}O_2$ was greater at the three fastest SF rates than at the other two ($P < 0.05$): differences among the three fastest or among the two slowest stroke frequencies were non-significant ($P > 0.05$).

The relation between SF and $\dot{V}E$ at the lowest and moderate exercise intensity tended towards curvilinearity (Table 1). However, only the slowest SF produced significantly lower $\dot{V}E$ values than the three fastest stroke rates ($P < 0.05$) which themselves did not differ significantly at any exercise intensity ($P > 0.05$). The highest $\dot{V}E$ peak was significantly related to the highest $\dot{V}O_2$ peak ($r = 0.966$).

The ANOVA established that varying the stroke frequency had a significant effect on heart rate only at the lowest exercise level ($P < 0.05$). The slowest SF produced lower HR values than the three fastest conditions, none of the other comparisons achieving a significant result ($P > 0.05$).

The mean power per stroke was found to vary as an 'inverted U' curvilinear function of SF. The highest power per stroke was generated at S_{opt} at all exercise intensities. The correlation between peak power per stroke at S_{opt} during high intensity exercise

Table 1. Physiological responses to variations in stroke rate at submaximal and maximal efforts

		Stroke Frequency				
		Slowest (34 ± 3)	Slow (38 ± 4)	Optimum (45 ± 2)	Fast (48 ± 2)	Fastest (53 ± 2)
$\dot{V}E$ (min⁻¹)	Low	38.0 ± 8.5	50.0 ± 14.0	57.6 ± 7.9	51.3 ± 10.5	58.1 ± 12.2
	Moderate	50.2 ± 18.5	54.1 ± 7.0	68.0 ± 11.1	64.1 ± 17.1	63.9 ± 10.8
	High	62.2 ± 13.5	66.4 ± 6.4	75.6 ± 7.1	80.0 ± 8.4	80.4 ± 11.8
$\dot{V}O_2$ (ml kg⁻¹ min⁻¹)	Low	15.1 ± 4.8	20.7 ± 3.6	23.0 ± 4.4	17.7 ± 6.4	17.7 ± 4.6
	Moderate	25.4 ± 3.2	27.3 ± 2.5	30.9 ± 2.6	30.1 ± 4.8	31.1 ± 4.9
	High	29.8 ± 4.6	32.2 ± 2.6	36.3 ± 3.1	36.2 ± 2.3	36.7 ± 4.4
Heart rate (beats min⁻¹)	Low	111 ± 9	118 ± 5	125 ± 6	124 ± 10	124 ± 12
	Moderate	127 ± 13	132 ± 16	135 ± 13	137 ± 15	134 ± 13
	High	136 ± 12	139 ± 13	151 ± 8	152 ± 10	147 ± 11
Power output (W stroke⁻¹ cycle⁻¹)	Low	2.47 ± 0.78	3.33 ± 0.59	3.76 ± 0.72	2.89 ± 1.05	2.89 ± 0.75
	Moderate	4.17 ± 1.44	3.97 ± 1.19	4.95 ± 1.13	3.81 ± 1.21	3.40 ± 1.42
	High	5.75 ± 1.49	6.06 ± 1.68	6.83 ± 0.83	5.92 ± 0.70	5.39 ± 0.69

and maximum swimming velocity was r = 0.879 (P < 0.000). This relationship was not significant for sub-maximal exercise levels. Total power output at S_{opt} was also related to maximum swimming velocity (r = 0.848; P < 0.01).

3.3 Arm-cycling and swim-bench ergometry

The $\dot{V}O_2$ peak values on the incremental swim-bench test were similar to the highest $\dot{V}O_2$ peak values of 38.2 ($\pm$ 3.4) ml kg^{-1} min^{-1} found during the experimental changes in SF. Mean values were significantly greater (P < 0.01) on the swim-bench for $\dot{V}O_2$ peak (38.7 $\pm$ 3.4 ml kg^{-1} min^{-1}) than on the arm-ergometer (36.7 $\pm$ 3.1 ml kg^{-1} min^{-1}). A similar difference was noted for heart rate, peak values being 167 $\pm$ 4 compared to 162 $\pm$ 6 beats min^{-1}. The difference in $\dot{V}E$ - 87.5 $\pm$ 19.2 vs 78.8 $\pm$ 24.5 l min^{-1} - was non-significant (P > 0.05). They were in good agreement with the highest $\dot{V}E$ peak values (80.4 $\pm$ 11.8 l min^{-1}) found during the experimental work on SF.

A significant correlation (r = 0.954: P < 0.001)) was observed between $\dot{V}O_2$ peak on arm-ergometry and on the swim bench. No relation was evident between maximum swimming velocity and $\dot{V}O_2$ peak for either the arm cycling or swim-bench ergometer tests.

4 Discussion

The studies of performance in the water confirmed earlier findings of a curvilinear relationship between stroke frequency and swim velocity (Reilly, 1990). The S_{opt} established in the present sample (45.1 $\pm$ 2.3) was almost identical to that (45.8 $\pm$ 2.6) found by Swaine and Reilly (1983). This was despite the faster swim velocities in the present swimmers - 1.45 ($\pm$ 0.05) m s^{-1} compared to 1.25 ($\pm$ 0.15) m s^{-1} over a similar distance. This underlines the importance of d/S in determining swim performance once S_{opt} has been established.

When responses to experimental variation of SF were monitored on the swim bench, the best relations with the water tests were observed for power production. This applied irrespective of whether power was expressed per stroke cycle or for the duration of the test. This extends earlier findings (Sharp et al., 1982; Reilly and Bayley, 1988) of a relation between swim sprinting and power output on a swim-bench over a short test.

In contrast the $\dot{V}O_2$ peak was not related to swim performance. This agrees with earlier findings (Swaine and Reilly, 1983). It suggests that although power output on a swim-simulator may be predictive of performance in the water, the $\dot{V}O_2$max may need to be measured in water tests to possess any predictive power. The highest heart rates reached 151 beats min^{-1} on average, almost identical to that reached on the swim-bench by the subjects of Swaine and Reilly (1983) and corresponding to 85% of the values attained during a $\dot{V}O_2$max test using the legs.

There seemed to be a number of influences on submaximal responses to exercise which include both the speed and the efficiency of the stroking actions. It has been shown that increasing pedalling speed for a constant power output does increase the metabolic loading (Hughes et al., 1982). This is due mainly to recruitment of more fast-twitch fibres as the cycling rate is increased. Beyond the S_{opt} power output tended to drop : nevertheless no fall was evident in $\dot{V}E$, $\dot{V}O_2$ or heart rate. This, in turn, suggests that mechanical efficiency falls when SF is increased beyond the freely-chosen stroke rate of the swimmer. At slow stroke frequencies the physiological strain is lower but power generation is adversely affected.

In conclusion, the relevance of monitoring responses to alterations in stroke parameters was evident mainly at maximal exercise intensities. A clearly defined peak was noted in power production whereas $\dot{V}O_2$, $\dot{V}E$ and heart rate showed a plateau over the fast stroke frequencies. It seems the ability to generate high power outputs was more important in simulations of the swim stroke than are the accompanying cardiorespiratory consequences.

5 References

Borg, G. (1982) Psychophysical bases of perceived exertion. Med. Sci. Sports Exerc., 14, 377.

Craig, A.B., Boomer, W.L. and Gibbons, J.F. (1979) Use of stroke rate, distance per stroke and velocity relationships during training for competitive swimming. In: Swimming III (eds J. Terauds and E.W. Bedingfield), University Park Press, Baltimore, pp. 265-274.

Hughes, E.G., Turner, S.C. and Brooks, G.A. (1982). Effects of glycogen depletion and pedalling speed on anaerobic threshold. J. Appl. Physiol., 52, 1598-1607.

Reilly, T. (1990) Swimming. In: Physiology of Sports (eds T. Reilly, N. Secher, P. Snell and C. Williams), E. and F.N. Spon, London, pp. 217-257.

Reilly, T. and Bayley, K. (1988) The relation between short-term power output and sprint performance of young female swimmers. J. Human Mov't Stud., 14, 19-29.

Sharp, R.L., Troup, J.P. and Costill, D.L. (1982) Relationships between power and sprint free-style swimming. Med. Sci. Sports Exerc., 14, 53-56.

Swaine, I. and Reilly, T. (1983) The freely-chosen swimming stroke rate in a maximal swim and on a biokinetic swim bench. Med. Sci. Sports Exerc., 15, 370-375.

VELOCITY, DISTANCE PER STROKE AND STROKE FREQUENCY OF HIGHLY SKILLED
SWIMMERS IN 50 M FREESTYLE SPRINT IN A 50 AND 25 M POOL

W. WIRTZ, K. WILKE and F. ZIMMERMANN
Deutsche Sporthochschule Köln, Germany

Abstract
This study compares distance per stroke, stroke frequency and mean
velocity of highly skilled swimmers (n = 7) having raced both in a
25 m and a 50 m pool. Videotapes of the European Championships 1989
(50 m pool) and the ARENA-Meetings (25 m) pool 1989 and 1990 were
analysed. Individual differences were found in the kinematic
profiles of the variables measured between and within groups. For
men, the shorter time in the 25 m pool results came mainly from the
better time between 0 and 30 m in the 25 m pool. For women, shorter
times in the 25 m pool results mainly from the better time between 20
and 30 m.
Keywords: Swimming, Kinematics, Field Study.

1 Introduction

Distance per stroke (d/S) and stroke frequency (SF) determine mean
velocity (v) of swimming. These parameters themselves are
individually influenced by other factors like anthropometry,
flexibility as well as psychological, technical and physical
conditions (Jähnig, 1983; Grimston and Hay, 1985; Ciccione and Lyons,
1987). Speed specific training in water and strength training
exercises grant the best adaptation in physical and psychological
performance (Gullstrand and Lawrence, 1987; Reischle, 1988; Sharp,
1986). Nevertheless the kinematic profile helps to find weak points
of some athletes and to eliminate them. This makes it worth knowing
how the different pool lengths influence mean velocity during a
swimming race.

2 Methods

2.1 Subjects
All swimmers swam at the ARENA-Meetings 1989 and 1990 (25 m pool) and
the European Championships 1989 (50 m pool) so that their 50 m races
are comparable on two different pool lengths within one year
(Table 1).

2.2 Measurements
The 50 m were divided into five sections of measurements and were
recorded by videocameras. In each section, time (t1-t5) and stroke

Table 1. 50 m times of the swimmers at the ARENA-Meeting and the
          European Championships

Subject	Sex	25 m pool	Time (s) 50 m pool	$\overline{X}$
1	m	21.76	22.76	22.26
2	m	22.21	22.64	22.43
3	m	22.27	22.89	22.58
4	m	22.60	22.67	22.64
5	f	25.83	25.94	25.89
6	f	25.97	25.87	25.92
7	f	25.64	26.13	25.89

frequency (SF2-SF5) were measured, the criterion used was the passing
of the head of the swimmer. Stroke frequency was calculated on the
basis of three cycles in frequency/min (SEIKO stop-watch) and neither
the first 10 m of each pool nor the turning section of the 25 m pool
were included. Time and frequency in each section were determined by
hand so that an error of 0.1 s for time and 2 strokes/ min for the
calculated frequency must be tolerated. In the last section of
measurement the swimming distance investigated was not really 10 m
(passing of the head is the criterion), because the last touch to the
wall reduces this distance. For that reason a correcting factor of
0.5 m was taken into account in calculating distance per stroke
(d/S5) for this part of the event.

3 Results and discussion

The results allow a kinematic profile of the events to be determined.
Besides individual differences, some more general behaviour could be
recognized (Table 2).

3.1 Events in the 25 m pool
For men, the time increased continuously (t1-t5). There was no
advantage of the turning section in relation to the fastest swimming
time (t2). For most swimmers SF decreased (except subject 3, who
increased SF in the last section (SF5) but the big loss in d/S5
caused the mean velocity to decrease also), d/S stayed on a
relatively steady level (d/S2-d/S4) and decreased enormously in d/S5.
    For women, after t1, the fastest swimming time was reached in
interval t2, decreased in t3, the rest (t4-t5) was relatively
constant. The stroke frequency (DF) decreased by a small amount and
d/S stayed relatively constant.

3.2 Events in the 50 m pool
For men, time increased until 30 m, then remained at a steady level
in t4 and increased in t5 once more. The stroke frequency decreased
after 20 m and stayed then on a relatively equal level (SF3-SF5); d/S
was on the same level until 40 m (d/S2-d/S4) and went down in the
last section (d/S5).
    For women, time increased until 30 m (t1-t3) and stayed until the
end on the same level. Both SF and d/S decreased less after 20 m

Table 2. Time, stroke frequency and distance per stroke of the
measured sections

		25 m pool												
		t (s)					SF (min^{-1})				d (m)			
n	sex	1	2	3	4	5	2	3	4	5	2	3	4	5
1	m	3.3	4.4	4.4	4.7	5.0	64	–	62	59	2.13	–	2.06	1.93
2	m	3.3	4.5	4.5	4.8	5.1	71	–	68	67	1.88	–	1.84	1.67
3	m	3.2	4.5	4.5	4.8	5.3	60	–	60	63	2.22	–	2.08	1.71
4	m	3.3	4.5	4.6	4.8	5.4	63	–	61	58	2.12	–	2.05	1.82
5	f	3.9	5.5	5.1	5.6	5.7	51	–	48	47	2.14	–	2.23	2.13
6	f	3.9	5.5	5.1	5.7	5.8	54	–	52	50	2.02	–	2.02	1.97
7	f	3.8	5.5	5.2	5.5	5.6	54	–	51	51	2.06	–	2.14	2.00
		50 m pool												
1	m	3.5	4.6	4.8	4.8	5.1	65	62	61	61	2.01	2.02	2.05	1.83
2	m	3.5	4.6	4.7	4.8	5.0	71	70	67	66	1.84	1.82	1.87	1.73
3	m	3.2	4.7	5.0	4.8	5.2	61	60	60	61	2.09	2.00	2.08	1.80
4	m	3.6	4.4	4.7	4.8	5.1	66	61	59	59	2.07	2.16	2.12	1.89
5	f	3.9	5.2	5.5	5.6	5.7	49	48	47	47	2.35	2.27	2.28	2.13
6	f	4.1	5.0	5.6	5.6	5.6	60	58	57	56	2.00	1.85	1.88	1.82
7	f	4.1	5.0	5.7	5.6	5.7	55	53	53	52	2.18	1.99	2.02	1.92

(SF3, d/S3) and stayed on an equal standard until the end.

3.3 Comparison between swimming in 25 and 50 m pool (Table 3)
For men, all swimmers were faster on the short course. They lost
their time on the long course until 30 m mainly by t1 and t3. The
biggest differences in time appeared in the last 10 m (t5). Both d/S
and SF in the comparable sections were nearly the same in each pool.
    For women, two of them had nearly the same result in time, but
only one of them was really faster (no. 7). Difference in time

Table 3. Differences for each subject between 50 and 25 m pool in
percentage (50 m = 100%)

		t section					SF section			d/S section		
n	sex	1	2	3	4	5	2	4	5	2	4	5
1	m	-5.7	-4.3	-8.3	-2.1	-2.0	-1.5	1.6	-3.3	6.0	0.5	5.5
2	m	-5.7	-2.2	-4.3	0.0	2.0	0.0	1.5	1.5	2.2	-1.6	-3.5
3	m	0.0	-4.3	-10.0	0.0	1.9	-1.6	0.0	3.3	6.2	0.0	-5.0
4	m	-8.3	2.3	-2.1	0.0	5.9	-4.5	3.4	-1.7	2.4	-3.3	-3.7
5	f	0.0	5.8	-7.3	0.0	0.0	4.1	2.1	0.0	-8.9	-2.2	0.0
6	f	-4.9	10.0	-8.9	1.8	3.6	-10.0	-8.7	-10.7	1.0	7.4	8.2
7	f	-7.3	10.0	-8.8	-1.8	-1.8	-1.8	-3.8	-1.9	-5.5	5.9	3.6

appeared less in t1 and more in t2 (faster on the long course; t3 was obviously better on the long course; SF2 to SF5 and d/S2 to d/S5 were nearly the same in each course, except subject no. 6 whose frequency (SF2 to SF5) was much smaller in the 25 m pool.

4 Conclusions

In this sample men gained more advantage from the 25 m pool than women (Table 1). Their first ten metres were extremely better on the short course and they took greater advantage of the distance between 20 and 30 m where the turn is executed. Women took their advantage mostly from the same sections, but they could not profit from it by a much better total time in the 25 m pool, because they lost time between 10 and 20 m where they were extremely slower on the short course (Tables 2/3). This field study demonstrates the very individual behaviour of top athletes who in different ways reach a good time both on the 25 and 50 m pools.

5 References

Ciccione, C.D. and Lyons, C.M. (1987) Relationship of upper extremity strength and swimming stroke technique on competitive freestyle swimming performance. **J. Human Mov't Stud.**, 13, 143-150.

Grimston, S.K. and Hay, J.G. (1986) Relationship among anthropometric and stroking characteristics of college swimmers. **Med. Sci. Sports Exerc.**, 18, 60-68.

Gullstrand, L. and Lawrence, S. (1987) Heart rate and blood lactate response to short intermittent work at race pace in highly trained swimmers. **Austr. J. Sci. Med. Sport**, March, 10-13.

Jähnig, W. (1983) Grunglegende Betrachtungen zum Verhältnis von Schwimmgeschwindigkeit, Frequenz und Zyklusweg. **Wiss. Z. DHFK Leipzig**, 24, 121-139.

Reischle, K. (1988) **Biomechanik des Schwimmens.** Sport Fahnemann Verlag, Bockenem.

Sharp, R.L. (1986) Muscle strength and power as related to competitive swimming. **J. Swimming Res.**, 2, 5-10.

ANALYSIS OF SWIMMING RACES IN THE 1989 PAN PACIFIC SWIMMING CHAMPIONSHIPS AND 1988 JAPANESE OLYMPIC TRIALS

K. WAKAYOSHI[*], T. NOMURA[+], G. TAKAHASHI[**], Y. MUTOH[++] AND M. MIYASHITO[++]
[*]Faculty of Health and Sport Sciences, Osaka University, Japan;
[+]Kyoto Institute of Technology, Japan; [**]University of Tsukuba,
Japan; [++]University of Tokyo, Japan.

Abstract
The purpose of this study was to determine the velocities (V) associated with the start phase, turn phase and stroke phase in the 100 m and 200 m swimming races, and to investigate the relationship between V, the stroke frequency (SF) and stroke length (SL) during the stroke phase. Swimming performances were analysed in the Pan Pacific Swimming Championships of 1989 and the 1988 Japanese Olympic Trials. The results of this study suggest that the swimmer's ability may be evaluated by determining the SF, SL and V of the three phases in the swimming races.
Keywords: Race Analysis, Velocity, Stroke Frequency, Stroke Length.

1 Introduction

Previous investigations of factors influencing competitive swimming events have been conducted by East (1970), Craig et al. (1985) and Wakayoshi (1988). These studies have all used video analysis in considering the relationships between SF, SL and mean V during competitive swimming.

The purposes of this study were (1) to determine the three average V values after the start (start phase), during the turn phase and in the period between the two phases (stroke phase) in the 100 m and 200 m swimming races, (2) to determine the relationships between V, SF and SL during the stroke phase and the V of the three phases, and (3) to compare the results on the above-stated items for the finalists in the Pan Pacific Swimming Championships (1989P) with those in the 1988 Japanese Seoul Olympic Trials (1988J).

2 Methods

In previous research into starting techniques, Wilson and Malino (1983) defined the start time as the time required to reach 10.93 m from the starting wall, whilst in a study of turning skills, Taskahashi (1983) defined the turn time as the time taken from 5 m before to 5 m after the turning wall, measured with respect to the swimmer's head. Taking this into consideration, the present study divided the race into three phases of the start, the turn and the stroke. The start phase was a period from the starting wall to the 10 m line, the turn phase was a period from 5 m before to 5 m after the turn wall, and the stroke phase was a period excluding the start and turn phases.

Four video cameras placed on the highest steps of the spectator stand opposite the starter were used for this experiment. Camera 1 (C1), Camera 2 (C2) and Camera 4 (C4) were positioned on the 5 m line, 10 m line and 45 m line from the starting wall and synchronized by switching on three small lights positioned in front of each camera (Figure 1). The light of the starting camera was videoed by C1, so that C1, C2 and C4 could be synchronized with the start. In the 100 m race, the lap times of 10 m (T10), 45 m (T45), 55 m (T55) and 95 m (T95) were measured by the three cameras (the phase used for this study was defined according to the passage of the swimmer's head).

In this way, V of each phase was calculated by the lap times in the 100 m race (the start phase: Vs, the turn phase: Vt, the stroke phase of first and second laps, V1 and V2, and average V of the stroke phase: Va).

Vs (m/s) $=^-$ 10 m/T10 s
$V1$ (m/s) $= 35$ m/(T45 - T10) s
Vt (m/s) $= 10$ m/(T55 - T45) s
$V2$ (m/s) $= 45$ m/(T95 - T55) s
Va (m/s) $= (V1 + V2)/2$

In the 200 m race, the average V of the four stroke phases and the three turn phases were indicated Va and Vta respectively (Figure 2).

Camera 3 (C3) was positioned on the 25 m line covering a shooting range of 15 m to the nearest lane from C3 (Figure 1). Stroke frequency (SF) was thus calculated by measuring the time taken for eight strokes in each lap (average SF:SRa).

SR (stroke/min) $=$ number of strokes/time taken.

SL was measured by dividing the V of the stroke phase by Sr (the average SL:SLa).

SL (m/stroke) $= V$ (m/s)/SF (stroke/min/60)

Finally, the average V in the 100 m race (Vr) was calculated from the official record (R).

Vr (m/s) $= 100$ m/R (s).

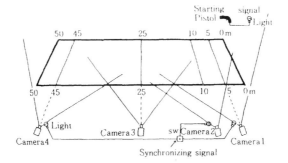

Fig. 1. Schematic illustration for the experiment.

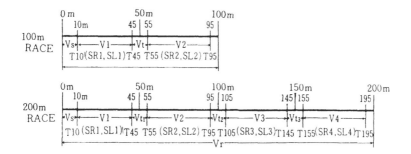

Fig. 2. Measures and definitions race analysis in the 100 m and 200 m races.

3 Results and discussion

The means and SD of the results for the finalists in all 100 m and 200 m races for 1989P and 1988J are presented in Tables 1 and 2 respectively. Significant differences were found for Vr in all strokes for men and women, and for Va in all strokes except 100 m backstroke for men and 200 m freestyle for women between the finalists of 1989P and 1988J. In Vt(Vta) of 14 strokes except 100 m breaststroke and 200 m BA for women, and in the Vs of 7 strokes of freestyle and butterfly, the finalists in 1989P were significantly higher than those in 1988J.

Figure 3 shows the relationship among SF and SL in all strokes for men and women finalists in 1989P and 1988J. For men, the higher V of the finalists in 1989P compared to those in 1988J were associated with a greater SL. For women, the finalists in 1989P had a tendency for a greater SF compared to those in 1988J. Even though it is thought that the stature of Japanese swimmers is smaller than those of the non-Japanese swimmers, it is considered that Japanese men who had a shorter SL should improve the stroke technique to produce a higher propulsive force, to increase muscular strength in response to the stroke technique, and to develop muscular endurance to prevent a decrease of SL in the race. The Japanese female swimmers who had a lower SF should work on arm cadence and speed work in order to producea faster stroke.

Figure 4 shows the relationship between Vs and Vr, Vt and Vr, and Vs and Vr in the 100 m freestyle for mean (n = 108) and women (n = 70) of 1989P and 1988J. There were significantly positive correlations (P < 0.001). From these relationships, it can be stated that those who deviated upward from the regression line could improve their swim times by improving their start and turn techniques.

Table 1. Means ± SD of finalists and comparison between the 1989 Pan Pacific Championships (1989) and the 1988 Japanese Olympic Trials (1988) in the 100 m races

Men

	N	Vs (m/s)	Vt (m/s)	Va (m/s)	SRa (stroke/min)	SLa (m/stroke)	Vr (m/s)
1989FR	8	2.68 ± 0.11	2.14 ± 0.05[a]	1.87 ± 0.04[a]	51.7 ± 2.2	2.18 ± 0.09	1.96 ± 0.04[a]
1988FR	8	2.59 ± 0.09	2.00 ± 0.06	1.80 ± 0.02	52.5 ± 3.0	2.06 ± 0.12	1.88 ± 0.02
1989BR	8	2.59 ± 0.15	1.75 ± 0.02[a]	1.47 0.02[a]	55.9 ± 1.8	1.58 ± 0.07	1.57 ± 0.02[b]
1988BR	8	2.49 ± 0.20	1.68 ± 0.02	1.44 ± 0.02	56.3 ± 4.7	1.54 ± 0.14	1.53 ± 0.03
1989BA	8	2.28 ± 0.10	1.88 ± 0.06[b]	1.67 ± 0.03	49.6 ± 2.4	2.02 ± 0.08	1.74 ± 0.03[b]
1988BA	8	2.15 ± 0.16	1.80 ± 0.07	1.64 ± 0.05	49.3 ± 2.9	2.00 ± 0.10	1.70 ± 0.05
1989FL	8	2.72 ± 0.08[a]	1.90 ± 0.04[a]	1.75 ± 0.03[a]	53.0 ± 2.3[a]	1.99 ± 0.07[a]	1.83 ± 0.03[a]
1988FL	8	2.53 ± 0.07	1.84 ± 0.03	1.70 ± 0.02	57.6 ± 3.5	1.77 ± 0.10	1.77 ± 0.01

Women

	N	Vs (m/s)	Vt (m/s)	Va (m/s)	SRa (stroke/min)	SLa (m/stroke)	Vr (m/s)
1989FR	8	2.33 ± 0.08[b]	1.90 ± 0.06[a]	1.68 ± 0.03[a]	52.2 ± 2.4	1.94 ± 0.10	1.76 ± 0.03[a]
1988FR	8	2.25 ± 0.05	1.81 ± 0.03	1.63 ± 0.02	51.2 ± 7.3	1.94 ± 0.24	1.70 ± 0.02
1989BR	8	2.08 ± 0.16	1.56 ± 0.03[a]	1.34 ± 0.02[a]	53.0 ± 6.6	1.54 ± 0.23	1.54 ± 0.02[a]
1988BR	8	1.98 ± 0.10	1.50 ± 0.03	1.27 ± 0.02	53.6 ± 3.4	1.43 ± 0.09	1.34 ± 0.01
1989BA	8	1.88 ± 0.04	1.63 ± 0.05	1.52 ± 0.02[a]	46.8 ± 3.3	1.96 ± 0.14	1.57 ± 0.01[a]
1988BA	8	1.85 ± 0.08	1.59 ± 0.04	1.48 ± 0.02	45.6 ± 4.0	1.96 ± 0.15	1.52 ± 0.02
1989FL	8	2.26 ± 0.06[a]	1.67 ± 0.05[a]	1.57 ± 0.01[a]	55.2 ± 2.1	1.71 ± 0.07	1.63 ± 0.02[a]
1988FL	8	2.12 ± 0.02	1.60 ± 0.05	1.53 ± 0.02	54.4 ± 4.7	1.69 ± 0.15	1.58 ± 0.02

FR - freestyle; BR - breaststroke; BA - backstroke; FL - butterfly
[a]$P < 0.01$; [b]$P < 0.05$

Table 2. Means ± SD of finalists and comparison between the 1989 Pan Pacific Championships (1989) and the 1988 Japanese Olympic Trials in the 200 m race

Men

	N	Vs (m/s)	Vt (m/s)	Va (m/s)	SRa (stroke/min)	SLa (m/stroke)	Vr (m/s)
1989FR	8	2.57 ± 0.10[a]	1.98 ± 0.04[a]	1.74 ± 0.02[a]	45.2 ± 2.1	2.31 ± 0.11	1.80 ± 0.02[a]
1988FR	8	2.39 ± 0.10	1.91 ± 0.04	1.67 ± 0.03	44.2 ± 2.2	2.27 ± 0.12	1.73 ± 0.03
1989BR	8	2.50 ± 0.12	1.63 ± 0.03[b]	1.39 0.02[a]	46.0 ± 4.5	1.83 ± 0.18	1.46 ± 0.02[a]
1988BR	8	2.38 ± 0.22	1.60 ± 0.02	1.34 ± 0.02	44.8 ± 4.5	1.82 ± 0.18	1.41 ± 0.03
1989BA	8	2.15 ± 0.09	1.75 ± 0.05[b]	1.57 ± 0.02[a]	41.3 ± 2.3[b]	2.28 ± 0.13	1.62 ± 0.02[a]
1988BA	8	2.15 ± 0.08	1.68 ± 0.05	1.52 ± 0.03	44.3 ± 2.8	2.06 ± 0.11	1.57 ± 0.03
1989FL	8	2.61 ± 0.09[a]	1.77 ± 0.03[a]	1.60 ± 0.02[a]	47.6 ± 2.0[a]	2.02 ± 0.09[a]	1.66 ± 0.02[a]
1988FL	8	2.50 ± 0.06	1.69 ± 0.04	1.56 ± 0.03	51.8 ± 2.5	1.81 ± 0.08	1.61 ± 0.03

Women

	N	Vs (m/s)	Vt (m/s)	Va (m/s)	SRa (stroke/min)	SLa (m/stroke)	Vr (m/s)
1989FR	8	2.27 ± 0.07[a]	1.79 ± 0.03[a]	1.57 ± 0.03[a]	47.1 ± 4.3	2.01 ± 0.16	1.63 ± 0.02
1988FR	8	2.16 ± 0.08	1.70 ± 0.04	1.52 ± 0.02	44.1 ± 2.9	2.07 ± 0.14	1.57 ± 0.02
1989BR	8	2.09 ± 0.18	1.47 ± 0.03	1.24 ± 0.01[a]	45.3 ± 5.6	1.67 ± 0.25	1.30 ± 0.02[a]
1988BR	8	1.93 ± 0.13	1.43 ± 0.05	1.20 ± 0.02	46.8 ± 3.6	1.55 ± 0.12	1.26 ± 0.03
1989BA	8	1.87 ± 0.04	1.56 ± 0.03[a]	1.44 ± 0.02[a]	39.6 ± 4.8	2.21 ± 0.30	1.48 ± 0.02[a]
1988BA	8	1.81 ± 0.05	1.49 ± 0.39	1.39 ± 0.02	39.7 ± 5.5	2.15 ± 0.34	1.43 ± 0.02
1989FL	8	2.15 ± 0.06[b]	1.57 ± 0.03[a]	1.46 ± 0.03	51.8 ± 3.2	1.70 ± 0.12	1.50 ± 0.02[b]
1988FL	8	2.09 ± 0.05	1.52 ± 0.03	1.44 ± 0.02	50.1 ± 5.2	1.74 ± 0.19	1.47 ± 0.02

FR – freestyle; BR – breaststroke; BA – backstroke; FL – butterfly
[a] $P < 0.01$, [b] $P < 0.05$

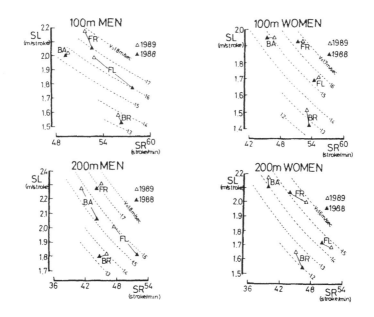

Fig. 3. The SF and SL in four competitive strokes of the finalists in the 1989 Pan Pacific Swimming Championships (1989) and 1988 Japanese Olympic Trials (1988). FR - freestyle; BR - breaststroke; FL - bufferfly.

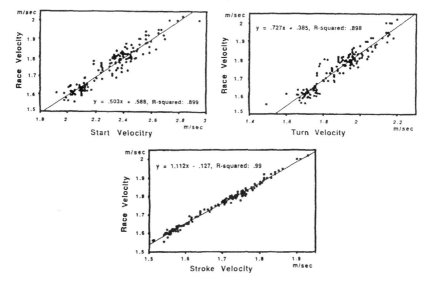

Fig. 4. Relationship between start velocity (Vs), turn velocity (Vt), stroke velocity (Va) and race velocity (Vr) in the 100 m freestyle of the 1989 Pan Pacific Championships and the 1988 Japanese Olympic Trials (total numbers = 178, 1989P: men = 16, women = 16; 1988J: men - 92, women = 54).

4 Conclusions

The results were summarized as follows:

1. The swimmer's ability in the swimming race could be evaluated by determining the SF and SL of the stroke phase, and V of three phases.

2. In all strokes, the V of the stroke phase of the 1988J group was lower than that of the finalists in 1989P. This was due to the slower SF compared to the finalists from the 1989P.

3. There were significant positive correlations between V of the start phase, V of the turn phase and the average V in the 100 m races.

5. References

Craig, A.B., Skehan, P.L., Pawelczyk, J.A. and Boomer, W.L. (1985) Velocity, stroke rate and distance per stroke during elite swimming competition. **Med. Sci. Sports Exerc.**, 17, 625-634.

East, D.J. (1970) Swimming: an analysis of stroke frequency, stroke length and performance. **New Zealand J. Health Phys. Educ. Recr.**, 3, 16-25.

Takahashi, G., Sakata, I., Tsubakimoto, S. and Ae, Y. (1983) A practical method for evaluation of swimming turn skill based on the movement structure. **Health and Sports Sci., Univ. of Tsukuba**, 6, 65-72.

Wakayoshi, K. (1988) Swimming techniques of Japanese elite swimmers. **1988 Seoul Olympic Scientific Congress, Abstracts**, 3, 319.

Wilson, D.S. and Marino, G.W. (1983) Kinematic analysis of three starts. **Swimming Technique**, 19, 30-34.

AN EVALUATION OF CHANGES IN THE CRAWL-STROKE TECHNIQUE DURING TRAINING PERIODS IN A SWIMMING SEASON

R. ARELLANO and S. PARDILLO*
INEF, Universidad de Granada, Granada, España; *Hospital S.A.S.,
Cádiz, España

Abstract
In an effort to determine changes in swimming stroke mechanics over
the seasonal training period, a study was initiated to evaluate the
degree of change following every mesocycle in the training season
(four-month macrocycle training period). Twenty-two average and high
level swimmers were evaluated after three different training periods.
The swimming movements in the crawl-stroke were recorded underwater
and digitized to determine kinematic parameters. The forces
generated during a tethered swimming test were sensed using a force
transducer. Other kinematic parameters measuring stroke length,
stroke frequency and average speed over 50 m of crawl-stroke were
analyzed. Analysis of variance with repeated measures showed
significant differences in 50 m time (T50), average speed (AV) and
maximal force during ten strokes and 30 s efforts. Our findings
support the suggestion that improvements in short distance results
are closely related to improvements in strength measured during
tethered swimming. This type of evaluation would help in effecting
better control of the adaptations brought about by specific strength
training.
Keywords: Biomechanics of Swimming, Computerized Analysis, Training,
Tethered Swimming, Swimming Technique, Quantitative Analysis.

1 Introduction

In an effort to determine changes in swimming stroke mechanics over
the seasonal training period, a study was initiated to evaluate the
degree of change following every mesocycle in the training season.
The four month macrocycle was divided in three mesocycles. The first
cycle was oriented to develop technique and stamina, the second was
designed to develop general and specific endurance and force
(dry-land and water), while the third constituted the tapering phase
ending with the regional championships.
    Differences between each of the training cycles were researched
using different methods of testing the crawl-stroke technique.

2 Methods

2.1 Subjects
The investigation was carried out between the September and December

1989 training period. Twenty-two male (n = 13, age mean = 14.6 ±
1.9) and female (n = 9, age mean = 15.3 ± 1.6) swimmers, members of
local swimming teams participated in the training, although not all
swimmers participated in each test as the group was selected from the
swimming population of Granada with swimming experience at
competitive levels.   All testing took place at the Instituto
Nacional de Educación Física (Universidad de Granada), on the dates:
September 14th, October 29th, December 6th. The pool measured 25 m ×
12.5 m with a depth from 1.2 m to 3.5 m.

2.2 Recording kinematic parameters of movement patterns
A SONY V88E (8 mm) video camera was placed in a plastic underwater
housing and interfaced to an external monitor. The plastic box was
held to the pool deck with a pivoting system, making it possible to
follow the swimmers' movements in a horizontal plane checking the
correct filming process while watching the monitor screen. The film
speed was set at 25 Hz with a shutter speed of 1/250 s (Fig. 1).
   Each subject swam 50 m (two lengths) at competitive speeds,
passing within 7 m of the camera. A stop watch was used to ensure
proper speed. The trial was repeated if not swum at the correct
speed. Filming began just before each swimmer started swimming the
50 m and ended after the 50 m was completed. Accepted trials for
analysis were those in which it was possible to digitize, keeping the
centre of the pool mark visible.
   The selected trials were projected using a VCR (8 mm) SONY
EV-S850PS controlling the frame by frame step with a special jog and
shuttle button on a SONY P14 monitor. A sonic digitizer (S.A.C.,
GP-7) was placed over the monitor screen and connected via RS-232 to
a Toshiba 1600 portable PC compatible computer. Each frame was
digitized. One complete underwater stroke of the right arm and the
left arm was digitized for each subject. For freestyle, digitizing
commenced when the hand was seen entering the water to begin an
underwater armstroke and continued until the hand left the water
repeating the process with the other arm stroke. The point selected
for analysis was the tip of the middle finger. In every frame two
reference marks were digitized to know exactly the hand position
since the camera was moving with the swimmer. Corrections for the
geometrical changes of the image due to panning were made using a
similar system as described by Persyn et al. (1989). The digitized
data were then analyzed with programs developed for an Apple
Macintosh SE 2.5/40.

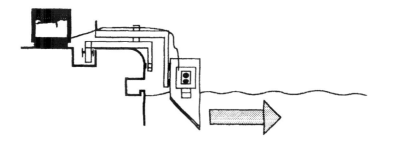

Fig. 1. Underwater video-recording system.

Following a similar process cited by Maglischo et al. (1987) to determine the reliability of the digitizing process, a film trial for a swimmer was digitized six times. Reliability was established by correlating the real coordinates of the tip of middle finger on one trial with the real coordinates for the additional five trials.

After digitizing the variables cited by Reischle (1979) the following were calculated for each arm: (i) distance between the point of entry and the end of the forward-downward phase (FI), (ii) distance between the point of the end of the forward-downward and the end of the backward-upward phase (FB), (iii) the deepest point (D) and (iv) the difference between FI and FB (R) (see Fig. 2).

2.3 Kinematic parameters of 50 m crawl-stroke
Each swimmer was video-recorded swimming 50 m crawl-stroke at maximal effort. Following the method developed for the biomechanical committee in the last European Championship (Bonn, 1989) a computer program was developed to obtain all kinematic parameters for each length. Only total time (T50), mean swimming speed (AV), stroke frequency (SF) and stroke length (SL) were analyzed.

2.4 Recording swimming force
The force recording was done using a dynamometer (strain gauge) made specially for our force recording research. This was connected to a Letica ISO-505 polygraph, the voltage was converted to digital by a DT-2801-A interface (12 bits) in a PC compatible computer (Fig. 3). A non-elastic metallic tube from the subject's belt was attached to the dynamometer. The system was calibrated each recording day before starting testing by hanging external weights (0.5, 3, 13, 23, 33 kg). Special programs control all the process and create ASCII files after statistical processing. Two different tests were carried out: average force during ten strokes (MF) and average force during 30 s effort (AF).

2.5 Measurement of flexibility
Only four flexibility measures: ankle flexion, ankle extension, shoulder upward extension and shoulder lateral abduction (each arm) were taken. During the training cycle little flexibility work was done by the swimming team, only that required for maintenance.

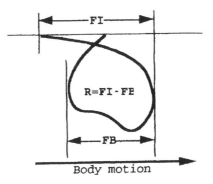

Fig. 2. Kinematic variables studied.

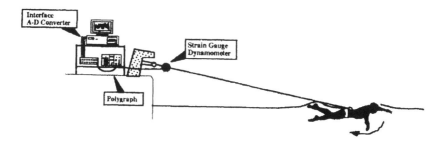

Fig. 3.   Swimming force recording system.

2.6 Statistics

The conventional statistics consisted of means and standard
deviations. The correlation coefficients were calculated between
variables. We distinguished between groups (male and female) as
means were different. We used the partial correlation to remove the
effect of age using the formula described by Thomas and Nelson
(1985).

In all cases, test results were analyzed using ANOVA with repeated
measures. The same dependent variables were measured three times
(within subjects' factor). The training in this study was the
independent variable with three levels (trials) and one only group.
Sometimes sex was considered as a grouping factor. In this case we
also check the interaction between sex trials.

3 Results

Reliability of the digitizing procedures produced correlations
ranging from 0.937 to 0.999 with the average being 0.986.
Reliability of quantitative analysis procedures produced correlations
ranging from 0.944 to 0.999 with the average being 0.956. All the
coefficient were significant (P < 0.01).

The results of this study are reported in Table 1. No significant
differences were found in the kinematic variables beyond the 0.01
level of confidence. In the force recording, the means for each test
in MF and AF across the three trials were significantly different,
$F_{2,20}$ = 4.688, P < 0.05 and $F_{2,18}$ = 13.857, P < 0.001 respectively.
At quantitative analysis level only T50 and AV showed significant
differences (T50: $F_{2,16}$ = 3.652, P < 0.05 and AV: $F_{2,16}$ = 5.37, P <
0.05). No differences in SF and SL were found. Flexibility showed
no changes during the different tests. Significant positive
correlations were seen between swimming velocity and force recording
during maximal and 30 s efforts only in the male group across the
three trials (see Table 2).

4 Discussion

Various studies have shown that the muscular strength of a swimmer
influences swimming performance, particularly over short distances

Table 1. Means of all variables studied

Variable type	Variable		N	Mean T1	Mean T2	Mean T3
Kinematic	FI	left arm	11	0.49	0.42	0.43
(m)		right arm	11	0.54	0.46	0.49
	FB	left arm	11	0.58	0.59	0.56
		right arm	11	0.58	0.59	0.56
	D	left arm	11	0.61	0.63	0.61
		right arm	11	0.61	0.58	0.60
	R	left arm	11	-0.09	-0.17	-0.13
		right arm	11	-0.07	-0.19	-0.06
Force	MF		12	111.92	117.19	128.09
(N)	AF		12	90.38	91.18	96.39
Kinematic of	T50 (s)		10	30.61	30.65	29.81
50 m	AV (m/s)		10	1.65	1.67	1.72
	SF (Hz)		10	0.86	0.86	0.89
	SL (m)		10	1.92	1.95	1.94
Flexibility	Ankle flexion		9	85	87	86
(degrees)	Ankle extension		9	156	161	158
	Should.upw.ext.		10	5	15	10
	Should.lat.ab.l		9	32	27	26
	Should.lat.ab.r		9	31	28	28

Table 2. Pearson correlation coefficients (r) between force recording and some quantitative tests

	N	Average force during ten strokes (MF)			Average force during 30 s effort (AF)		
		T1	T2	T3	T1	T2	T3
Male							
AV(T1)	9	0.889**			0.848**		
AV(T2)	8		0.813*			0.946***	
AV(T3)	9			0.855**			0.848**
Female							
AV(T1)	6	ns			0.828**		
AV(T2)	5		ns			ns	
AV(T3)	7			ns			ns

*P < 0.05; **P < 0.01; ***P < 0.001; ns: not significant

(Adams et al., 1982, Costill et al., 1983). Other studies have found that tethered swimming propulsion strength was positively correlated with swimming velocity (Keskinen, 1989; Montpetit, 1981; Onoprienko and Bartaszuk, 1973; Ria et al., 1986; Yeater et al., 1981). The present data reveal a positive relation between AV and MF, and between AV and AF, in the male group. The absence of a relationship in the female group may be explained by the fact that this group was less homogeneous than the male group.

Other authors recommend recording tethered-swimming strength as a means for evaluating the effects of training on swimmers (Boulgakova, 1990; Platonov, 1988; Rasulbekov et al., 1986; Rohra et al., 1990), and have stated that changes effected at strength levels better explain the progression of competition results than the measurement of other physiological variables (Gullstrand and Holmer, 1983). Our results show parallel improvement between strength recording and the increase in swimming velocity. The other systems (kinematics) used were not susceptible to changes in such a short training period or were not sensitive enough. Other physical trainable characteristics such as force, which is developed more quickly than the previous variables, show an increase, as the changes in T50, AV, MF and AF demonstrate. These variables also show differences between sex.

An individual and qualitative analysis was conducted for each subject and for each of the variables studied (similar to those used by Bollens et al., 1988). This type of analysis showed that the data collected for each particular subject revealed in some cases modifications in the recordings and trajectories greater than those measures obtained for the group as a whole.

The differences in the strength recording and two-dimensional propulsion trajectory seen individually make it possible to give more practical recommendations to each subject.

5 Conclusions

The present results support the following conclusions: (i) The tethered swimming force (MF and AF) was positively correlated to MV, showing the close relationship between force production and swimming velocity, (ii) the former relationship is maintained throughout the different training cycles, showing improvements essentially after the period of specific "dryland" and "wet" strength development, (iii) the individualized analysis of strength recordings and videotapes can help the coach in addressing more effectively possible modifications in the technique the swimmer needs.

6 References

Adams, T.A., Martin, R., Yeater, R.A. and Gilson, K.A. (1983) Tethered force and velocity relationships. **Swimming Technique**, 20, 21-28.
Bollens, E., Annemans, L., Vaes, W. and Clarys, J.P. (1988) Peripheral EMG comparison between fully tethered and free front crawl swimming, in **Swimming Science V** (eds B.E. Ungerechts, K. Wilke and K. Reischle), Human Kinetics Books, Champaign, Ill.
Boulgakova, N. (1990) **Sélection et Préparation des Jeunes Nageurs.** (Editions Planeta, Trans), Vigot, Paris.
Christensen, C.L. and Smith, G.W. (1987) Relationship of maximum spring speed and maximal stroking force in swimming. **J. Swimming Res.**, 3, 18-20.
Costill, D.L., King, D.S., Holdren, A. and Hargreaves, M. (1983)

Spring speed vs swimming power. **Swimming Technique**, 20, 20-22.

Gullstrand, L. and Holmer, I. (1983) Physiological characteristics of champion swimmers during a five-year follow-up period, in **Fourth International Symposium of Biomechanics in Swimming and the Fifth International Congress on Swimming Medicine** (eds P.A. Hollander, P.A. Huijing, and G. de Groot), Human Kinetics Publishers, Amsterdam, pp. 258-262.

Keskinen, K.L., Tilli, L.J. and Komi, P.V. (1989) Maximum velocity swimming: interrelatioships of stroking characteristics, force production and anthropometric variables. **Scand. J. Sports Sci.**, 11, 87-92.

Maglischo, C.W., Maglischo, E.W. and Santos, T.R. (1987) The relationship between the forward velocity of the center of gravity and the hip in the four competitive strokes. **J. Swimming Res.**, 3, 11-17.

Montpetit, R.R. (1981) Maximul voluntary propelling force in swimming, in **American Swimming Ass. World Clinic** (ed J. Leonard), American Swimming Coaches Ass., pp. 279-283.

Onoprienko, B.I. and Bartaszuk, W.J. (1973) Indice del peso específico y de la fuerza de tracción de los nadadoes. **Sport Wyczynowy**, 11, 60-61.

Persyn, U.J.J., Hoeven, R.G.C. and Daly, D.J. (1979) Evaluation centre for competitive swimmers, in **Swimming III - Third Int. Symp. of Biomechanics in Swimming** (ed T.A. Bedingfield), University Park Press, Baltimore, pp.

Platonov, V.N. (1988) **L'Entrainement Sportif** (trans N. Jonco, D. Water and J.R. Lacour), Revue EPS, Paris.

Rasulbekov, R.A., Fomin, R.A., Chulkov, V.U. and Chudovsky, V.I. (1986) Explosive strength in pulling. **National Strength and Conditioning Ass. J.**, 8, 30-32.

Reischle, K. (1979) A kinematic investigation of movement patterns in swimming with photo-optical methods, in **Swimming III - Third Int. Symp. of Biomechanics in Swimming** (ed T.A. Bedingfield), University Park Press, Baltimore, pp. 127-136.

Ria, B., Van-Praagh and Falgairette, G. (1986) Forces maximales propulsives et coordination motrice des sprinters en nage libre. **Cinésiologie**, 25, 121-126.

Rohrs, D.M., Mayhew, J.L., Arabas, C. and Shelton, M. (1990) The relationship between seven anaerobic tests and swim performance. **J. Swimming Res.**, 6, 15-19.

Thomas, J. and Nelson, J. (1985) **Introduction to Research in Health, Physical Education, Recreation and Dance.** Human Kinetics Publishers, Champaign, Ill.

Yeater, R.A., martin, R.B., White, M.K. and Gilson, K.H. (1981) Tethered swimming forces in the crawl, breast and backstrokes and their relationship to competitive performance. **J. Biomech.**, 14, 527-537.

INTRA-STROKE VELOCITY FLUCTUATIONS IN PACED BREASTSTROKE SWIMMING

P.K. MANLEY and J. ATHA*
Eton College, Windsor, England and *Department of Human Sciences,
Loughborough University, England

Abstract
In an attempt to explain how inter-stroke periodicity and velocity
patterns modify the mean swimming pace in breaststroke, the swimming
profiles of skilled teenage competititve breaststroke swimmers, four
County and four National standard (n = 8), were recorded continuously
during three independent trials at each of three different paced
swims. Digitally coded on-line velocity profiles over the final 12 m
of the pool length were analysed to determine intra-stroke maximum
and minimum velocities, leg-arm transitional (glide) velocity, stroke
period and mean stroke velocity. At all levels of pace the boys
produced larger intra-stroke mean velocities (1.14 m/s), peak velocities (2.14 m/s), and shorter stroke periods (1.30 s) than the girls
(1.03 m/s, 2.05 m/s, and 1.47 s respectively). The girls produced
higher mean leg-arm transitional velocities (1.19 m/s) than the boys
(1.10 m/s) and the minimum stroke velocity of all swimmers was
observed to vary little with sex or pace. The arm action, building
on the velocity produced by the leg action, generated the peak velocities while the recovery of the legs led to the minimum intra-stroke
velocity. The duration of the leg-arm transition varied greatly,
being a marked and extended discontinuity at slow speed, and a smooth
transition at maximum speed. The velocity-time profile increasingly
approximated to an isosceles triangle as pace increased, from which
it may be postulated, on the grounds of simple geometry, that an
individual swimmer exhibits a high level of swimming skill when the
mean swimming velocity equals half peak velocity. Unless a swimmer
introduces qualitative changes in technique, a decrease in stroke
period will necessarily follow the generation of higher peak velocities. In skilled swimming the mean stroke velocity is held to be
independent of stroking rate for any given peak velocity. For any
given mean stroke velocity shorter stroke periods may only be
achieved by cutting the stroke cycle, thereby increasing the accelerations and decelerations and hence the effort expended. Optimisation
of stroke period for a given peak velocity is, therefore, important
in energy conservation, making in this way its contribution to overall competitive swimming performance.
Keywords: Swimming, Breaststroke, Velocity, Tachometer, Pace,
Intra-stroke.

1 Introduction

An attempt has been made to determine how pacing affects the intra-stroke velocity profile of competitive breaststroke swimmers. The pulsatile nature of the breaststroke velocity is well known and has been quantified (Karpovich and Karpovich, 1970; Miyashita, 1970; Kent and Atha, 1975) but the sequential variation in this velocity profile has received little attention. Difficulties in recording long series of stroke cycles are faced when using photographic and related techniques. These difficulties have been avoided by the use of a self-contained device which continuously records velocity on-line. This swimming tachometer is a more sensitive version of a device previously reported (Manley and Atha, 1976; Atha et al., 1985).

2 Methods

Eight competitive breaststroke swimmers, four boys and four girls, aged 14-16 years, took part in this study. Two boys and two girls had County or District representative experience and two boys and two girls were members of their National youth squads. Each swimmer swam one practice followed by three recorded 12 m trials at each of three assigned paces: A = 50% maximum, B = 100% maximum, C = acceleration over the 12 m from 50% to 100% maximum. The order AB was alternated with the order BA in successive subjects, after assigning the first subject randomly to one of the two orders. In each case C was scheduled third. The two middle cycles in each stroke series were selected for analysis. Records for swims at pace A and B were displayed to determine whether the two median cycles were consistent with the two cycles which preceded and succeeded them. Very occasionally six strokes were found not to have been encompassed within the 12 m recording zone, leaving on these occasions only one stroke available for analysis. To prevent these rare losses unbalancing the results a procedure of random discard of a single stroke was adopted across the other conditions. The three trials thus provided for analysis fifteen stroke cycles for each swimmer. With condition C the middle two strokes were selected for analysis to provide a maximum effort but an intermediate pace at approximately 75% maximum speed. The analysis that follows is, therefore, of data from a total of five stroke cycles gathered from three independent swims for each of three conditions of pace for all eight subjects, yielding a total of 120 stroke cycles. Each stroke cycle consisted of over 2000 discrete velocity-time measurements.

Observations of the displayed velocity traces, of which a typical example can be seen in Figure 1, demonstrate well established features. The traces have three distinctive points, a peak velocity, a minimum velocity, and a secondary, sometimes indeterminate, transitional velocity. Between these points the velocity trace is essentially a linear function of time. The minimum velocities recorded between each stroke are approximately constant for a given swimmer irrespective of pace. The inter-stroke period (t) measured between these minima varies little at any given pace but varies appreciably between pace conditions. The well defined peak velocity (vmax) occurs at the end of the arm pull and varies appreciably with pace. The inter-stroke period (t) measured between these minima

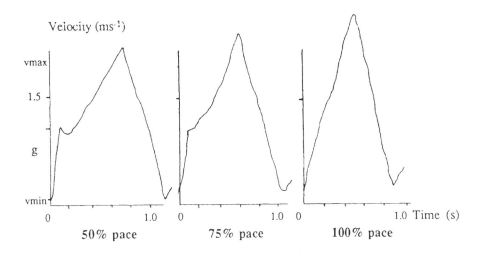

Velocity (ms⁻¹)

vmax

1.5

g

vmin

0   1.0   0   1.0   0   1.0 Time (s)

50% pace   75% pace   100% pace

Fig. 1.   Intra-stroke velocity profiles for three different
conditions of pace.

varies little at any given pace but varies appreciably between pace
conditions. The much lower mid-stroke secondary peak (g) occurs at
the transition between the end of the leg kick and the start of the
arm pull. This transition may be marked by a slightly rising or
falling velocity plateau, which in more leisurely days, was defined
as the glide phase.

This leg-arm transitional phase shortened as the speed increased.
Five measurements were thus sufficient to provide a summary definition of the intra-stroke velocity curve, namely peak velocity (vmax),
minimum stroke velocity (vmin), stroke period (t), mid-stroke
secondary peak (g), and mean stroke velocity (v̄). This latter value
was obtained by integrating the velocity-time trace for each stroke
and dividing by the stroke period (t). It should be remembered,
however, that these values relate to the movements at the hip and
that minor corrections are needed to transform them to reflect the
movements of the centre of gravity of the swimmer.

At the conclusion of the period of testing, the eight swimmers
were timed over a maximal breaststroke swim of two lengths of the
pool (50 m) under race conditions.

An additional set of records consisting of four maximum speed
breaststroke cycles were obtained from one male Olympic gold
medallist. These data provided background for comparison and
tentative generalisation.

2.1 Measurement system

Swimming speed was measured by a swimming tachometer, a small
diameter (25 mm) eight bladed, brass, impeller which rotated as a
function of distance as it was drawn through the water by the
swimmer. A thin brass rim projected 5 mm from the outer edge of the
impeller blades and passed between a photodiode and transistor
elements of an infrared photocell. Twenty holes of 3 mm diameter
were equally spaced around the rim. As holes and rim passed through

the photodiode/photocell arrangement, the IR light path was
interrupted, at a rate proportional to the velocity of the impeller's
movement through the water. The resulting small pulsatile voltage,
which varied as a function of water speed, was conditioned by a
Schmitt trigger and used to drive a monostable housed in a waterproof
box carried by the swimmer. The transducer unit was mounted on a 80
mm boom attached to a waterproof box (120 × 80 × 60 mm) containing
elecronic circuits, switches, battery and optical signal generator.
The whole assembly was mounted on a shaped perspex plate and strapped
firmly against the lower abdomen of the swimmer by a broad nylon belt
around the pelvis. The unit and belt were 0.5 kg negatively buoyant
and subjects reported that it did not interfere with their normal
swimming movements.

The output voltage from these circuits was used to drive a second
photodiode connected via fibre-optic cable to the poolside. On the
poolside the incoming intermittent signal was converted into a voltage signal and held in a FIFO buffer. This queuing system allowed
the real time intervals between successive pulses to be measured and
converted by means of calibration data into a velocity reading by a
standard BBC B micro-computer, without loss of any data. A program
was written to present graphically these transient velocities as a
function of time.

At maximum velocity, when the greatest rates of change were being
produced, data were received at a rate of some 5000 Hz. As the
intra-stroke velocity decreased the rate of data generation also
decreased. The advantage of having precision when needed and data
economy at other times was a welcome feature of the device.

2.2 Calibration

The device was calibrated in three ways, one was a static procedure,
the other two were dynamic methods. The device's response to laminar
flows was linear for the range of velocities (0.3 m/s to 2.2 m/s)
generated in the flume at Loughborough University. At these velocities impeller frequencies ranging from 24 to 176 Hz were recorded
providing an intermittent light output ranging from 480 to 3520 Hz.
The least squares conversion from rotor frequency (RF) to flume water
velocity (FV) is given by:

$$RF = 80.41FV - 0.30 \qquad\qquad (1)$$

Variations in the tachometer's response at two constant flume velocities (1.0 m/s and 2.0 m/s) were measured as the central axis of the
impeller was swung at increasing angles of pitch and yaw to the
centre of flow of the flume. No discernible decrease in response was
noted for angular off-sets of < 15°, a tolerance considered adequate
to cover the angular movements of the pelvis of the most skilled
breaststroke swimmers.

The linear relationship between water speed and the tachometer's
response was dynamically tested in the circular flume of the
Hydraulics Research Establishment, Wallingford. The total number of
impeller revolutions was recorded for a known distance of travel
(3 m) at eight constant and eight non-constant velocities (0.4 m/s to
1.2 m/s). The impeller revolution count (n) was compared with the
number of revolutions for a 3 m displacement calculated from the

Loughborough calibration experiments (240.3 rev). At the eight
constant flow velocities the mean rotor revolution count was (n) =
235.9 (SD = 5.1) rev while the mean count under non-constant flow
velocities was (n) = 236.8 (SD = 3.2) rev.

Possible eddy and boundary layer effects on the tachometer
response, when worn by a swimmer, were investigated by pulling a
swimmer a known distance in various held configurations of arms and
legs, and comparing the total number of blade passages occurring over
this fixed distance (12 m). No postural influence on device response
was identified. Ten trials were conducted by moving the device 12 m
by hand through the water at non-uniform speeds exaggerating the
velocity surges found in breaststroke swimming. The total number of
hole passages per metre impeller displacement was found to be 1601
(SD = 26) i.e. 80.1 revolutions of the impeller occurred per metre of
impeller displacement. This pool calibration procedure was repeated
periodically during the experimental sequence.

3 Results

The mean intra-stroke velocity for all five strokes at each of the
three levels of pace for every subject are presented in Table 1. It
may be seen that as the mean stroke velocity ($\bar{v}$) increases, peak
velocity (vmax) and the leg-arm transitional velocity (g) increase,
there is an expected and corresponding reduction in the stroke period
(t). Although a residual minimum stroke velocity (vmin) is always
present in each stroke cycle this parameter is relatively constant
whatever the pace of swim.

The boys (swimmers 1 to 4) produced faster mean and peak intra-
stroke velocities than the girls (swimmers 5 to 8) at all levels of
pace. The boys also produced shorter stroke periods (t) and
unexpectedly lower arm-leg transitional velocities (g) than the girls
at each pace. The difference between the National and the County
swimmers can be assessed from their maximal 50 m sprint times. The
National swimmers produced the largest peak velocities, confirming
the expected relationship between level of performance and intra-
stroke peak velocity. It is observed that for this group of subjects
the mean intra-stroke velocity ($\bar{v}$) is close to 50% of the peak intra-
stroke velocity (vmax). As pace increases from the slower to the
faster conditions there is an increasing tendency for this ratio to
move towards the 50% value for all swimmers. Thus it ranges from
54.0% at half pace, 51.0% at three-quarter pace, to 50.4% at maximum
pace.

Regression techniques were applied to determine the nature of the
relationship between the mean stroke velocity and all other measurement variables. For the intra-stroke parameters selected here the
relationship is best described (F = 221; P < 0.01) by the equation:

$$\bar{v} = 0.817 + 0.239vmax - 0.1999t + 0.201vmin + 0.039sex \qquad (2)$$

which accounts for 89% of the variance in $\bar{v}$.

However, further analysis showed the mean stroke velocity to be
independent of the leg-arm transitional velocity (g) while sex and
minimum velocity only contributed in a minor, though positive, way to
the mean velocity variance.

155

Table 1. Mean intra-stroke summary parameters

			50% pace			
Swimmer	$\bar{v}$ (m/s)	vmax (m/s)	t (s)	g (m/s)	vmin (m/s)	
1	1.21	2.22	1.46	1.13	0.53	
2	1.12	1.99	1.37	1.05	0.08	
3	0.70	1.16	2.13	0.86	0.11	
4	0.89	1.53	1.83	1.08	0.07	
5	0.86	1.69	1.74	0.99	0.06	
6	0.86	1.69	1.74	0.99	0.06	
7	0.89	1.68	1.87	1.39	0.12	
8	0.94	1.72	1.80	1.06	0.07	
All boys	0.98	1.72	1.70	1.03	0.20	
All girls	0.89	1.71	1.81	1.14	0.08	
All swimmers	0.93	1.72	1.76	1.08	0.14	

			75% pace			
Swimmer	$\bar{v}$ (m/s)	vmax (m/s)	t (s)	g (m/s)	vmin (m/s)	
1	1.38	2.97	1.16	1.11	0.17	
2	1.22	2.16	1.16	1.17	0.12	
3	1.04	1.86	1.25	1.12	0.08	
4	1.09	2.16	1.15	1.12	0.08	
5	1.14	2.32	1.22	0.95	0.11	
6	1.03	1.94	1.37	1.15	0.09	
7	1.00	1.98	1.57	1.53	0.10	
8	0.99	1.98	1.59	1.20	0.09	
All boys	1.18	2.29	1.18	1.13	0.11	
All girls	1.04	2.06	1.44	1.18	0.10	
All swimmers	1.11	2.18	1.31	1.15	0.11	

			100% pace			
Swimmer	$\bar{v}$ (m/s)	vmax (m/s)	t (s)	g (m/s)	vmin (m/s)	50 m time (s)
1	1.36	2.96	1.13	1.10	0.09	33.98
2	1.24	2.17	1.12	1.22	0.14	36.87
3	1.22	2.20	0.91	1.07	0.09	39.01
4	1.18	2.32	0.96	1.17	0.08	40.07
5	1.22	2.57	1.04	1.04	0.11	37.42
6	1.23	2.20	1.04	1.19	0.09	37.62
7	1.17	2.41	1.27	1.69	0.09	37.62
8	1.06	2.34	1.33	1.11	0.11	41.22
All boys	1.25	2.41	1.02	1.14	0.10	37.48
All girls	1.17	2.38	1.17	1.26	0.10	39.17
All swimmers	1.21	2.40	1.10	1.20	0.10	38.58
Olympian	1.50	3.03	1.12	1.25	0.15	

As the peak intra-stroke velocity increases the expected decrease occurs in stroke period. The decrease is expected, of course, because the limbs must accelerate in order to produce this larger peak velocity. The reverse is, however, not necessarily true, for faster arm and leg movements do not of themselves increase peak velocity, traction being lost if they are moved too quickly. An optimum stroke period should be found for each mean stroke velocity for any given swimmer. Linear, quadratic and higher order regression techniques were applied to test for the suspected optimisation of the relationship between stroke period and peak velocity. The relation-ship was found to be best described by the quadratic:

$$vmax = -1.865 + 8.972/t - 4.699/t^2 \qquad (3)$$

from which the stroke period is shown to be optimal at 1.05 s (F = 101; P < 0.01). As the stroke period is a function of the peak velocity this variable, together with sex and minimum stroke velocity, were excluded from the regression analysis to arrive at a simplified equation which accounted for almost all the equivalent amount of observed variance (79%; F = 449, P < 0.01):

$$\bar{v} = 0.297 + 0.376vmax \qquad (4)$$

Contraining this equation to pass through the origin since it is not possible to have a non-zero mean velocity without a non-zero peak velocity:

$$\bar{v} = 0.512vmax \qquad (5)$$

Thus, as the equation shows, the mean velocity for these swimmers is estimated as 51.2% of the peak velocity.

To compare the stroke periods of National and County standard swimmers at similar mean speeds, it was necessary to compare National standard subjects at their intermediate three-quarter pace with the County swimmers at their maximal pace. National performers recorded a mean stroke period of 1.23 s at three-quarter pace, whereas the less expert County swimmers recorded a mean stroke period of 1.12 s at maximal pace. The National swimmers swam at a mean average stroke velocity of 1.19 (SD = 0.16) m/s, whereas their County colleagues recorded a result of 1.16 (SD = 0.09) m/s. Thus it may be summarised that the expert swimmers swam 0.03 m/s (2.7%) faster than the less expert, while stroking 0.11 s (9.8%) more slowly. The highly skilled performers were thus able to produce a longer stroke period for a given mean stroke velocity. Results from the Olympic breaststroke medallist underline this observation. He combined the fastest mean stroke velocity (1.50 m/s) with the long stroke period, relative to this speed, of 1.12 s.

4 Discussion

The mean speed of a competitive breaststroke swimmer is a function of the effective (residual unbalanced) propulsive forces generated by the legs and arms during each stroke cycle. However, the legs and the arms differ characteristically in their size, strength and speed of movement. The legs are relatively massive, stronger and slower, whereas the arms are less massive, weaker and faster. Harnessing these two limb systems to the single task of achieving maximum swimming speed poses a coordination problem solved by breaststroke swimmers in a smooth summation of movements, the legs first accelerating the body from near rest to a transitional velocity at which time, after a pause of variable duration, the arms take over and accelerate the body to its peak velocity. The recovery actions return the velocity to near zero again. The legs, with a restricted maximum speed of extension, and always having to start from approximately the same minimum velocity, produce a fairly constant velocity whatever the pace of the swim. The arms, however, have a reserve capacity and can move faster if called upon to accelerate the body to a higher velocity. They can also be timed to take over from the legs smoothly as the legs achieve their maximum velocity, so reducing the duration of the leg-arm transitional phase. Differences in upper body strength alone may well account for most of the observed differences between male and female intra-stroke velocities. The girls recorded higher leg-arm transitional velocities than the boys, but seemed unable to convert this good base of leg generated velocity into as great an arm produced peak velocity as the boys. The smooth transition from leg to arm velocity is illustrated in the specimen traces shown in Figure 1. The velocity profiles increasingly approximate to an isosceles triangle. As mean stroke velocity ($\bar{v}$) increases the distance (d) covered per stroke cycle is given by an area under the velocity triangle:

$$d = 1/2 . vmax . t \qquad\qquad (6)$$

so mean velocity for the stroke

$$\bar{v} = d/t = 1/2 . vmax \qquad\qquad (7)$$

This implies that an individual swimmer's capacity to swim a single stroke of breaststroke quickly depends solely on the production of a high peak velocity and is independent of the duration of the stroke.

To increase his peak velocity the swimmer has either to improve his movement pattern or to move his limbs faster through well practised pathways without reducing their traction. Radical technique changes are a theoretical possibility within the laws of breaststroke swimming. To be successful such changes would have to square off the triangle without unduly reducing the magnitude of the peak and how this might be achieved is not easily seen given the results here recorded. The alternative of moving limbs faster would decrease the stroking period and produce the observed increase in peak velocity as long as the effectiveness of the limbs could be preserved. If effectiveness were to be lost the stroke period would continue to be shortened by the overstroking, with the swimmer either shortening his stroke, or slipping water. If peak velocity is linearly dependent on stroke period the latter manoeuvre should still be effective in increasing peak velocity. However, for the 120 stroke cycles considered in this study the relationship between stroke period and peak velocity was found to be non-linear and optimised when t = 1.05 s. An optimum value for the stroke period means that a shorter stroke period does not necessarily result in a higher mean stroke velocity.

As the swimmer strives to increase velocity there is an increasing danger of a breakdown in established movement patterns. Thus, the highly skilled swimmer produces higher mean velocities for each chosen stroke period, thereby reducing the number of strokes required to cover any given distance. A reduction in the total number of strokes results in a reduction in the number of the velocity surges. The slower stroking rate is advantageous, therefore, because, having fewer energy consuming accelerations and decelerations, it is more economical. Improvements in competitive swimming performance, arising from the foregoing, should be sought from the calculated optimisation of stroke period and increased peak velocity.

5 Conclusions

(a) In skilled breaststroke swimming mean stroke velocity varies as a simple function of peak intra-stroke velocity.

(b) Mean stroke velocity is independent of stroking rate for strokes of constant peak velocity.

(c) There is an optimum stroke period below, or above, which peak velocity is decreased.

(d) A successful competitive swimmer, in contrast to his less skilled colleague, combines more effectively a high intra-stroke peak velocity with relatively longer stroke periods.

6 References

Atha, J., Harris, D., West, G. and Manley, P.K. (1985) Monitoring performance using a real-time biodynamic feedback device. **Int. J. Sport Biomech.**, 4, 348-353.

Karpovich, P.V. and Karpovich, G.P. (1970) Magnetic tape natograph. **Res. Quart. Am. Ass. Hlth. Phys. Educ.**, 41, 119-122.

Kent, M.R. and Atha, J. (1975) A device for the on-line measurement of instantaneous swimming velocity. **Proceedings of the Second International Symposium on Biomechanics in Swimming II** (eds J.P. Clarys and L. Lewillie), University Park Press, Baltimore, pp. 58-63.

Manley, P.K. and Atha, J. (1976) A new on-line tachometer. **Presentation to the Carnegie Conference on the Analysis of Human Performance, Leeds Polytechnic, Leeds (September).**

Miyashita, M. (1970) An analysis of fluctuations of swimming speed. **Proceedings of the First International Symposium on Biomechanics in Swimming** (eds L. Lewillie and J.P. Clarys), Vrije Universiteit Brussel, Brussels, pp. 53-58.

COMPARATIVE ANALYSIS OF STUDIES OF SPEED VARIATIONS WITHIN A BREASTSTROKE CYCLE

C. TOURNY, D. CHOLLET, J.P. MICALLEF and J. MACABIES
Unit of Formation and Research in Sciences and Technique of the
Physical and Sportive Activities, University of Montpellier, France

Abstract
The analysis of the speed variations within a breaststroke cycle
gives information about the manner in which the different phases of
the cycle contribute to swimmer's movement. This study underlines
the technical changes in the breaststroke during the last fifteen
years and compares the recordings of the speed variations with the
curve of the women's 100 m breaststroke champion in the Seoul Olympic
Games 1988.
Keywords: Breaststroke, Biomechanical, Speed Variations, Top Level
Swimmers.

1 Introduction

The speed variations within a breaststroke cycle are the result of
the actions of acceleration and deceleration exerted on the body by
the propulsive movements and by fluid resistances. Persyn et al.
(1989) statistically showed that the amplitudes of these variations
during certain phases of the stroke are linked to the degree of skill
of the swimmer. After having been subjected to regular modifications, the breaststroke is technically still evolving. Currently
three styles of breaststroke are found at a competition level:
(i) the "flat" style which is characterized by a flat position of
the body, with the hips of the swimmer remaining flat on the surface
of the water, the pelvis in a fixed position and the shoulders
constantly immersed,
(ii) the "vertical" style which is characterized by the vertical
emergence of the torso, the swaying of the shoulders and the
occurrence of a vertical half-beat of the legs from bottom to top,
(iii) the "wave" style which is a logical step in the progress of
the breaststroke, involving a wave-like action of the body, the head
dipping below the surface of the water and the growth in amplitude,
from top to bottom, of the diving movements of the arms and legs.
The aim of this report is to compare the recorded speed variations
of the body (considered at the hip's level) from the "waving" style
represented by Bogomilova-Dangalakova (women's 100 m breaststroke
gold medallest in Seoul Olympic Games 1988) with those of different
authors (from 1975 to 1990).

2 Methods

The methods of recording speed were similar between the authors used. The procedures consisted of fixing a belt to a swimmer attached via a cable to an electric generator. The generator gave an electrical voltage proportional to the swimmer's speed. A cinematographic camera (type 16 mm) or a video (VHS) synchronized with the information of the instantaneous speed, recorded the stroke cycle. D'Acquisto et al. (1988) point out that a computerized system, based on both speed and video has a correlation of 0.95 with the digitalization of the film. Persyn et al. (1989) confirmed this correlation by comparing the accuracy of the video analysis compared with the 16 mm film. The films allowed the calculation of the speed at each stage of the cycle.

2.1 Authors' data used

Kent and Atha (1975) recorded the speed variations of an Olympic British swimmer (the contraction "KEN" will be used in this report). Bober and Czabanski (1975) carried out the recording for a national recordholder from Poland at different swimming frequencies (BOB). Wilkie and Juba (1986) interpreted the speed variations of Wilkie who was the 100 m breaststroke world champion in 1975 (WIL). D'Acquisto et al. (1988) compared the speed variations according to sex and the degree of skill of 17 male and female swimmers (DAC). Craig et al. (1988) analysed the speed variations with regard to the swimming frequency from four groups of swimmers (CRA). Reischle (1988) determined the speed variations in a German national level swimmer (REI). Van Tilborgh et al. (1987) recorded the speed variations in order to estimate both resistance and propulsion forces of the breaststroke (VAN). Our study recorded the speed variations of the Seoul (1988) 100 m womens' breaststroke champion (Bogomilova-Dangalakova). These data characterize the current "wave" breaststroke style (TOU).

3 Results

The graphic speed-time of each of the authors' data used allowed the more characteristic speed data within a breaststroke cycle to be determined. For each speed we can identify a precise phase of the cycle. The stroke cycle starts when the swimmer is in the gliding phase; it ends at the end of the legs' action. An explanatory scheme (Fig. 1) presents the speed information gathered, associated with a temporal scale.

3.1 Statistical analysis

Firstly, we performed an analysis of the main component in order to identify the more relevant characteristics of our data tables. The correlation matrix allowed a determination of the relationships which exist between time and frequency speed parameters. The study of the individuals over the main axes allowed comparison of authors' data and placed the TOU style in the sample.

Secondly, we performed an analysis with each significant correlation ($P < 0.02$) in order to determine each authors' influence on the correlation matrix.

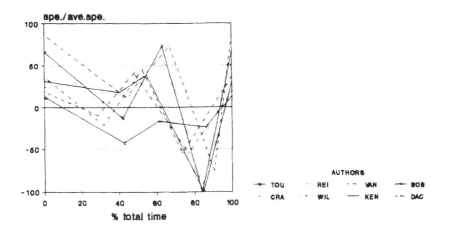

Fig. 1. Explanatory scheme.

The correlation analysis between the speed variables, between the frequency and defined time highlighted possible relations on the graphs including the relative values (Table 1) and 36 possible relations on the graphs including the absolute values (Table 2). After crossing the variables, it appears that five correlations were significant over the relative values and that eight correlations were significant over the absolute values. We therefore define a significant correlation when the reliability coefficient went beyond 50% (r = 0.71).

The correlation analysis between the speed variables, between the frequency and defined time highlighted 45 possible relations on the graphs including the relative values (Table 1) and 36 possible relations on the graphs including the absolute values (Table 2). After crossing the variables, it appears that five correlations are significant over the relative values and that eight correlations were significant over the absolute values. We therefore define a significant correlation when the reliability coefficient went beyond 50% (r = 0.71).

4 Discussion

4.1 Breaststroke styles study

The representation of the individuals on the main axes (X,Y,Z) produces 91.5% of the total variation. The TOU style was well represented in the graphic representation ($\Sigma \cos^2$ = 0.63). The BOB style was different from the others where the swimmer probably used a flat style. The VAN, WIL and CRA subjects formed a group representing the reference style (TOU). The VAN, WIL and CRA styles probably have the same characteristics to the vertical style. The DAC, REI and KEN subjects exhibited wide variations and were difficult to analyse.

Table 1. Speed variations according to the breaststroke cycle time

	AS*	S1	S2	S3	S4	FRE*	T1	T2	T3	T4	TT*
TOU	1.50	1.30	2.60	0.00	2.60	39.4	0.64	0.32	0.32	0.24	1.52
REI	1.12	1.27	1.73	0.11	1.39	26.6	1.03	0.42	0.45	0.35	2.25
VAN	1.31	1.20	1.85	0.60	1.55	45.1	0.38	0.26	0.38	0.31	1.33
BOB	1.44	0.83	1.20	0.34	1.58	31.2	0.82	0.35	0.48	0.25	1.92
CRA	1.25	1.32	1.75	0.20	1.95	53.5	0.35	0.19	0.38	0.20	1.12
WIL	1.10	0.87	1.6	0.5	1.5	37.9	0.50	0.33	0.33	0.41	1.58
KEN	1.41	1.66	1.95	0.00	1.85	55.5	0.45	0.17	0.34	0.17	1.13
DAC	0.97	1.09	1.68	0.24	1.81	27.2	0.96	0.51	0.52	0.22	2.20

*AS: Average speeed in m/s; FRE: Frequency in cycle/min;
TT: Total time in seconds

S1: minimum speed before the action of the arms
S2: maximum speed associated with the action of the arms
S3: minimum speed before the action of the legs
S4: maximum speed associated with the action of the legs
T1: decreasing time between S4 and S1 (glide)
T2: acceleration time between S1 and S2 (action of the arms)
T3: decreasing time between S2 and S3 (recovery of the arms and legs
T4: acceleration time between S3 and S4 (action of the legs)

Table 2. Speed variations (percentages) with respect to the average speed and time variation with respect to the total time

	S1	S2	S3	S4	T1	T2	T3	T4
TOU	−13.4	+73.3	−100	+66.6	42.0	63.0	84.0	99.7
REI	+14.2	+54.5	−90.1	+24.1	45.7	64.4	84.4	99.9
VAN	−9.4	+41.2	−54.2	+18.3	28.6	48.1	76.7	100
BOB	−42.3	−16.6	−23.6	+12.8	42.7	60.9	85.9	98.9
CRA	+5.6	+40.0	−84.0	+56.0	31.2	48.2	82.1	99.9
WIL	−20.9	+45.4	−54.5	+36.4	31.6	52.5	73.4	99.3
KEN	+17.7	+38.3	−100	+31.2	39.8	54.8	84.8	99.8
DAC	+12.4	+74.2	−75.3	+86.6	43.6	66.8	90.4	100

4.2 Interpretation of the correlations

A relationship existed for 77% (r^2 relative value) to 86% (r^2 absolute value) of the swimmers between the decreasing time due to the gliding phase (T1) and the acceleration time due to the action of the arm (T2). Among the reports taken into consideration, seven of those are in the correlation. Only the data from Kent et al. (1975) make the degree of reliability of the relation fall. A relationship existed for 56 to 64% of the swimmers between the decreasing time due to the glide (T1) and the decreasing time due to the recovery of the arms and the legs (T3). A relationship existed for 52 to 64% of the swimmers between the maximum speed associated with the action of the arms

Table 3. Correlation analysis

	Relative values (Table 1)	Absolute values (Table 2)
T1/T2	r = 0.88*	r = 0.93*
T1/T3	r = -0.75*	r = 0.80*
S2/S4	r = 0.80*	r = 0.72*
FRE/S2	r = -0.95*	r = -0.77*
S1/T4	r = -0.55	r = 0.85*
S2/S3	r = -0.51	r = -0.73*
S2/T4	r = -0.22	r = 0.73*
S1/S3	r = -0.65	r = -0.79*
FRE/T1	r = -0.90*	r = -0.61

*Significant

(S2) and the maximum speed associated with the action of the legs
(S4). Even if this correlation was significant, five studies did not
support the finding. Indeed the correlation between S2 and S4 did
not exist either with respect to the relative values, or to the
absolute values. Being cautious, we should limit the meaning of this
relation and not assign a meaningful interpretation to this. A
relationship existed for 59 to 90% of the swimmers, between the
stroke frequency (FRE) and the acceleration due to the action of the
arms (T2). The correlation means that the stroke frequency is great
when the acceleration time is short. In contrast, Wilkie and Juba
(1986) and our study (TOU) did not support this relationship.

5 Conclusions

Our analysis leads to the following six points:
    (a) The "wave" style, illustrated by the speed variations plotting
of the 100 m breaststroke Olympic champion is characterized by great
speed variations within the cycle.
    (b) The arm's movement and the distance covered within the phase
by the Olympic champion represent almost 40% of the total distance
covered within a cycle.
    (c) The swimming frequency is linked to the acceleration time due
to the action of the arms.
    (d) The acceleration time due to the action of the arms shows a
relationship with the decreasing time of the glide phase.
    (e) The decrease in time due to the recovery of the arms and the
legs is associated with the decrease in time due to the glide.

6 References

Bober, T. and Czabanski, B. (1975) Changes in breaststroke techniques
    under different speed conditions, in Swimming II (eds J.P. Clarys
    and L. Lewillie), University Park Press, Baltimore, pp. 188-193.
Craig, A.B., Jr., Boomer, W.L. and Skehan, P.L. (1988) Patterns of
    velocity in competitive breaststroke, in Swimming V (eds B.E.
    Ungerechts, K. Wilke and K. Reischle), Human Kinetics Books,
    Champaign, Ill., pp. 73-77.

D'Acquisto, L.J., Costill, D.L., Gehlsen, G.M., Wong-Tai Young and Lee, G. (1988) Breaststroke economy, skill and performance: study of breaststroke mechanics using a computer based "velocity-video" system. **J. Swimming Res.**, 4, 2, 9-13.

Kent, M.R. and Atha, J. (1975) Intracycle kinematics and body configuration changes in the breaststroke, in **Swimming II** (eds J.P. Clarys and L. Lewillie), University Park Press, Baltimore, pp. 125-129.

Persyn, U. and Colman, V. (1989) Suivi informatique de la technique de nage, in **Actes of Third Colloque of the Association Reflexion Natation,** Canet, np.

Reischle, K. (1988) **Biomechanik des Schwimmens.** Sport Fahnemann, Bockenem.

Tilborgh, L.M. van, Stijnen, U.V. and Persyn, U.J. (1987) Using velocity fluctuations for estimating resistance and propulsion forces in breaststroke swimming, in **Biomechanics XB** (ed B. Johnsson), Human Kinetics Publishers, Champaign, Ill., pp. 779-784.

Wilkie, D. and Juba, K. (1986) **The Handbook of Swimming.** Pelham Books, London.

APPLICATION OF KNOWLEDGE GAINED FROM THE COORDINATION OF PARTIAL MOVEMENTS IN BREASTSTROKE AND BUTTERFLY SWIMMING FOR THE DEVELOPMENT OF TECHNICAL TRAINING

A. HAHN and T. KRUG
Sektion Sportwissenschaft, Martin-Luther-University, Halle, Germany

Abstract
The aim of this study was to biomechanically analyse the coordination of partial movements in breaststroke and butterfly within different load ranges. By obtaining objective information about the coordination of partial movements, improvements in technical training could be achieved. For technique training a relatively complex procedure has been developed and experimentally tested. The profiles of velocity in breaststroke and butterfly swimming has provided important findings about the criteria for effectiveness of swimming techniques. This has allowed technical models of coordination in these swimming styles to be considerably improved. The results concerning the specificity of coordination in load ranges such as basic endurance and competition specific endurance, as well as under conditions of exhaustion, are informative. This knowledge is the basis of the present development of a specific training technique for breaststroke and butterfly. The measuring capability of speedography has allowed us to pinpoint problem areas and focus on these during training.
Keywords: Technique Training, Coordination, Breaststroke, Butterfly, Cinematography, Speedography.

1 Introduction

In swimming research efforts are being made to increase propulsion either by raising the number of impulses per unit time or by increasing the effect of mechanical energy of the individual impulses in the movement cycle. In this respect we must consider that:

(1) the number of propulsion impulses per unit time cannot be increased indefinitely;

(2) when increasing the number of impulses within the movement cycle only a part of the invested energy can be transformed into propulsion, because a part of the energy expenditure will not be effective.

(3) the mechanisms of energy supply summoned up by swimmers are used almost to their fullest limits.

Therefore, the coordination of partial movements is essential for the reduction of fluctuations in velocity. It is especially important for the stroke patterns involving synchronous arm and leg movements, as the greatest differences in velocity within the movement cycle are recorded in these styles. Another important aspect of coordination deals with different load ranges employed in swim training. Most swim training focuses on basic endurance. It can be taken for granted that the actual technique of movement in basic endurance differs from the preferred technique in competition specific endurance. Therefore if the competitive technique is not carried through during the bulk of training there is a danger of negative transfer (Hahn, 1988). For this reason it is important to find alternatives. The increase of propulsive force by coordination of partial movements has been recognised as a performance reserve and consequently has been studied in detail. This study led to the development a form of technique training. The essential point in this process is the transfer of the biomechanical parameter of motion into learning information. The starting point of this approach is the principle formulated for endurance events in which acceleration phases should be as long as possible and given preference over short intermittent phases (Hochmuth, 1986).

2 Methods

2.1 For the basic research

The procedure consisted of cinematography, tensography (four strips were fixed to the extremities to obtain the time structures and the water resistance; deformation due to the fluctuation of pressure is proportionally transformed into fluctuation of voltage); and speedography (by means of an impeller attached to the swimmer's abdomen). These techniques were employed whilst subjects were swimming in a training session at a steady submaximal pace (i.e. basic endurance).

2.2 For the training research

This procedure consisted of speedography incorporating computerized recording and synchronized video films. By checking the velocity record, the effect of the power used by the swimmers was indirectly assessed (Figure 1). These techniques were also employed during swim training, but with the swimmers working at race pace (i.e. competition specific training).

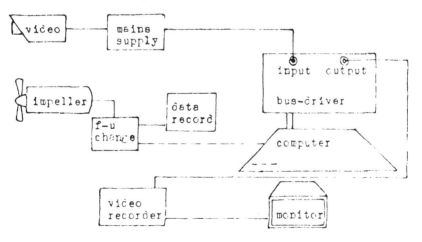

Fig. 1. Configuration of apparatus.

3 Results and discussion

A number of parameters of swimming techniques in breaststroke and butterfly have been evaluated in relation to coordination in basic endurance and competitition specific endurance and have been compared with each other. In comparison with other swimming styles a great fluctuation of velocity during the breaststroke cycle is shown. The first decrease in velocity is achieved during the recovery of the legs (V = 0.4 m/s). This can be influenced only trivially as it is limited by the rules of competition. On account of the squared influence of velocity on the resistance to movement of the legs in the direction of swimming, this has to be performed slowly. As there is a direct dependence in the reduction of velocity on the duration of the propulsion lag, the recovery of the legs has to be performed relatively quickly. In our opinion the legs should be drawn up when the second part of the push with the hand is done. Therefore the legs can be moved slowly in the direction of swimming and the propulsive lag is kept short.

The swimming velocity drops again at the end of the cycle. At this time there are great differences between the swim speeds on account of the different techniques for movement coordination. The level of the average velocity achieved depends on the type of coordination. In addition the average swimming velocity determines the degree of fluctuation, the minimum-maximum difference decreases with increasing velocity (r = -0.74) (Figure 2).

The examinations of swimmers in basic endurance indicate that the peaks of velocity are not significantly different from those for competition specific endurance although the greater fluctuation of velocity leads to a lower average swimming velocity (Table 1). This lower average velocity is due to the difference in coordination techniques between the two swim speeds.

Table 1. Swimming velocity in breaststroke at the end of a cycle (m/s)

	Average V_{max}	Average V_{min}	Average fluctuation
Basic endurance	1.24	0.66	0.58
Competition specific endurance	1.31	0.90	0.31

In basic endurance swimming the temporal relation of the brake phase to the push phase is 1:3 whereas it is 1:1.5 in competition mode.

In the bufferfly stroke the average fluctuation of velocity connected with a push lag of 0.55 s is 1.0 m/s. Research with tensography has shown that the first leg kick in the cycle is the strongest. The difference in intensity between both initial kicks is most pronounced. The difference in intensity between kicks depends on the swimming velocity. In basic endurance the difference is considerable. The first kick is performed with an intensity characteristic of higher velocities.

From the pedagogical and psychological view a symmetrical

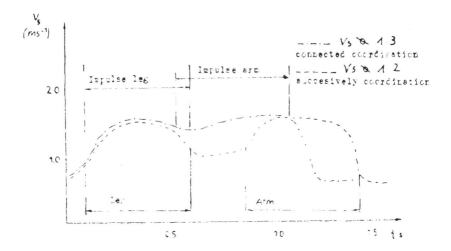

Fig. 2. Graph of swimming velocity in breaststroke versus time for two styles of coordination.

performance of the kick should be demanded from the swimmer. The temporal coordination of the first kick is also dependent on the range of velocity. The first kick is performed at the beginning of the underwater motion of the hand. Here there is a difference between the sexes. Male swimmers perform this first kick 0.1 s later than in the competition range whereas females perform this kick 0.12 s earlier than in the competition range. The proportion of underwater to overwater movement during the cycle amounts to 60:40 and does not depend on the range of velocity. This means that the arms both under and over water are moved more slowly in the basic endurance context so that the time of the cycle increases.

The longer partial cycles make the optimal temporal coordination of the first kick difficult. When breathing is observed it is seen that in the butterfly the coordination of the breathing cycle and the non-breathing cycle place different demands on the swimmer. Breathing, in which the head is lifted out of the water, demands an additional control of movement resulting in a decrease in velocity. The results demonstrate that the highest velocity is obtained in the non-breathing mode (V = 1.6 m/s). During breathing swimming velocity is at a minimum (V = 1.5 m/s).

Two reasons for the low swimming velocity are the greater angle of the body during inhalation (about ten degrees greater than in the non-breathing cycle) and the longer 'push still' (movement over the water by the arms). The 'push still' is about 0.1 s longer in the respiratory cycle. The movement over the water also leads to an earlier first kick in relation to the underwater motion by the arms during the next cycle. Another result concerns the relation of respiration to the intensity of the first kick of a cycle. The tensograms show that the first kick after respiration is weaker than the kick following the recovery phases of the arms without respiration.

4 Conclusions

Taking the velocity profiles of top swimmers as an ideal, the technique training can be improved by removing a typical drop in velocity. The algorithm for our training technique is as follows:

1. establishment of the starting level of swimming technique (by means of video and speedography);
2. designation of the aims of any change;
3. elaboration of methodical influence of the mistake diagnosed or technical reserve and formulation of counteractive steps;
4. use of visual aids, language and motivation to activate receptive and perceptive processes;
5. control exercise in water by means of video and speedography, and use of the methodical steps formulated in point 3;
6. stabilization of the style of coordination and development of adaptability to different conditions.

Following this procedure the technique of young swimmers may be influenced positively by minimizing velocity fluctuations.

5 References

Hahn, A. (1988) To coordination of partial movements in breaststroke and butterfly in different load range and their improvement to increasing the performance of impulse. Diss A., MLU Halle-Wittenberg.

Hochmuth, B. (1986) Contribution of biomechanics to higher effectiveness of technique training, in **Theorie und Praxis des Leistungssports**, Berlin 24, 3.

SWIMMING SKILL CANNOT BE INTERPRETED DIRECTLY FROM THE ENERGY COST OF SWIMMING

J.C. CHATARD[*], J.M. LAVOIE[**] and J.R. LACOUR[*]
[*]Laboratoire de Physiologie, GIP Exercise, Université de
Saint-Etienne, France; [**]Département d'Education Physique, Université
de Montréal, Canada

Abstract
The purpose of this study was to determine if swimming skill could be
interpreted directly from the energy cost of swimming (C_s) per unit
distance at a given velocity. A total of 101 males were studied.
Three performance levels were determined from the slower (A) to the
faster (B, C) times over a 400 m swim. For a given velocity, there
were no statistical differences in C_s between the three levels.
However, at level C and at 1.1 m/s, C_s was reduced by 55% and 25%
when compared to levels A and B and when calculated per unit of
surface area and hydrostatic lift. To evaluate the specific
influence of arm length two groups of long- and short-armed swimmers
were selected among swimmers of similar height and performance. The
C_s was significantly (P < 0.05) higher by 12 ± 3.3% for short-armed
than long-armed swimmers. To evaluate the influence of different
types of swimming technique two other groups of similar performance
and anthropometric characteristics were selected. The C_s was significantly higher by 15 ± 3.8% for swimmers preferentially using their
legs than their arm (P < 0.05). The C_s of the sprinters was 16.5 ±
3% higher than that of the long-distance swimmers. For all the
groups, C_s increased with velocity on average by 10% every 0.1 m/s.
Thus, technical ability cannot be interpreted directly from C_s.
Perfor-mance levels, body size, type of swimming technique and
velocity must also be taken into account.
Keywords: Anthropometric Size, Energy Cost, Buoyancy, Performance,
Swimming.

1 Introduction

The energy cost of swimming (C_s) per unit distance at a given velocity varies to a large extent from one swimmer to another. This
variation is thought to depend mainly on swimming skill (Holmer,
1974; Montpetit et al., 1983; Pendergast et al., 1977; Van Handel et
al., 1988). Pendergast et al. (1978) reported that competitive swimmers were twice to three times more economical than poor swimmers.
However, this relationship, established by comparing different groups
of swimmers, is somewhat imprecise because the exact level of performance is unquantifiable. Furthermore, direct interpretation of C_s is
difficult because height, mass and buoyancy affect C_s (Chatard et
al., 1985; Costill et al., 1985; Montpetit et al., 1983; Pendergast
et al., 1977). Swimming technique should also affect C_s because arm

173

swim is more economical than leg or whole stroke swim (Holmer et al., 1974, Hollander et al., 1988). Thus, the swimmers who preferentially use their arm during swimming should be more economical than the swimmers preferentially using their legs. However, in the literature, there are no data concerning individual differences in C_s of the arm and leg swimmers as there is no information concerning sprinters specialized in 100 m versus long-distance swimmers specialized in 1500 m.

This study was designed to examine the relationship between C_s of a large population of male swimmers and various performance levels of timed performances to determine if swimming skill could be interpreted directly from C_s. The 400 m event was chosen as a reference because it is a common distance that can be swum by all swimmers - sprinters, middle or long-distance swimmers. As body size and type of swimming technique may affect this relationship, specific attention was given to anthropometric and technique variations among the swimmers.

2 Methods

A group (GI) of 101 males was studied. Three performance levels were determined: level A, n = 37, when the velocity of a 400 m swim (V-400) measured in competition was less than 1.35 m/s, level B, n = 41, when V-400 was between 1.36 and 1.55 m/s, level C, n = 23, when V-400 was between 1.56 and 1.76 m/s. Among the swimmers, a group (GII) of 20 swimmers, characterized by almost the same mean height and performance and other variables but different arm lengths were selected and identified as two sub-groups, long (n = 10) or short (n = 10) arm. In the same way, two other groups of 20 swimmers (GIII and GIV) characterized by the same physical characteristics and performance but different types of swimming technique were selected by three coaches of a team, i.e. arm (n = 10) or leg (n = 10) swimmers (GIII) and sprinters (n = 10), specialized in 100 m, or long distance (n = 10) swimmers (GIV), specialized in 1500 m.

Oxygen uptake was measured in a 50 m pool, at increasing speed, each 200 m step, until exhaustion. Effective velocity sustained at each stage was measured over 40 m within two points which were 5 m distant from each end of the pool to eliminate the influence of the turn velocity. Subjects were fitted with a mouthpiece connected to a valve. Expired gases were collected during the last 30 s of each 200 m in a Douglas bag attached to a trolley which followed the swimmer. Oxygen and carbon dioxide fractions were determined using Beckman gas analyzers. Energy cost (C_s), expressed in millilitres of oxygen per metre, was calculated from the oxygen uptake measured at 1.10, 1.20, 1.30, 1.40 m/s and expressed respectively by $C_s 1.1$, $C_s 1.2$, $C_s 1.3$, $C_s 1.4$. Body surface area was estimated from the standing height and mass. Arm length (AL) was measured from the acromion to the extremity of the third finger. The hydrostatic lift (HL) was measured at the end of a maximal inspiration when swimmers were floating. Lead masses, varying from 0.1 to 1 kg, were applied on their back. The hydrostatic lift (HL) was the load necessary to maintain the swimmer in a balanced position just under water.

2.1 Statistical analysis

Means and standard deviations were computed for all variables. ANOVA comparisons were used to test for significant differences in main characteristics and C_s at different velocities between the three performance levels and between groups of long or short arms, between arm or leg swimmers and between sprinter and long-distance swimmers. Stepwise regressions were calculated between C_s 1.1 and anthropometric variables (height, mass, body surface area and hydrostatic lift) using StatView 512+ program, developed by Brain Power Inc., Calabasas. In all statistical analyses, the 0.05 level of significance was taken. Only the variables which added significantly to prediction ($P < 0.05$) were included in the final regression equation. Thus, coefficient values of all these variables were calculated and related to their standard error of estimate (SEE) to calculate the critical P values.

3 Results

For GI, results of anthropometric data, V-400 and C_s are presented in Table 1. The higher the performance level the greater the body size and the longer the duration of training. For a given velocity, there are no statistical differences in C_s between levels A, B and C.

The best single predictor of C_s 1.1 was SA (r = 0.50, $P < 0.01$). Incorporation of HL in the stepwise regression, as a second variable, significantly improved the accuracy of the regression to r = 0.56 (P < 0.01, equation 1).

$$C_s 1.1 = 21.88SA - 2.15HL + 5.9 \tag{1}$$

Statistical differences ($P < 0.05$) appeared in levels A, B and C when C_s 1.1 was calculated per unit of SA and HL (Figure 1). For GII,

Table 1. Main characteristics of group GI at levels A, B, and C (mean and standard deviation)

		Level A	Level B	Level C
n		37	41	23
Age	(years)	14±1.4	17±3.7*	17±1.6
Height	(cm)	164±12	173±9*	178±5**
Arm length	(cm)	73±6	78±5*	82±3**
Mass	(kg)	52±14	63±11*	69±6**
Surface area	(m²)	1.55±0.24	1.75±0.19*	1.86±0.10**
Hydrostatic lift	(kg)	1.7±0.7	2.1±0.8*	3±0.7**
Duration of training	(h/week)	8±3	12±5*	19±6**
V400	(m/s)	1.21±0.10	1.45±0.06*	1.62±0.05**
C_s1.1	(ml/m)	39.5±6.3	39.8±7	38±5.6
C_s1.2	(ml/m)	43.3±5.7	44±7.4	42.5±6.5
C_s1.3	(ml/m)	–	47.2±5.4	46.8±6.8
C_s1.4	(ml/m)	–	48.6±4.3	49.2±7

* Significant differences at $P < 0.05$ between level A and level B.
**Significant differences at $P < 0.05$ between level B and level C.

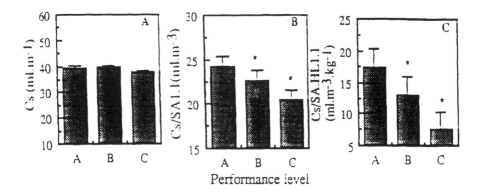

Fig. 1. Mean and standard error of estimate of $C_s 1.1$ of different performance levels; in absolute values (Fig. 1A), per unit of surface area (C_s/SA) (Fig. 1B) and hydrostatic lift ($C_s/SA.HL$) (Fig. 1C). Significant differences, $P < 0.05$ (ANOVA test) between level A and level B, and between level B and level C are marked*.

long and short arm swimmers differed only in arm length (82 ± 4 cm compared to 78 ± 3 cm, $P < 0.01$, Table 2). The C_s of long arms was lower than short arms at the four velocities by 12 ± 3.3% ($P < 0.01$, Fig. 2A). For GIII, C_s was lower for arm than for leg swimmers by 15 ± 3.8% ($P < 0.01$, Fig. 2B). For GIV, C_s was lower for long-distance swimmers than for sprinters by 16.5 ± 3% ($P < 0.01$, Fig. 2C). For all groups, C_s increased significantly ($P < 0.05$) between each velocity. At level A, between 1.1 and 1.2 m/s, C_s increased by 10%. At level B, between 1.1 and 1.3 m/s, C_s increased by 20%. At level C, between 1 and 1.4 m/s, C_s increased by 30%.

Table 2. Main characteristics of groups GII, GIII and GIV.   Mean ± SD

	Group II		Group III		Group IV	
	Long arm	Short arm	Arm swimmers	Leg swimmers	Sprinters	Long-distance
n	10	10	10	10	10	10
Age (years)	17 ± 3	17 ± 2	16 ± 2	17 ± 2	18 ± 4.6	17 ± 3.4
Height (cm)	175 ± 6	179 ± 5	175 ± 8	178 ± 4	178 ± 5	178 ± 10
Arm length (cm)	82 ± 4	78 ± 3*	80 ± 6	81 ± 2	80 ± 3	80 ± 7
Mass (kg)	64 ± 8	67 ± 8	65 ± 9	68 ± 8	70 ± 8	65 ± 13
Hydrostatic lift (kg)	2.7 ± 0.9	2.7 ± 0.9	2.9 ± 0.9	2.8 ± 0.8	2.2 ± 1	2.9 ± 1.3
Training (h/week)	16 ± 6	14 ± 6	19 ± 6	18 ± 7	14 ± 7	14 ± 8
V400 (m/s)	1.54 ± 0.1	1.48 ± 0.1	1.59 ± 0.1	1.60 ± 0.1	1.53 ± 0.1	1.53 ± 0.2

*Significant difference at $P < 0.05$ between short and long arm swimmers

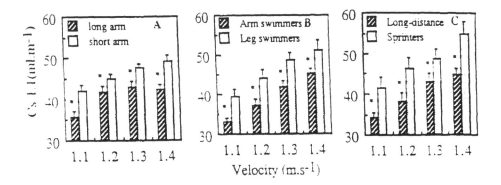

Fig. 2. Mean and standard error of estimate of C_s of the long and
short arm (Fig. 2A), arm and leg swimmers (Fig. 2B),
sprinter and long-distance swimmers (Fig. 3C) at
different velocities and performance levels. Significant
differences, $P < 0.05$ (ANOVA test) are marked *.

4 Discussion

On average, C_s values of the present study are in agreement with
other observations (Holmer, 1974; Montpetit et al., 1983; Pendergast
et al., 1977; Van Handel et al., 1988). However, no differences in
C_s was found between the three performance levels. Apparently, these
data contrast with those of other studies comparing swimmers of
different levels (Cazorla and Montpetit, 1988; Costill et al., 1985;
Holmer, 1974; Montpetit et al., 1983; Pendergast et al., 1977; 1978).
However in these studies anthropometric data were homogeneous whereas
in the present study, anthropometric data of subgroups A, B and C
were very different. A superior body size hid a part of the greater
swimming skill of group C compared to B and A. Thus, when C_s was
related to given body dimensions (SA and HL) the differences between
C_s and the three performance levels appeared, confirming that it is a
prerequisite for success in swimming performance (Holmer, 1974;
Montpetit et al., 1983; Pendergast et al., 1977; Van Handel et al.,
1988).
Anthropometric data, such as SA and HL, represented 31% of the C_s
variability. The C_s increases with the body surface area. Thus
bigger individuals are penalized. A greater body size induces
greater body drag (Tilborgh et al., 1983; Chatard et al., 1990). It
explains why successful distance swimmers are smaller and lighter
than others, as reported by Lavoie and Montpetit (1986). However, in
sprint swimming, swimmers with greater muscle mass and larger body
height swim faster because they can produce a greater anaerobic
energy output and cover a shorter distance in race. Moreover, in
this study, arm length had a specific effect on C_s where a variation
of 4 cm resulted in a 12% gain.
The present study also revealed that the variability of C_s was
related to the types of swimming technique used. Arm swimmers were
more economical than leg swimmers. Kicking requires a proportionally
greater oxygen uptake but contributes little to propulsion. Long-
distance swimmers were more economical than sprinters, although they
were characterized by almost the same physical characteristics and

400 m performances. Most of the sprinters use a six-beat kick versus a two-beat kick for the long-distance swimmers explaining, perhaps, why they were less economical.

Another major feature of this study was that C_s increased with velocity. It was probably due to the relationship between the energy output and drag. Holmer (1974) demonstrated that $\dot{V}O_2$ is a linear function of body drag. This is not in agreement with data obtained by Pendergast et al. (1977) showing that C_s was independent of velocity. However, the velocities, from 0.4 to 1.20 m/s, and the practice level of the subjects they studied were very different. These relationships raise the question whether assessing swimming skill from C_s is reasonable. Moreover, factors such as the underwater torque (Pendergast et al., 1977), joint laxity (Chatard et al., 1990), hand surface (Toussaint et al., 1983) and maybe others influence C_s.

In summary, the wide individual variability of C_s must not be interpreted as being related only to the technical ability. Performance levels, anthropometric data, types of swimming technique and velocity should also be taken into account. Further experiments are required to determine the role of other factors (hand surface area, shaving, apparatus and so on) to evaluate the exact variability of C_s due to swimming skill.

5 References

Cazorla, G. and Montpetit, R. (1988) Metabolic and cardiac responses of swimmers, modern pentathletes and water polo players during freestyle swimming to a maximum, in **Swimming Science V** (eds B.E. Ungerechts, K. Wilke and K. Reischle), Human Kinetics Books, Champaign, Ill., pp. 251-257.

Chatard, J.C., Bourgoin, B. and Lacour, J.R. (1990) Passive drag is still a good evaluator of swimming aptitude. **Eur. J. Appl. Physiol.**, 59, 399-404.

Chatard, J.C., Padilla, S., Cazorla, G. and Lacour, J.R. (1985) Influence of body height, weight, hydrostatic lift and training on the energy cost of the front crawl. **N.Z. J. Sports Med.**, 12, 82-84.

Costill, D.L., Kovaliski, J., Porter, D., Fielding, R. and King, D. (1985) Energy expenditure during front crawl swimming: predicting success in middle distance events. **Int. J. Sports Med.**, 6, 266-270.

Holmer, I. (1974) Physiology of swimming man. **Acta Physiol. Scand.** Suppl. 407, 1-55.

Hollander, A.P., Groot, G. de, van Ingen Schenau, G.J., Kahman, R. and Toussaint, H.M. (1988) Contribution of the legs to propulsion in front crawl swimming, in **Swimming Science V** (eds B.E. Ungerechts, K. Wilke and K. Reischle), Human Kinetics Books, Champaign, Ill., pp. 38-44.

Lavoie, J.M. and Montpetit, R. (1986) Applied physiology of swimming. **Sports Med.**, 3, 165-189.

Montpetit, R., Lavoie, J.M. and Cazorla, G. (1983) Aerobic energy cost of the front crawl at high velocity in international class and adolescent swimmers, in **Biomechanics and Medicine in Swimming** (eds A.P. Hollander, P.A. Huijing and G. de Groot), Human

Kinetics Publishers, Champaign, Ill., pp. 228-234.

Pendergast, D.R., di Prampero, P.E., Craig, A.B, Wilson, D.R. and Rennie, D.W. (1977) Quantitative analysis of the front crawl in men and women. **J. Appl. Physiol.**, 43, 475-479.

Pendergast, D.R., di Prampero, P.E., Craig, A.B, Wilson, D.R. and Rennie, D.W. (1978) The influence of selected biomechanical factors on the energy cost of swimming, in **Swimming III** (eds B. Eriksson and F. Furberg), University Park Press, Baltimore, pp. 367-378.

Toussaint, H.M., van der Helm, H.C.T., Elzerman, J.R., Hollander, A.P., Groot, G. de, van Ingen Schenau, G.J. (1983) A power balanced applied to swimming, in **Biomechanics and Medicine in Swimming** (eds A.P. Hollander, P.A. Huijing and G. de Groot), Human Kinetics Publishers, Champaign, Ill., pp. 165-172.

Van Handel, P.A., Katz, A., Morrow, J.R., Troup, J.P., Daniels, J.T., and Bradley, P.W. (1988) Aerobic economy and competitive performance of US elite swimmers, in **Swimming Science V** (eds B.E. Ungerechts, K. Wilke, K. Reischle), Human Kinetics Books, Champaign, Ill., pp. 219-227.

Van Tilborgh, L., Daly, D. and Persyn, V. (1983) The influence of some somatic factors on passive drag, gravity and buoyancy forces in competitive swimmers, in **Biomechanics and Medicine in Swimming** (eds A.P. Hollander, P.A. Huijing and G. de Groot), Human Kinetics Books, Champaign, Ill., pp. 207-214.

SEX DIFFERENCES IN KINEMATICS AND TEMPORAL PARAMETERS OF THE GRAB START

I. KOLLIAS[*], V. BALTZOPOULOS[**], K. CHATZINIKOLAOU[*], D. TSIRAKOS[*] and I. VASILIADIS[*]
[*]Department of Sport Science, University of Thessaloniki, Greece,
[**]Department of Movement Science and Physical Education, University of Liverpool, England

Abstract
The purpose of this study was to examine sex differences in the kinematic and temporal parameters of the grab start using two-dimensional analysis. The main findings of the study are that male swimmers develop a higher take-off speed without significant delay on the block and the angle of projection is usually above the horizontal. This results in a longer flight period but improved horizontal displacement compared to the start of female swimmers.
Keywords: Swimming, Start, Kinematics, Technique.

1 Introduction

The starting technique in swimming is an important performance factor, especially in short-distance events. Biomechanical comparisons of various techniques have shown that the grab start is superior to other starting techniques in competitive swimming using different criterion measures (Bloom et al., 1978; Bowers and Cavanagh, 1975). Other studies, however, indicate that there is no difference between the starting techniques (Lewis, 1980). Havriluk (1983) suggested that the results of the above comparisons are only dependent on the particular criterion measure used in a study and do not indicate overall superiority of the grab start. This type of start, however, is the most widely used starting technique in competitive swimming (Havriluk and Ward, 1979).

Despite the participation of both male and female swimmers in the above studies there is no detailed examination of the sex differences in the performance of the swimming start. The purpose of this study was to compare the grab start of male and female elite swimmers by examining the kinematic and temporal parameters of the start.

2 Methods

2.1 Subjects and procedures

Six male (age 15.3 $\pm$ 1.5 yrs, mass 68.5 $\pm$ 10.3 kg, height 174.9 $\pm$ 7.2 cm), and six female (age 16.4 $\pm$ 0.8 yrs, mass 57.3 $\pm$ 3.4 kg, height 162.7 $\pm$ 4.2 cm) elite swimmers signed informed consent and volunteered to participate in this study. All subjects were members of the Greek national swimming team in their respective age groups.

Testing was conducted in an official 50 m swimming pool in a single testing session. Each swimmer performed a grab start after a 10 min swimming warm-up and two trial starts. The official starting command procedure was followed and in order to simulate competitive conditions the swimmers were asked to perform the start as part of a 25 m freestyle sprint.

2.2 Instrumentation
The starts were filmed using an electrically driven 16 mm Locam camera fitted with a zoom lens. The film speed was set at 100 Hz. The film in the camera was marked using a time light generator at constant intervals of 0.1 s. The camera was placed perpendicular to the plane of movement which was considered parallel with the swimming pool edge at a distance of 20 m from the starting block, 1.8 m in front of the starting line and 1.8 m above the surface of the water. The field of view in the movement plane was approximately 4 x 3 m. The starting gun was connected to an electric bulb that was in the field of view of the camera in front of the starting block. The camera was started with the preliminary starting command to ensure that the film was running at the set rate at the firing of the starting gun. Two dimensional film analysis was performed using a Complot 7000 digitiser connected to a Stride 440 microcomputer for data analysis.

2.3 Data analysis
The centre of mass (CM) of the swimmers was computed using a 14 segment model and the anthropometric data by Dempster (1955). Position-time data were filtered using a two-pass, fourth order Butterworth digital filter (Winter et al., 1974) with a cut-off frequency of 6 Hz. The cut-off frequency was computed using the procedure suggested by Lesh et al. (1979). Linear velocities of the CM were computed using numerical differentiation of the filtered data (Miller and Nelson, 1976).

The following temporal parameters were determined from the film analysis: block time (BT): the time from the starting stimulus until take-off from the block, flight time (FT): the time from take-off until the first contact of the swimmer with the water, total time

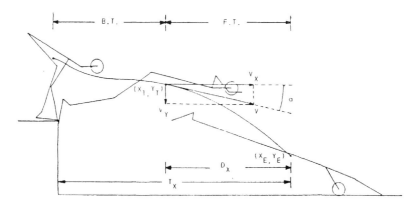

Fig. 1. Temporal and kinematic parameters of the grab start.

(TT): the sum of block and flight time (Figure 1). The kinematic parameters determined were horizontal (V_y) and vertical (V_z) linear velocity of the CM at take-off, angle of projection (a), position of CM at take-off (Y_T, Z_T) and entry (Y_E, Z_E), horizontal (D_y) displacement of CM during flight and total starting distance (T_y) (Fig. 1).

Sex differences in the above parameters were examined using Student's t-ratios and relationships between temporal and kinematic parameters were examined using correlation techniques. Significance was accepted at the 95% level.

3 Results and discussion

The correlation coefficients between temporal and kinematic parameters are presented in Table 1. Temporal parameters of the start are presented in Table 2. These results indicate that although there was no significant difference in the block and total time, the flight duration of male swimmers was 0.08 s longer ($P < 0.05$). The total start time was approximately 1 s for both groups (Table 1).

Table 1. Relationship between temporal and kinematic parameters of the grab start

	FT	TT	V_y	V_z	V	a	D_y	T_y
BT	0.08	0.67*	-0.25	0.21	-0.25	0.19	-0.06	-0.20
FT		0.79*	-0.34	0.93*	-0.30	0.93*	0.81*	0.92*
TT			-0.41	0.82*	-0.38	0.81*	0.64*	0.48
V_y				-0.395	0.99*	-0.40	-0.02	0.24
V_z					-0.38	0.99*	0.86*	0.71*
V						-0.39	0.28	0.01
a							0.86*	0.72*
D_y								0.93*

*$P < 0.05$

The kinematic parameters of the start are presented in Table 2. There was no significant difference in the take-off speed and angle of projection between the two groups although the take-off speed of male swimmers was approximately 0.3 m/s faster. It is important to note, however, that the mean angle of projection was below the horizontal for female and above the horizontal for male swimmers (Table 2). Groves and Roberts (1972) reported that the optimum angle of projection for maximisation of the horizontal component of the take-off velocity is approximately 0.23 rad below the horizontal. The difference in take-off speed, however, was not significant when the angle of projection was above the horizontal.
The results of the present study further indicate that V_y is not a significant factor for the total start time and horizontal displacement during the flight. On the contrary, the vertical component of the take-off velocity was a significant factor for a longer flight period ($P < 0.05$) and therefore improved total displacement during the start ($P < 0.05$) (Table 1). Furthermore there was a significant positive relationship between angle of projection and flight time and

Table 2. Comparison of temporal and kinematic parameters in male and female swimmers

	Male $\bar{x}$ ($\pm$ SD)	Female $\bar{x}$ ($\pm$ SD)
BT (s)	0.62 ($\pm$ 0.04)	0.64 ($\pm$ 0.07)**
FT (s)	0.39 ($\pm$ 0.07)	0.31 ($\pm$ 0.05)*
TT (s)	1.01 ($\pm$ 0.11)	0.96 ($\pm$ 0.08)**
V (m/s)	4.05 ($\pm$ 0.27)	3.70 ($\pm$ 0.49)**
V_y (m/s)	4.01 ($\pm$ 0.44)	3.67 ($\pm$ 0.45)**
V_z (m/s)	0.38 ($\pm$ 0.44)	-0.26 ($\pm$ 0.47)**
a (rad)	0.10 ($\pm$ 0.11)	-0.06 ($\pm$ 0.11)**
D_y (m)	1.44 ($\pm$ 0.20)	1.05 ($\pm$ 0.13)*
T_y (m)	2.45 ($\pm$ 0.16)	2.03 ($\pm$ 0.08)*

*$P < 0.05$, **$P > 0.05$

total displacement ($P < 0.05$). The optimum angle of projection for maximum horizontal displacement was 0.63 ($\pm$ 0.04) rad for males and 0.65 ($\pm$ 0.07) rad for females. The deviation from the optimum angle was larger in female swimmers, which perhaps explains the significant difference in total starting distance (Table 2). The results of this study suggest that although an angle of projection above the horizontal has a positive effect on TT ($r = 0.81$, $P < 0.05$), it also has a positive effect on both D_y ($r = 0.86$, $P < 0.05$) and T_y ($r = 0.72$, $P < 0.05$).

4 Conclusions

The main conclusions within the limitations of the present study are that male swimmers develop a higher take-off velocity without significant delay on the block and the angle of projection is usually above the horizontal. This results in a longer flight period but improved horizontal displacement compared to the start of female swimmers.

5 References

Bloom, J.A., Hosler, W.W. and Disch, J.G. (1978) Differences in flight, reaction and movement time for the grab and conventional starts. **Swimming Technique,** 15, 34-36.
Bowers, J.A. and Cavanagh, P.R. (1975) A biomechanical comparison of the grab and conventional sprint starts in competitive swimming, in **Swimming II** (eds J.P. Clarys and L. Lewillie), University Park Press, Baltimore, pp. 43-45.
Dempster, W.T. (1955) Space requirements for the seated operator (WADC-TR-55-159). Wright-Patterson Air Force Base, OH: Aerospace Medical Research Laboratory.
Havriluk, R. (1983) A criterion measure for the swimming start, in **Biomechanics and Medicine in Swimming** (eds P. Hollander, P. Huijing and G. de Groot), Human Kinetic Publishers, Champaign, Ill., pp. 89-95.

Havriluk, R. and Ward, T. (1979) A cinematographic analysis of three grab starts. **Swimming Technique,** 16, 50-52.

Groves, R. and Roberts, J. (1972) A further investigation of the optimum angle of projection for the racing start in swimming. **Res. Quart.,** 35, 81-82.

Lesh, M.D., Mansour, J.M. and Simon, S.R. (1979) A gait analysis subsystem for smoothing and differentiation of human motion data. **J. Biomed. Engng.,** 10, 205-212.

Lewis, S. (1980) Comparison of five swimming starting techniques. **Swimming Technique,** 16, 124-128.

Miller, D. and Nelson, R. (1976) **Biomechanics of Sport: A Research Approach,** Lea and Febiger, Philadelphia.

Winter, D.A., Sidwall, H.G. and Hobson, D.A. (1974) Measurement and reduction of noise in kinematics of locomotion. **J. Biomech.,** 7, 157-159.

PART FIVE

TRAINING

ADAPTATIONS TO INTERVAL TRAINING AT COMMON INTENSITIES AND DIFFERENT WORK:REST RATIOS

A. BARZDUKAS, P. FRANCIOSI, S. TRAPPE, C. LETNER and J.P. TROUP
U.S. Swimming, International Center for Aquatic Research, Colorado
Springs, Colorado, USA

Abstract
Interval training sets are commonly used in competitive swimming
programmes. It is unclear, however, how different work:rest ratios
used in interval training affect aerobic and anaerobic energy
systems. The purpose of this study, therefore, was to determine
which work:rest ratio (1:2 or 1:1/2) was more effective in improving
400 m specific race performance. Relative energy delivery (anaerobic
vs aerobic) was also examined. Two groups of swimmers participated
in five weeks of training with a major set of 10 × 100 freestyle at
an intensity of 110% of $\dot{V}O_2$max: Group 1:2 at a work:rest ratio of
1:2, and Group 1:1/2 at a work:rest ratio of 1:1/2. Results indicate
that, at the same intensity, a work:rest ratio of 1:2 is more
specific to anaerobic work and a work:rest ratio of 1:1/2 is more
conducive to aerobic development. Because swimming performance is
dependent on optimal anaerobic and aerobic energy delivery, it is
recommended that both modes of training be utilized.
Keywords: Interval Training, Swimming Economy, Oxygen Deficit,
Physiology.

1 Introduction

Swimming performance is dependent on energy released from both
aerobic and anaerobic sources. Thus, training which enhances either,
or both, means of energy delivery is beneficial for swimming
perfomance. Nomura (1983) reported that swim training increased
$\dot{V}O_2$max, or aerobic capacity. Medbø and Burgers (1990) reported
increased anaerobic capacity after six weeks of sprint training.
 Thus, the purpose of this study was to determine the effect of
swim training on aerobic and anaerobic energy delivery. Because
interval training sets are commonly used in competitive swim
training, 10 × 100 m freestyle was selected as the training set. Two
work:rest ratios were also selected to examine the effect of length
of rest on relative energy delivery.

2 Methods

2.1 Subjects
Fifteen (n = 15) trained female college swimmers participated in this

controlled training study. Each swimmer signed an informed letter of
consent. Group age and selected physiological characteristics are
presented in Table 1.

Table 1. Subject characteristics: Mean ($\pm$ SD)

Age (yrs)	Height (cm)	Weight (kg)	Body fat (%)
18.92 $\pm$ 1.73	166.42 $\pm$ 4.32	58.04 $\pm$ 2.0	21.4 $\pm$ 3.7

All testing was conducted at the International Center for Aquatic
Research on the grounds of the United States Olympic Training Center
in Colorado Springs, Colorado. The 10 $\times$ 100 m freestyle training set
was completed, with respective work:rest ratios, three times a week
for five weeks in the subjects' training facility (25 yard pool).

2.2 Study design
Subjects were randomly assigned to one of two training groups for a
five week training cycle. All subjects trained five times per week:
mean training volume per session = 2732 $\pm$ 1093 m; swimming intensity
= < 80% of $\dot{V}O_2$max. In addition to the above training regimen, three
times a week the two training groups performed a set of 10 $\times$ 100 m
freestyle at an intensity of 110% of $\dot{V}O_2$max. Group 1:2 (n = 8)
completed the set at a work:rest ratio of 1:2. Group 1:1/2 (n = 7)
completed the set at a work:rest ratio of 1:1/2.

2.3 Measurements
All measurements were performed prior to and following the five week
training cycle. All swimming measurements were performed in a
swimming treadmill, or flume, as described by D'Aquisto et al.
(1989).

2.3.1 Swimming economy
The swimming economy profile consisted of four sub-maximal swims
followed by a maximal effort. To determine steady state conditions
in which O_2 uptake fully delivered the energy need, all sub-maximal
efforts were performed at intensities of less than 60% $\dot{V}O_2$max. A
progressive intensity/velocity protocol in which swimmers swam until
volitional exhaustion was used to elicit $\dot{V}O_2$max.
The linear relationship between $\dot{V}O_2$ and swimming intensity was
represented by the formula:

$$\dot{V}O_2 = a + b.v^3$$

In this formula "a" represents $\dot{V}O_2$ in l/min at a swimming speed of
0 m/s. "$b.v^3$" represents the energy cost above the resting level
(Hollander, 1990a).

2.3.2 Training velocities/$\dot{V}O_2$ demand
The relationship described above was extrapolated to 100% of $\dot{V}O_2$max
(Troup, 1986) to determine training velocities and O_2 demand. Total
O_2 demand was determined for each swim by multiplying the O_2 demand

by the time required to complete the swim.

2.3.3 Test sets/accumulated O_2 uptake/accumulated O_2 deficit

Test sets consisted of 6 x 100 m freestyle on-line swims in a flume at the prescribed intensity for the given work:rest ratio. The test sets were completed at the same absolute workload prior to and following the five week training period.

Accumulated O_2 uptake was determined from continuous on-line measurements at 10 s increments. Relative power delivery was calculated by the formula (Medbø et al., 1988):

$$O_2 \text{ demand} - O_2 \text{ uptake} = O_2 \text{ deficit}$$

Subtracting accumulated O_2 uptake from total O_2 demand gave an estimation of accumulated O_2 deficit (Hermansen and Medbø, 1984). Relative energy delivery was thus calculated by the formula (Medbø et al., 1988):

$$\text{Total } O_2 \text{ demand} - \text{accumulated } O_2 \text{ uptake} = \text{Accumulated } O_2 \text{ deficit}$$

Calculating O_2 in this way has previously been shown to be an accurate estimation of anaerobic energy production (Medbø et al., 1988; Hollander, 1990b; Bangsbo et al., 1990).

2.3.4 Biochemistry

Resting muscle biopsies of the posterior deltoid were analyzed for lactate dehydrogenase (LDH: an enzyme which catalyzes the reaction converting lactic acid back into a usable energy substrate), phosphofructokinase (PFK: a glycolytic rate limiting enzyme), and citrate synthase (a catalyst for synthesis of citrate from acetyl CoA and oxaloacetate) (McArdle et al., 1986; Rawn, 1989). Blood lactate, obtained 2 min post-swim by means of a finger prick and base excess immediately post-swim were measured upon completion of the test set.

2.4 Statistics

An ANOVA was used to evaluate within and between group differences. Regression analysis was used to analyze within and between group swimming economy differences. A probability level of $P < 0.05$ was selected for statistical significance. Significance was analyzed using Tukey's post-hoc test.

3 Results

3.1 Swimming economy

Swimming economy improved significantly in Group 1:1/2. Pre- and post-economy variables are found in Table 2.

3.2 O_2 demand

The ANOVA for O_2 demand indicated a significant difference between pre- and post-training O_2 demand values. Post-hoc analysis revealed that Group 1:2 had improved O_2 demand (pre-training: 1025 watts vs post-training: 993 ± 18 watts, $P < 0.05$). Consequently, 400 m race specific pace (110% of $\dot{V}O_2$max) also improve significantly in Group 1:2 (pre-training: 1.22 ± 0.01 m/sec vs 1.26 ± 0.02 m/sec, $P < 0.05$).

Table 2. Pre- and post-training swimming economy profiles of trained female swimmers

Variable	Group	
	1:2	1:1/2
Constant: Pre-	0.649 ± 0.543	0.760 ± 0.472
Post-	0.685 ± 0.447	0.747 ± 0.462
Coefficient: Pre-	0.741 ± 0.159	0.753 ± 0.226
Post-	0.756 ± 0.214	0.689 ± 0.109*

*P < 0.05

3.3 Test sets

The ANOVA, and subsequent post-hoc analysis, indicated that at the same absolute workload for the test set, O_2 demand fell in group 1:1/2 following the five week training period. The percent anaerobic contribution also increased significantly in Group 1:1/2 (see Table 3).

Table 3. Pre- and post-training test set O_2 demand, relative energy delivery, accumulated $\dot{V}O_2$, and accumulated O_2 deficit values

Variable	Group	
	1:2	1:1/2
O_2 demand (l/min)		
Pre-	2.82 ± 0.30	2.79 ± 0.16
Post-	2.88 ± 0.27	2.41 ± 0.29*
Percent anaerobic		
Pre-	32.20 ± 7.75	20.10 ± 6.33
Post-	34.35 ± 4.23	34.57 ± 5.17*
Accumulated $\dot{V}O_2$ (litres)		
Pre-	15.57 ± 1.42	18.93 ± 2.90
Post-	15.44 ± 1.52	13.39 ± 2.91
Accumulated O_2 deficit (l)		
Pre-	7.53 ± 2.50	4.86 ± 1.96
Post-	8.09 ± 1.30	7.19 ∝ 2.84

*P < 0.05

3.4 Biochemistry

The ANOVA revealed significant variance in post-training test set blood lactate, base excess, and citrate synthase values. Subsequent post-hoc analysis indicated where significant differences occurred. Post-training test-set blood lactate values fell significantly in Group 1:2. Post-training test-set base excess values increased in Group 1:2. Citrate synthase values increased in Group 1:1/2. Biochemistry results are found in Table 4.

Table 4. Pre- and post-training post-test set blood lactate, base excess, and citrate synthetase values

Variable	Group	
	1:2	1:1/2
Blood lactate (mM)		
Pre-	8.92 ± 0.38	9.41 ± 1.15
Post-	7.38 ± 0.40*	8.55 ± 0.92
Base excess		
Pre-	-15.30 ± 0.20	-14.20 ± 0.30
Post-	-13.60 ± 0.10*	-13.90 ± 0.20
LDH		
Pre-	15.84 ± 13.81	18.34 ± 9.29
Post-	18.12 ± 11.50	13.80 ± 4.56
PFK		
Pre-	7.03 ± 4.93	3.75 ± 1.60
Post-	5.13 ± 3.17	3.66 ± 1.21
Citrate synthase ($\mu M/min/g$)		
Pre-	32.12 ± 7.82	35.80 ± 6.01
Post-	25.05 ± 8.99	42.04 ± 1.52*

*$P < 0.05$

4 Discussion

In summary, these data suggest that, for 400 m specific race intensity, work:rest ratios of 1:1/2 result in aerobic energy delivery improvements and that work:rest ratios of 1:2 result in increased anaerobic energy delivery. Thus, appropriate utilization of both modes of training should result in enhanced performance for 400 m specific race intensity.

Medbø and Burgers (1990) reported that anaerobic capacity, when expressed by maximal accumulated O_2 deficit, can be improved 10% within six weeks by proper training. The results of the present study confirm these findings in that longer, or more sprint orientated, work:rest ratios resulted in improved anaerobic energy delivery, or sprint capacity.

A work:rest ratio of 1:1/2 led to improvements in swimming economy suggesting that shorter intervals are more conducive to aerobic training. According to Hollander (1990a), change in swimming economy is the result of change in propelling efficiency. Thus, a work:rest ratio of 1:1/2 may be more conducive to improving propelling efficiency than larger work:rest ratios.

A work:rest ratio of 1:2 also led to decreases in post-test set lactate values suggesting that adaptation had occurred to the anaerobic specific nature of this work:rest ratio. Base excess values also suggest that training at larger work:rest ratios may enhance lactate removal processes.

Citrate synthase values rose in Group 1:1/2. This may indicate that work of a shorter work:rest ratio may enhance aerobic metabolism.

5 Conclusions

In summary, these data suggest that longer work:rest ratios appear to emphasize anaerobic adaptation while short work:rest ratios enhance aerobic adaptation. Thus, when training for a 400 m swimming event both types (long and shorter) of work:rest ratios, relative energy delivery, biomechanical factors affecting swimming, and performance needs to be examined further to determine specific modes of training for different swimming events.

6 References

Bangsbo, J., Gollnick, P.D., Graham, T.E., Juel, C., Kiens, B., Mizuno, M. and Saltin, B. (1990) Anaerobic energy production and O_2 deficit-debt relationship during exhaustive exercise in humans. **J. Physiol.**, 422, 539–559.

D'Acquisto, L., Troup, J. and Holmberg, S. (1989) **Description and water velocity characteristics of a new swimming treadmill.** Paper presented at the VIII World Federation Internationale de Natation Amateur (FIA) Medical Congress, London, UK, September.

Hermansen, L. and Medbø, J.I. (1984) The relative significance of aerobic and anaerobic processes during maximal exercise of short duration. **Medicine, Sport and Science,** 17, 56–57.

Hollander, A.P. (1990a) Economy regression lines and their meaning. Unpublished manuscript (Vrije Universiteit, Amsterdam).

Hollander, A.P. (1990b) O_2 deficit and energy stores. Unpublished manuscript (Vrije Universiteit, Amsterdam).

McArdle, W.D., Katch, F.I. and Katch, V.L. (1986) **Exercise Physiology: Energy, Nutrition and Human Performance** 2nd edition. Lea & Febiger, Philadelphia.

Medbø, J.I. and Burgers, S. (1990) Effect of training on the anaerobic capacity. **Med. Sci. Sports Exerc.,** 22, 501–507.

Medbø, J.I., Mohn, A.C., Tabata, I., Bahr, R., Vaage, O. and Sejersted, O.M. (1988) Anaerobic capacity determined by maximal accumulated O_2 deficit. **J. Appl. Physiol.,** 64, 50–60.

Nomura, T. (1983) The influence of training and age of O_2max during swimming in Japanese elite age group and Olympic swimmers, in **Biomechanics and Medicine in Swimming** (eds A.P. Hollander, P.A. Huijing and G. de Groot), Human Kinetics Publishers, Champaign, Ill., pp. 251–258.

Rawn, J.D. (1989) **Biochemistry.** Carolina Biological Supply Company, Burlington.

Troup, J.P. and Daniels, J. (1986) Swimming economy: An overview. J. **Swimming Res.** 2, 1–7.

PHYSIOLOGICAL ADAPTATIONS TO 60 VS 20 MINUTES OF SWIM TRAINING AT 76% $\dot{V}O_2$max

L.J. D'ACQUISTO, A.P. BARZDUKAS, P. DURSTHOFF, C. LETNER and
J.P. TROUP
U.S. Swimming, International Center for Aquatic Research, Colorado
Springs, Colorado, USA

Abstract
The intent of this project was to evaluate the benefits of swim
training at $76 \pm 2\%$ $\dot{V}O_2$max for 60 vs 20 min duration would have on
submaximal and maximal swimming performances. Moderately trained
swimmers (n = 17) were divided into two groups. The GRP1 (n = 7)
trained for 60 min while GRP2 trained 20 min per session. Both
groups worked at the same intensity ($76 \pm 2\%$ $\dot{V}O_2$max) and frequency (5
sessions per week). The duration of the study was 5 weeks. The
primary findings of this study included: (1) 60 min of moderate
intensity swimming resulted in enhanced perfomance (91.44 and
365.88 m), increased aerobic power and swimming efficiency ($P <$
0.05); (2) 20 minutes of work was adequate in maintaining aerobic
power and improving swimming efficiency, but did not result in faster
swimming; (3) 60 and 20 min of work at $76 \pm 2\%$ $\dot{V}O_2$max resulted in a
decrease of muscle CS and PFK activity.
Keywords: Physiology, Muscle Enzymes, Blood Enzymes, Aerobic Power.

1 Introduction

The physiological adaptations associated with endurance training, as
reflected by increases in aerobic power ($\dot{V}O_2$max) and submaximal
exercise endurance, are increases both in cardiovascular and muscular
capacity (Nadel, 1985; Saltin and Rowell, 1980). Enhancements in
endurance capacity usually require emphasis on aerobic oriented work.
The minimal amount of aerobic work necessary to achieve peak endurance capacity in swimming has received little research attention.
The purpose of this project was to examine the physiological adaptations for moderate aerobic work when training 20 vs 60 min while
maintaining intensity and frequency constant.

2 Methods

2.1 Experimental design
Moderately trained male swimmers (n = 17) participated in this study
after being informed of the possible risks and benefits associated
with the project. Subjects were assigned to one of two groups. Both
groups trained at the same intensity ($76 \pm 2\%$ $\dot{V}O_2$max) and frequency
(5 sessions/week) for a 5 week period. A GRP1 (n = 7) group trained
60 min per session while GRP2 (n = 10) trained 20 min per session.

Subject characteristics for GRP1 and GRP2 were (mean ± SE):
GRP1, wt = 73.8 ± 2.5, % body fat = 10.5 ± 0.5; GRP2, wt = 75.9 ±
2.5, % body fat = 13.9 ± 1.7. Subjects were tested pre (P; 4 days
prior to start of study) and post training (PT; 2 days following the
completion of the study for submaximal and maximal swim tests
(economy and $\dot{V}O_2$max swims). Blood draws (06:00–08:00 hours) were
conducted at P, immediately following wk1, wk2, wk3, wk4, and PT.

2.2 Testing procedure
Performance/body composition. Swimmers performed a 25 (22.86 m), 100
(91.44) and 400 (365.8 m) yard time trial from a push-off start.
Trials were performed at P and PT. Body weight and percent body fat
were determined (P and PT) using a Health-o-meter clinical weighing
scale and skinfold measurements, respectively (Behnke and Wilmore,
1969).
Metabolic: Subjects performed a swimming economy (4 submaximal
swims) and $\dot{V}O_2$max test in a swimming treadmill at P and PT. Blood
lactate and heart rate were determined for each swim (refer to
D'Acquisto et al., 1990, for procedure). Four submaximal swims
determined the $\dot{V}O_2$ vs velocity (m.s) curve (economy profile). For
regression analysis the velocity values (0.8, 0.9, 1.0 and 1.1 m/s)
were cubed in order to increase the r^2 value and reduce the standard
error about the regression line (Hollander et al., 1990). To
determine changes in swimming efficiency between P and PT the slopes
of the economy curves were compared.
Biochemistry: A resting morning blood sample from an antecubital
vein was taken at each point of testing. Creatine phosphokinase
(CPK) and lactate dehydrogenase (LDH) serum activities were
quantitated (Spectrophotometry, ABOTT-Spectrum) to assess muscle
membrane damage with the different training regimens.
Muscle biopsy: A muscle biopsy was performed at P and PT on the
posterior deltoid (Bergstrom, 1962; Costill et al., 1984). Muscle
activity of citrate synthase (CS), and phosphofructokinase (PFK) were
determined (Lowry and Passoneau, 1972).
Statistics: A MANOVA (SPSS) was used to analyze the data with the
level of significance set a priori at 0.05. A post hoc test was
utilized when appropriate (Tukey LSD). Results are presented as mean
± SE.

3 Results

3.1 Anthropometric measures and performance
There were no significant differences in body weight (kg) or percent
body fat for GRP1 and GRP2 with the respective training regimens.
The only significant improvement in performance occurred with GRP1
(60 min) for 91.44 and 365.88 m freestyle performance (91.44, P =
1.47 ± 0.01 vs PT 1.51 ± 0.02 m/s; 365.88, P = 1.20 ± 0.02 vs PT =
1.29 ± 0.03).

3.2 Submaximal and maximal swimming
Regression equation (mean ± SE) results of the economy curves
(l O_2/min vs velocity^3) for P vs PT were the following (*P < 0.05):

GRP1:
    Pre-study $\dot{V}O_2 = 1.09(V^3) + 0.77$
                         (0.05) (0.03)

    Post-study $\dot{V}O_2 = 0.35(V^3) + 0.80$
                       $*(0.10)$ (0.06)

GRP2:
    Pre-study $\dot{V}O_2 = 1.18(V^3) + 0.90$
                         (0.06) (0.04)

    Post-study $\dot{V}O_2 = 0.47(V^3) + 0.64$
                       $*(0.08)$ $*(0.05)$.

Significant improvements occurred for slope values between P and PT
for GRP1 and GRP2, whereas the intercept value significantly changed
only for GRP2. Between P and PT, $\dot{V}O_2$max (l/min) improved for GRP1,
2.91 (0.21) vs 3.48 (0.17), by 16.4%^{2} (P < 0.05), while GRP2 did not
significantly enhance aerobic power, 2.89 ± 0.27 vs 3.13 ± 0.13, an
increase of 7.7% (P = 0.12).

3.3 Serum creatine phosphokinase and lactate dehydrogenase activity
There was a significant change in total serum activity of CPK during
the 5 week training period for GRP2. The difference was found
between P vs wk1 (117.5 ± 11.9 vs 162.14 ± 41.3 IU/l), wk1 vs wk2
(162.1 ± 41.3 vs 105.4 ± 13.6 IU/l), and wk4 vs PT (113.3 ± 20.0 vs
261.1 ± 53.9 IU/l). No difference in LDH was noted for GRP2 (P =
0.10). GRP1 experienced no session effect for CPK and LDH, P = 0.20
and P = 0.62, respectively.

3.4 Muscle activity of citrate synthase, and phosphofructokinase
A decrease (P < 0.05) in skeletal muscle CS and PFK activity for GRP2
was noted between P vs PT (Table 1). There was a decrease for GRP1
(P < 0.05) in PFK activity with no change in CS.

Table 1. Citrate synthase and pyruvate dehydrogenase activity

Group	Pre	Post
1 (60 min)		
CS	27.7 ± 4.0	26.6 ± 5.0
PFK	39.3 ± 3.3	33.1 ± 1.5*
2 (20 min)		
CS	35.1 ± 2.0	29.1 ± 2.5*
PFK	44.1 ± 2.1	32.5 ± 3.1*

Muscle CS and PFK (μmoles/gram/min).

4 Discussion

The magnitude of a training effect is dictated by the manipulation of
frequency, duration and intensity of the exercise regimen. The
intent of this study was to study the effects of training volume on
submaximal and maximal swimming performance. The variance was some-

what maximized in that GRP1 swam for 60 min whereas GRP2 swam for 20 min. Performance (91.44 and 365.88 m) improvements were only noted in GRP1 (P < 0.05). This suggests that training at a moderate intensity (76 $\pm$ 2% $\dot{V}O_2$max) for 20 min per session, 5 sessions a week was inadequate in promoting performance enhancements.

The improvements in performance for GRP1 can be explained by enhanced aerobic power, as illustrated by a 16.4% increase in $\dot{V}O_2$max (P < 0.05). The second group had a 7.7% increase in $\dot{V}O_2$max, but this change was not significant (P = 0.12). The slope of the economy regression equation decreased significantly for GRP1. This suggests that for a given increase in velocity the VO_2 (l/min) change became less, implying an improvement in swimming efficiency. The improvement in swimming efficiency also explains, in part, the enhancement of swimming performance.

Swimmers in GRP2 also became more efficient as indicated by a drop in the slope value of the regression economy equation with training (P < 0.05). This improvement in swimming efficiency for GRP2 was not sufficient in enhancing swimming performance. These data suggest that not one variable enhances swimming performance, but rather a combination of factors, i.e. aerobic power, swimming efficiency, motivation.

Significant reductions in CS and PFK muscle activity did not result in a deterioration of performance or decrease in $\dot{V}O_2$max for GRP2. A significant reduction in PFK muscle activity was found for GRP1, but this did not appear to compromise performance. It is possible that the intensity and duration of swim training for these subjects was not adequate in promoting enhancements of CS and PFK activity. Therefore, either a higher intensity or duration of training (or both) is necessary for enhancing CS and PFK activity in skeletal muscle.

Serum CPK and LDH activities have been known to fluctuate depending on the training load (Noakes, 1987). GRP2 was found to have significant CPK activity fluctuations. During the first week of training CPK activity increased significantly, suggesting muscle membrane damage (Noakes, 1987). With continued training (second week) CPK levels significantly dropped suggesting an adaptive response took place such that the muscle was more resistive to any damage and/or that any damage that did take place was repaired faster (Clarkson and Tremblay, 1988). The CPK levels following the final week of training rose dramatically (P < 0.05) for GRP2. Swimmers in GRP1 experienced no significant fluctuations of serum enzyme activities throughout the study, although during the final week of training there was a tendency for CPK to rise (P = 0.20). There is no clear answer as to why the CPK levels were significantly elevated following the study in GRP2. These data suggest that there is great variability in muscle damage that occurs with training and that these markers may not always be a sensitive indicator of the training stress.

5 Conclusions

In conclusion, this study has illustrated that when moderately trained swimmers are subjected to a workload of 76 $\pm$ 2% $\dot{V}O_2$max for 60 min, 5 times a week, significant improvements in performance, aerobic power, and swimming efficiency are possible. Although 20 minutes of training did not result in significant improvements in swimming performance, this was adequate in maintaining aerobic power and enhancing efficiency.

6 References

Behnke, A.R. and Wilmore, J.H. (1969) An anthropometric estimation of body density and lean body weight in young men. **J. Appl. Physiol.**, 27, 25-31.

Bergstrom, J.. (1962) Muscle electrolytes in man. **Scand. J. Clin. Lab. Invest.** (Suppl.), 68, 1-15.

Clarkson, P.M. and Tremblay, I. (1988) Exercise-induced muscle damage, repair and adaptation in humans. **J. Appl. Physiol.**, 65, 1-6.

Costill, D.L., Fink, W.J., Van Handel, P.J., Miller, J.M., Sherman, W.M., Watson, P.A. and Witzmann, F.A. (1984) **Analytical Methods for the Measurement of Human Performance** (ed D.L. Costill), Ball State Univ., Muncie, Ind.

D'Acquisto, L.J., Bone, M., Takahashi, S., Langhans, G., Barzdukas, A.P. and Troup, J.P. (1990) Changes in aerobic power, swimming economy, and rating of perceived exertion as a result of reduced training volume. VIth International Symposium on Biomechanics and Medicine in Swimming, Liverpool.

Hollander, P.A., Troup, J.P. and Toussaint, H. (1990) Linear vs exponential extrapolation in swimming research. VIth International Symposium on Biomechanics and Medicine in Swimming, Liverpool.

Lowry, O.H. and Passoneau, J.V. (1972) **A Flexible Systems of Enzymatic Analysis.** Academic Press Inc., New York, pp. 120-128.

Nadel, E.R. (1985) Physiological adaptations to aerobic training. **American Scientist,** 73, 334-343.

Noakes, T.D. (1987) Effect of exercise on serum enzyme activities in humans. **Sports Med.,** 4, 245-267.

Saltin, B. and Rowell, B.L. (1980) Functional adaptations to physical activity and inactivity. **Fed. Proc.,** 39, 1506-1513.

CHANGES IN AEROBIC POWER AND SWIMMING ECONOMY AS A RESULT OF REDUCED TRAINING VOLUME

L.J. D'ACQUISTO, M. BONE, S. TAKAHASHI, G. LANGHANS, A.P. BARZDUKAS
and J.P. TROUP
U.S. Swimming, International Center for Aquatic Research, Colorado
Springs, Colorado, USA

Abstract
This investigation examined the metabolic changes for submaximal and
maximal swim efforts during a period of reduced training volume
(taper). Well trained high school swimmers were assigned to one of
two groups: GP1 (n = 7) and GP2 (n = 6) averaged 32 000 and 64 000
metres/week, respectively, for the month preceding the study. The
GP1 did not experience a reduction in training volume until wk3 and
wk4, whereas GP2 decreased their volume on a weekly basis for four
weeks. Subjects were tested pre- (P), mid- (M and post-study (PT).
Both GP1 and GP2 were able to maintain aerobic power (1 O_2/min) (P <
0.05) and improve performance (100 m and 200 m) (P < 0.05) despite an
approximate 65% (wk2 vs wk4) and 90% (P-wk4) reduction in training
volume, respectively. The aerobic demand (ml O_2/min/kg) for four
submaximal efforts decreased (P < 0.05) following the respective
tapers. Greatest shift in economy occurred between M and PT for GP1,
P and M for GP2. In conclusion: (1) a taper regimen which reduced
training volume and maintained previous intensity and frequency
resulted in enhancement of performance, no deterioration of aerobic
power and improved economy (2) the 2 wk taper was similar in
effectiveness to the 4 wk taper.
Keywords: Swimming, Taper, Economy, Aerobic Power.

1 Introduction

A common practice prior to major swimming competition is a reduction
in training volume and intensity, also known as taper (Costill et
al., 1985; Van Handel et al., 1988). It is felt that such practice
results in enhanced physiological and psychological preparation,
resulting in optimal performance (Costill et al., 1985). The purpose
of this investigation was to examine the physiological changes that
accompany a swim taper period in which training volume is reduced
while intensity and frequency of training remain constant.

2 Methods

2.1 Subjects and experimental design
Thirteen (males = 11, female = 2) well trained high school swimmers
(Table 1) participated in this investigation after signing an
informed letter of consent. Swimmers were assigned to one of two

groups, depending on previous training history. Group 1 (GP1; n = 7) and group 2 (GP2; n = 6) averaged approximately 32 000 and 64 000 metres per week, respectively, for the month preceding the study. The duration of the study was four weeks. For weeks 1 and 2, GP1 trained at approximately the same training volume as the previous month (mean = 30 miles/wk). Weeks 3 and 4 required that the training volume be reduced to 17 300 and 9 900 metres/wk, respectively. Group 2 swimmers reduced their training volume each week of the four week study, wk1 = 53 700, wk2 = 36 100, 2k3 = 22 500, wk4 = 11 400 metres/ wk. Groups were tested pre- (P; 2 days prior to wk1), mid- (M; immediately after wk2), and post-taper (PT; 2 days after the fourth week of taper).

A swimming economy profile ($\dot{V}O_2$ vs velocity) was determined for each subject. From these curves and review of training logs for the month prior to the taper, it was determined that of the total training volume, approximately 5% was swum at >120% of $\dot{V}O_2$max, 15% at 100-120% $\dot{V}O_2$max, 50% at 80-99% $\dot{V}O_2$max and the balance at < 80% of $\dot{V}O_2$max. Training frequency was six to seven sessions per week. Throughout this study workouts were evaluated weekly to ensure that overall intensity and frequency were maintained constant. The subjects had been tested in previous projects during the prior 12 months and consequently completely familiar with the testing procedures.

2.2 Testing procedures
Performance/training. One hundred and 200 m freestyle time trials (s) from a push-start were conducted pre- and post-taper.

Table 1. Characteristics of subjects - Mean $\pm$ SE

Group	Age (yrs)	Ht (cm)	Wt (kg)	Fat (%)
1	18.44 ± 0.96	176.66 ± 2.77	68.89 ± 3.31	11.56 ± 1.40
2	16.17 ± 0.94	179.49 ± 4.48)	67.85 ± 1.88	11.79 ± 1.29

Performance and training were supervised by two research assistants and a coach.

Metabolic. A swimming economy profile and $\dot{V}O_2$max were conducted P, M and PT. Prior to each session, body weight (kg) was measured, and percent body fat was determined from skinfolds (Behnke et al., 1969). All economy profiles were conducted in a flume (D'Acquisto et al., 1989).

Statistical analysis. Statistical comparisons were made using a MANOVA (SPSS) with the level of significance set a priori at $P < 0.05$. Post-hoc comparisons were performed using the Tukey LSD test.

3 Results

3.1 Antropometric measures
For Group 1, body weight and percent body fat were not significantly different between P, M and PT. Body weight (kg) was 69.89 ± 9.95, 68.56 ± 8.22 and 71.03 ± 9.45 for P, M and PT respectively. Percent

body fat was 11.56 ± 4.21, 12.61 ± 4.45 and 12.78 ± 4.19% respectively.

For Group 2, body weight and percent body fat were not significantly different between P, M and PT. Body weight (kg) was 67.85 ± 4.61, 67.30 ± 5.43 and 67.33 ± 4.93 for P, M and PT respectively. Percent body fat was 11.79 ± 3.17, 13.20 ± 4.25 and 12.66 ± 2.78% for P, M and PT, respectively.

3.2 Performance
In Group 1, performance for 100 m and 400 m, as measured at P and PT, improved 8 and 4%, respectively ($P < 0.05$). Time (s) (pre- vs post-taper) for performance swims were the following: 100 m, 64.11 ± 3.10 vs 59.01 ± 4.49; 400 m, 304.22 ± 8.76 vs 292.06 ± 14.47.

In Group 2, performance for 100 m and 400 m freestyle, as measured at P and PT, improved 7.7 and 6.4%, respectively ($P < 0.05$). Time (s) for performance swims were the following: 100 m, 60.58 ± 3.95 vs 57.28 ± 3.70; 400 m, 279.67 ± 14.65 vs 265.68 ± 16.94.

3.3 Maximal swim
The $\dot{V}O_2$max values for Group 1 were 3.59 ± 0.13, 3.49 ± 0.10, 3.78 ± 0.10 l/min, for P, M and PT, respectively, for GP1, $P < 0.05$. Peak lactate values (mM) for P, M and PT were: 8.89 ± 1.07, 8.89 ± 1.07, and 8.83 ± 0.95, respectively ($P z 0.05$). Maximal heart rates (beats/min) were 190 ± 3, 192 ± 3 and 187 ± 4 for P, M and PT. The PT HR max was significantly different from P and M.

For Group 2, the P, M and PT $\dot{V}O_2$max (l/min) values were the following: 3.48 ± 0.02, 3.45 ± 0.07 and 3.30 ± 0.09, respectively ($P < 0.05$). The mean peak lactate value for GP2 was found to be 42 percent higher for P vs PT measurements; however, because of great variability in the values this was a non-significant increase (5.11 ± 0.63, 7.35 ± 1.64 and 8.80 ± 2.54 mM for P, M and PT, respectively). Maximal HR (beats/min) values were 198.0 ± 2.19, 194.0 ± 3.10 and 185.0 ± 2.86 for P, M and PT, respectively. The PT HR max was significantly different from P and M.

3.4 Swimming economy
A downward shift in the economy curve occurred in Group 1 between M and PT. The greatest decrease in the economy profile was noted for M vs PT values. At 1.0, 1.1, 1.2 and 1.3 m/s a 4.9, 11.7*, 15.62* and 7.3* difference was found (*$P < 0.05$). Heart rate at 1.1, 1.2 and 1.3 m/s was found to decrease for M vs PT measurements (2.9, 3.0, 2.0 and 2.5%). The largest drop in lactate occurred at 1.2 and 1.3 m/s for M vs PT (15.1 and 26.1%, respectively). However, no session effect for heart rate and lactate at a given submaximal effort was noted. The peak lactate value between P vs M was 6.52 ± 1.76 vs 9.89 ± 3.03 mM ($P < 0.05$) with no further change between M vs P (8.83 ± 2.52 mM).

For Group 2, a downward shift in $\dot{V}O_2$ (ml/kg/min) values occurred at 1.0, 1.1, 1.2 and 1.3 m/s between P vs M. Differences were as follows: 16.4, 8.5, 16.7 and 15.6%, respectively. Although the session by swim percent difference is large, statistical significance was not reached, $P = 0.45$. No observable differences were noted in economy for M vs PT values at all four velocities. Between P-M, heart rate (beats/min) at 1.1, 1.2 and 1.3 m/s decreased by 2.9, 10.6 and 8.3% ($P < 0.05$ at 1.2 and 1.3 m/s), respectively with little shift occurring between M-PT. The lactate curve shifted downward at all velocities. The difference between M-PT lactate measurements for 1.0, 1.1, 1.2 and 1.3 m/s was 32.6, 26.6, 27.9 and 25.60%, respectively ($P > 0.05$).

4 Discussion

This study examined whether a 2 wk and 4 wk swim taper regimen which maintained previous training intensity and frequency while reducing volume would result in a deterioration or enhancement of swimming performance. Both groups were able to maintain aerobic power ($P < 0.05$) and improve performance ($P < 0.05$) during their respective taper despite an approximate 65% (wk2 vs wk4) and 80% (P vs wk4) reduction in training volume for GRPS 1 and 2, respectively. Studies have shown that about a 70% reduction in training results in no loss of conditioning and enhanced performance (Crossman et al., 1987) provided that the training intensity is maintained, which supports the findings of this investigation.

During tapering in swimmers in which the total distance swum progressively declined (7,500 yd, d1 to 3,500 yd, d13), performance (50 to 1650 yd) was found to improve an average of 3.1% (Costill et al., 1985). This improvement was attributed to significant improvement in muscular power. For GP1 and GP2, performances for 100 and 400 m improved 8 and 4%, 7.7 and 6.4%, respectively. Apparently, the tapers employed in the present study provided sufficient "rest", perhaps allowing the swimmers to develop better stroke mechanics, which was reflected by enhanced swimming economy.

In general, it is found that a "talented" swimmer is able to consume less oxygen at a given submaximal intensity than a "less talented" swimmer, primarily as a result of better mechanics (Holmer et al., 1980; Holmer et al., 1983). The taper in this study resulted in large downwards shifts in the economy curves for both groups, illustrating that the energy required at a given submaximal effort became less. The greatest change in the economy profile occurred when the training volume was initially decreased (wk2 vs wk4 for GRP1; pre-taper vs wk2 for GRP2), suggesting that changes in economy were dependent on volume.

5 Conclusions

In conclusion, coaches and athletes are often concerned that any major reduction in training volume may induce a detraining effect. This investigation has illustrated that a swim taper which maintains previous training intensity and frequency while reducing training volume results in enhanced swimming performance for 100 and 400 m. Furthermore, no deterioration of aerobic power occurred and swimming economy was improved despite large decreases in training volume.

6 References

Behnke, A.R. and Wilmore, J.H. (1969) An anthropometric estimation of body density and lean body weight in young men. **J. Appl.**

Physiol., 27, 25-31.

Costill, D.L., Fink, W.J., Hargreaves, M., King, D.S., Thomas, R. and Fielding, R.A. (1985) Metabolic characteristics of skeletal muscle during detraining from competitive swimming. **Med. Sci. Sports Exerc.**, 17, 339-343.

Costill, D.L., King, D.S., Thomas, R. and Hargreaves, M. (1985) Effects of reduced training on muscular power swimmers. **Physician Sportmed.**, 13, 91-101.

Crossman, J., Jamieson, J. and Henderson, L. (1987) Responses of competitive athletes to lay-offs in training: exercise addiction or psychological relief? **J. Sports Behav.**, 10, 28-38.

D'Acquisto, L.J., Troup, J. and Holmberg, S. (1989) Description and water velocity characteristics of a new swimming treadmill. **Proc. VIII World FINA Medical Congress on Aquatic Sports**, London, England, pp. 11-15.

Holmer, I. (1980) Physiology of swimming man, in **Exercise and Sport Sciences Reviews** (eds S.R. Hutton and I.D. Miller), pp. 87-123.

Holmer, I. (1983) Energetics and mechanical work in swimming, in **Biomechanics and Medicine in Swimming** (eds A.P. Hollander, P.A. Huijing and G. de Groot), Human Kinetics Publishers, Champaign, Ill., pp. 154-164.

Montpetit, R.R., Lavoie, J.M. and Cazorla, G.A. (1983) Aerobic energy cost of swimming the front crawl at high velocity in international class and adolescent swimmers, in **Biomechanics and Medicine in Swimming** (eds. A.P. Hollander, P.A. Huijing and G. de Groot), Human Kinetics Books, Champaign, Ill., pp. 228-267.

Neufer, P.D., Costill, D.L., Fielding, A.R., Flynn, G.M. and Kirwan, J.P. (1988) Effects of reduced training on muscular strength and endurance in competitive swimmers. **Med. Sci. Sports Exerc.**, 18, 486-490.

Van Handel, P.J., Katz, A., Troup, J.P., Daniels, J.T. and Bradley, P.W.L (1988) Oxygen consumption and blood lactic response to training and taper, in **Swimming Science V** (eds B.E. Ungerechts, K. Wilke and K. Reischle), Human Kinetics Books, Champaign, Ill., pp. 269-275.

Yamamoto, Y., Mutoh, Y. and Miyashita, M. (1988) Hematological and biochemical indices during the tapering period of competitive swimmers, in **Swimming Science V** (eds. B.E. Ungerechts, K. Wilke and K. Reischle), Human Kinetics Books, Champaign, Ill., pp. 243-249.

PHYSIOLOGICAL ADAPTATIONS TO SWIM TRAINING IN UNTRAINED FEMALE SWIMMERS

L.J. D'ACQUISTO, P. DURSTHOFF, S. SPRY, C. LETNER, S. BADGER and
J.P. TROUP
U.S. States Swimming, International Center for Aquatic Research,
Colorado Springs, Colorado, USA

Abstract
The effects of a 13 week swim training period were studied in
untrained high school females (n = 11, 16.1 ± 1.3 years). Dramatic
improvements in swimming performance, 91.44 and 182.88 m) occurred
throughout the entire season (P < 0.05). These improvements were
explained, in part, by enhanced aerobic power (P < 0.05) and an
increase in maximal stroke frequency (P z 0.05). Indirect markers of
muscle membrane damage, creatine phosphokinase (CPK), lactate
dehydrogenase (LDH) and serum oxaloacetate transaminase (SGOT) were
found to be sensitive indicators of the training load. Furthermore,
a drop in volume of training during the first two weeks of the three
week taper (66%), and a 37% drop in frequency, while maintaining
intensity (90-100% HR max) of training, did not decrease aerobic
power and resulted in an enhancement of swimming performance. This
is of importance to the coach and athlete who feel that reductions in
the training load late in the season may lead to a detraining effect.
Keywords: Physiology, Muscle Membrane Damage, Aerobic Power, Training
Volume.

1 Introduction

A systematic training regimen is important and usually involves
periodization, which is a process of dividing the training season
into phases. Studies have examined the interrelationship between
swimming performance and physiological adaptations to swim training
over prolonged periods of time (Eriksson et al., 1977). Few studies
have provided insight into the adaptations which occur within phases
of the swim season especially in young inexperienced female swimmers.
  Additionally, if the athlete fails to recover and adapt properly
from the training overload (Kuipers and Keizer, 1988) and performance
is not enhanced or deteriorates, then the athlete is overtrained.
During overtraining plasma activities of muscle enzymes may be
increased (Kuipers and Keizer, 1988; Noakes, 1987). Investigators
have concluded that the levels of these markers, such as increased
serum activity of creatine phosphokinase and lactate dehydrogenase
provide information regarding the status of the muscle cell membrane.
Information regarding the effect of swim training on the fluctuation
of serum markers of overtraining during various phases of the season
is minimal.
  In view of the above the purposes of the following investigation

were to answer the following: (1) what basic physiological changes occur during various phases of the swim season in individuals who have had little swim training and (2) are serum markers of muscle membrane damage sensitive markers of the training load?

2 Methods

2.1 Experimental design

Thirteen females with minimal swim training experience participated in this study after being informed of the risks associated with the project and signing an letter of informed consent. Subject characteristics were age (mean $\pm$ SE) 16 $\pm$ 1.3 years, height 163.1 $\pm$ 5.0 cm, weight 54.82 $\pm$ 1.82, percent adipose tissue 19.01 $\pm$ 0.37). The swim season was 13 weeks in duration. Subjects were tested pre-season (P), mid (M, following 7 weeks of training, mainly averaging 60-70% HR max, 4400 m per session (ses), 9 ses/wk), pre-taper (PT) (after three weeks of intense training, major workouts at 90-100% HR max, 6900 m/ses, 8 ses/wk), and post-season (PS) (following 3 weeks of taper in which volume was reduced by 66% during the first two weeks), frequency was reduced by 37%, and intensity maintained as the previous 3 weeks of training. A workout log was kept by the coach and reviewed weekly by coach and research staff.

2.2 Testing procedures

Performance/body composition. Swimmers performed a 100 yd (91.44 m) and 200 yd (181.88 m) time trial from a push-off start. Time trials were performed at each test period (P, M, PT, PS). Body weight and percent body fat were determined using a Health-o-meter clinical weighing scale and skinfolds, respectively (Behnke and Wilmore, 1969). Measurements were done by the same individual throughout the study.

Metabolic. Subjects performed a submaximal swim (0.9 m/s) and a maximal swim for the determination of $\dot{V}O_2$max in a swimming treadmill using an on-line metabolic system (Ametk Metabolic Analyzers; Rayfield). The submaximal swim was five minutes in duration. Subjects swam at 0.9 m/s for the first two minutes of the max test, thereafter the velocity of the water was increased 0.05 m/s every 30 s until volitional exhaustion (5-7 min).

Blood analysis. A resting morning blood sample from an antecubital vein was taken between 06:00-07:00 hours of each measurement period. To standardize the procedure, subjects were informed to fast 12 hours preceding the blood draw. In addition, swimmers completed a workout of moderate intensity on the day prior to all blood draws. To indirectly assess muscle membrane status the following variables were measured: creatinine phosphokinase (CPK) (IU/l), lactate dehydrogenase (LDH) (IU/l), serum glutamic oxaloacetic transaminase (SGOT) (IU/l) (Spectrophotometry, ABBOTT-Spectrum). Haemoglobin (Hb, g/dl), haematocrit (Hct, %), and red blood cell count (RBC) (1.10^{-6}/μl) measurements were done on a Sysmex Particle Counter.

Statistics. A MANOVA (SPSS) for repeated measures with the level of significance set a priori at $P < 0.05$ was used to determine a session effect. Post-hoc comparisons were performed using the Tukey LSD test. Data are presented as mean $\pm$ SE.

3 Results

3.1 Anthropometric/performance.
There were significant changes in body weight (kg) and percent body fat throughout the season (Table 1). Significant improvements were also noted for both 100 (91.44 m) and 200 (181.88 m) yd performance swims (P < 0.05, Table 1).

Table 1. Body composition and performance changes

Variables	P	M	PT	PS
Body wt (kg)	54.82	53.33*	52.76*	53.77
	± 1.82	± 1.68	± 1.65	± 1.56
Body fat (%)	19.0	16.5*	15.8*+	15.2*+
	± 0.4	± 0.4	± 0.4	± 0.2
91.44 m (s)	80.5	79.5	76.7*	73.7*+o
	± 1.54	± 1.33	± 1.08	± 0.86
181.88 (s)	189.1	174.8*	164.5*+	159.2
	± 4.0	± 2.2	± 1.8	± 1.6

*P < 0.05, vs P; +P < 0.05, vs M; °P < 0.05, vs PT

3.2 Maximal and submaximal swimming
Refer to Table 2 for mean ± SE values. The $\dot{V}O_2$max progressively improved during the first three measurement periods (P < 0.05) with no further improvement between PS vs PT. Maximum heart rate (beats/min) was found to decrease between P vs M and increase after very intensive training (M vs PT) with no further change between PT and P. Heart rate for a submaximal swim was found to decrease significantly (P vs M) and increase after intense training. With taper the heart rate response returned to mid season values. The blood lactate level for a submaximal effort decreased between P and M, with no further change during the remainder of the season.

Table 2. Metabolic change during swim training

Variables	P	M	PT	PSW
$\dot{V}O_2$ (1 O_2/min):				
Maximal	2.16	2.36*	2.62*+	2.72*+
	± 0.10	± 0.10	± 0.09	± 0.05
Submaximal	1.58	1.55	1.66	1.55
(0.90 m/s)	± 0.04)	± 0.06	± 0.05	± 0.03
Heart rate (beats/min):				
Maximal	185.3	177.7*	191.4+	191.0+
	± 3.2	± 2.0	± 2.7	± 4.2
Submaximal	154.8	141.4*	149.4+	140.0*o
(0.90 m/s)	± 2.6	± 3.9	± 3.6	± 2.9
Lactate (mM):				
Maximal	7.49	6.82	6.95	8.43
	± 0.32	± 0.49	± 0.58	± 0.64
Submaximal	4.06	2.70*	2.18*	2.70*
	± 0.32	± 0.26	± 0.19	± 0.22

*P < 0.05, vs P; +P < 0.05, vs M; °P < 0.05, vs PT

3.3 Indirect serum markers of muscle membrane damage

A significant decrease in CPK (IU/l) occurred between P vs M, with no change in LDH (IU/l). With intense swim training CPK and LDH were found to increase, M vs PT, followed by a decrease after three weeks of taper, PT vs PS, $P < 0.05$ (CPK: P = 164.6 $\pm$ 22.9, M = 109.9 $\pm$ 13.4), PT = 144.3 $\pm$ 18.7, PS = 72.6 $\pm$ 5.8 IU/l; LDH: P = 162.1 $\pm$ 12.2, M = 149.0 $\pm$ 6.6, PT = 176.6 $\pm$ 6.8, PS = 135.0 $\pm$ 4.3). SGOT was found to decrease between P vs M (P < 0.05; 26.3 $\pm$ 3.3 vs 22.4 $\pm$ 3.1 respectively), and rise (25.0 $\pm$ 2.9) toward P values during intense training (P > 0.05). Following taper SGOT dropped to 21.2 $\pm$ 2.6, significantly different from P and M values.

3.4 Haematology

The Hb and Hct values were found to significantly decrease between P vs M and PT, with a return to P values following a three week taper. The PS values were significantly different from M and PT (Hb: P = 14.8 $\pm$ 0.2, M = 14.2 $\pm$ 0.2, PT = 14.3 $\pm$ 0.3, and PS = 15.0 $\pm$ 0.2; Hct: P = 43.9 $\pm$ 0.6, M = 41.4 $\pm$ 0.7, PT = 41.2 $\pm$ 0.8, PS = 44.6 $\pm$ 0.7). The RBC (1.10/μl) did not change significantly throughout the season, P = 4.85 $\pm$ 0.08; M = 4.65 $\pm$ 0.05; PT = 4.67 $\pm$ 0.08; PS = 4.79 $\pm$ 0.08.

4 Discussion

Swimming performance for 100 (91.44 m) and 200 (181.88 m) yd freestyle improved during each macrocycle of the season. These improvements can be explained, in part, by the significant increases in aerobic power ($\dot{V}O_2$max). Despite the dramatic decreases in training volume over the final three weeks, $\dot{V}O_2$max (1 O_2/min) was maintained while performance continued to improve. Training frequency was also reduced during the taper (37%) while intensity was maintained the same (90–100% max HR). This suggests that a three week period of reducing training volume did not compromise aerobic power or performance.

The $\dot{V}O_2$ at a given submaximal effort remained unchanged throughout the season while the heart rate response significantly decreased, suggesting an increase in stroke volume (Brooks and Fahey, 1984). An explanation for no improvement in swimming economy may be the selection of the 0.90 m/s speed. With training, this pace became "very easy", resulting in a pace which was not within the normal intensity of training (for 0.90 m/s, P = 75% vs PS = 55% $\dot{V}O_2$max). A pace of 0.90 m/s, therefore, did not allow for the measurement of any true changes in swimming economy midway and late into the season. The blood lactate level (mM) at 0.90 m/s significantly decreased after seven weeks of training with no further change over the next six weeks. This implied that major adaptations of those processes which enhance the body's ability to remove lactate from the blood, i.e. clearance of lactate by the liver (Donovan and Brooks, 1983), and use of lactate as fuel substrate (Brooks, 1988), occurred during the first phase of the season.

During the first seven weeks of training, the level of enzyme activities of CPK, LDH and SGOT fell. A subsequent three week period of intense training resulted in significantly elevated activities of CPK and LDH relative to M. A three week taper resulted in a decrease in serum activities of CPK, LDH and SGOT, relative to PT. Despite the elevated CPK levels following three weeks of intense training, swimming performance times improved ($P < 0.05$). During the intense training period, swimmers were complaining of feeling heavy, sluggish, and generally tired. Therefore, it should be considered that elevated indirect markers of muscle membrane damage may not always necessarily indicate an overtrained condition. The elevation of these markers appears to be a normal response to the intense training load.

This study also illustrated a sports anaemia if one compares M and PT haemoglobin and haematocrit values to P values (Yoshimura et al., 1970). However, these values are all within the normal physiological range. The RBC count did not change during this time frame, suggesting that the decreases in Hb and Hct may have been due to a plasma volume expansion (Williams, 1983). During taper Hb and Hct values were found to return P values. Return of these values to P level seems to be dependent on training volume, since this was the primary factor manipulated during the taper. This supports the earlier discussion on plasma volume expansion based on reduced heart rate response for submaximal swimming (0.90 m/s) without any corresponding change in $\dot{V}O_2$ requirement.

5 Conclusions

In conclusion, a 13 week swim season resulted in dramatic swimming performance improvements. An elevation of indirect markers of muscle membrane damage did not indicate an overtrained state but more of an overworked state. In addition, a decrease in haemoglobin and haematocrit within the normal physiological range did not compromise performance, but appeared to be a normal response to training.

6 References

Behnke, A.R. and Wilmore, J.H. (1969) An anthropometric estimation of body density and lean body weight in young men. **J. Appl. Physiol.**, 27, 25-31.

Brooks, G.A. and Fahey, T.D. (1984) **Exercise Physiology: Human Bioenergetics and its Application.** John Wiley and Sons, New York, pp. 330-336.

Brooks, G.A. (1988) Blood lactate acid: Sports "Bad Boy" turns good. **Sports Gatorade Exchange,** Gatorade Sports Science Institute, Chicago, Ill., 1, April.

Costill, D.L., Flynn, M., Kirwan, J.P., Houmard, J.A., Mitchell, J.B., Thomas, R. and Sun Han Park (1988) Effect of repeated days of intensified training on muscle glycogen and swimming performance. **Med. Sci. Sports Exerc.**, 20(3), 249-254.

Donovan, C.M. and Brooks, G.A. (1983) Training affects lactate clearance, not lactate production. **Am. J. Physiol.**, 244, E83-E92.

Eriksson, B.O., Holmer, I. and Lundin, A. (1977) Physiological effects of training in elite swimmers, in **Swimming Medicine IV** (eds B. Eriksson and B. Furberg), University Park Press, Baltimore, MD, pp. 177-187.

Eriksson, B.O., Berg, K. and Taranger, J. (1977) Physiological analysis of young boys starting intensive training in swimming., in **Swimming Medicine IV** (eds B. Eriksson and B. Furberg), University Park Press, Baltimore, MD, pp. 147-160.

Gullstrand, L. and Holmer, I. (1983) Physiological characteristics of champion swimmers during a five-year follow-up period, in **Biomechanics and Medicine in Swimming** (eds A.P. Hollander, P.A. Huijing, G. de Groot), Human Kinetics Publishers, Champaign, Ill., pp. 258-262.

Kuipers, H. and Keizer, H.A. (1988) Overtraining in elite athletes: Review and directions for the future. **Sports Med.**, 6, 79-92.

Millard, M., Zauner, C., Cade, R. and Reese, R. (1985) Serum CPK levels in male and female world class swimmers during a season of training. **J. Swimming Res.**, 1(2), 12-16.

Noakes, T.D. (1987) Effect of exercise on serum enzyme activities. **Sports Med.**, 4, 245-267.

Nomura, T. (1983) The influence of training and age on $\dot{V}O_2$ max during swimming in Japanese elite age group and Olympic swimmers, in **Biomechanics and Medicine in Swimming** (eds A.P. Hollander, P.A. Huijing and G. de Groot), Human Kinetics Publishers, Champaign, Ill., pp. 251-257.

Ryan, A.J., Brown, R.L., Frederick, E.C., Falsetti, H.L. and Burke, R.E. (1983) Overtraining of athletes; a round table. **Physician Sportsmed.**, 11 (6), 93-110.

Toussaint, H.M. (1988) Mechanics and energetics of swimming. Doctoral Dissertation. Vrije Universiteit, Amsterdam.

Williams, M.H. (ed) (1983) **Ergogenic Aids in Sports.** Human Kinetics Publishers, Champaign, Ill., p. 31.

Yoshimura, H. (1970) Anaemia during physical training (sports anaemia). **Nutr. Rev.**, 28, 251-253.

ANALYSIS OF DELAYED TRAINING EFFECTS IN THE PREPARATION OF THE WEST GERMAN WATER POLO TEAM FOR THE 1988 OLYMPIC GAMES

A. HOHMANN
University of Stuttgart, Germany

Abstract
This study investigated the variations in the timescale of adaptation to endurance training using the German national water polo players preparing for the Fifth World Championships in 1986. Regression analysis was used on the training and performance data collected, and this highlighted the fact that four players peaked from endurance training in the days immediately prior to the championships whereas four others peaked after the championships. A repeat analysis performed on these players in preparation for the 1988 Olympic Games produced similar results, thus verifying the stability of this training adaptation.
Keywords: Water Polo, Endurance Training, Adaptation.

1 Introduction

In order to optimize training for effective sports performance, there is a need to perform detailed analysis on each individual to determine any possibility of a delayed training effect (Werchoshanskij, 1988). The athlete should train to reach peak performance at the required time. This study was designed to investigate the likelihood of a delayed training effect (DTE) following endurance training using German national water polo players. A repeat, follow-up study was performed two years after the initial investigation in order to check for stability of the training response.

2 Methods

A computer aided training documentation (CTD) was obtained for eight male players of the German national water polo squad both in preparation for the 1986 World Championships and for the 1988 Olympic Games (Fig. 1). The CTD involved recording all the training details as well as the performance details in terms of official games and daily scrimmages over a three month period prior to the championships. The collected data were then subjected to regression analysis. The dependent variable, game performance index (GPI), was assessed using the game observation system for water polo (Hohmann, 1985). The first stage involved production of individual graphs of the GPI and the daily total training load (TTL) as depicted in Fig. 2.

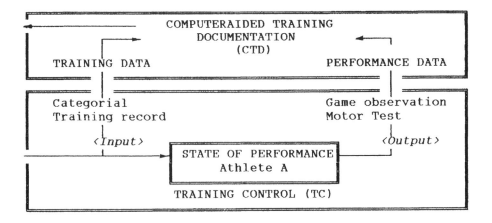

Fig. 1. Training control (TC) by training record and game observation resp. motor test as basis of the CTD.

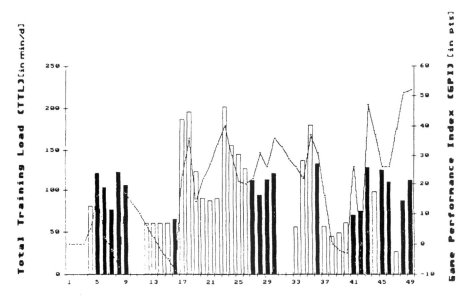

Fig. 2. Time series of the GPI and TTL of player ST in the course of preparation for the 1986 World Championships (from Hohmann, 1988) .

The second stage involved the statistical explanation of the GPI using TTL on a certain number of preceding days as independent variables. Equation (1) results from a regression analysis of time series and provides information on the GPI for player ST on any day of competition (DOC) on the basis of a polynomial distributed lag model (Pindyck and Rubinfeld, 1986). In the following example the analysis includes the TTL of the previous seven days (with t statistics in parentheses):

$$GPI_{DOC} = -57.357 + 0.11TTL^{0}_{DOC} + 0.86TTL^{0-1}_{DAY} + 0.67TTL^{0-2}_{DAY}$$
$$(-2.92) \qquad (3.71) \qquad\quad (3.85) \qquad\qquad (3.85)$$
$$+ 0.57TTL^{0-3}_{DAY} + 0.55TTL^{0-4}_{DAY} + 0.61TTL^{0-5}_{DAY} + 0.77TTL^{0-6}_{DAY}$$
$$(2.94) \qquad\quad (2.85) \qquad\qquad (3.18) \qquad\qquad (3.45)$$
$$+ 0.10TTL^{0-7}_{DAY}$$
$$3.27$$
$$(R^2 = 0.42; \ DW = 2.00) \tag{1}$$

3 Results and discussion

The results for the investigated Partial Training Load in swimming endurance training (PTL$_{end}$) led to players being assigned to two groups (Fig. 3, a,b). The first group showed an "early" delayed training effect (DTE) and consisted of players HU, JA, ST and OT. The second group of "late" DTEs included the players OS, EH, TH and FE. In the five days immediately before important games, the first training group showed positive adaptations to high volumes of endurance swim training. It seems that these players have higher aerobic abilities. The players in the second group exhibited a decrease in game performance over the same period. Hence positive adaptations after high volumes of endurance training should follow later. However, this was only verified for the player OS between the preceding 7th to 13th day. It was assumed that the players of the second group have lower aerobic abilities, or take longer to adapt.

On the basis of the results from the 1986 analysis the eight players who remained in the Olympic Team, were separated into two training groups with different partial training loads in swimming endurance (PTL$_{end}$) and game training (PTL$_{game}$). It was assumed that the determination of the individual characteristics of an early or late DTE on the findings of only one single training process did not lead to conclusive results. Thus the investigations were repeated in the course of the preparation for the 1988 Olympic Games. The success of the practical application of these findings together with the results of the repeated study on the individual DTE in swimming endurance training confirm:

(a) a high stability over a long time period, and
(b) a high stability against different models of training structure.

All four national players with an early DTE in swimming endurance training before the 1986 World Championships could also be assigned to the same group in 1988. Of the three players with a late DTE in swimming endurance training in 1986 two showed nearly identical results in 1988.

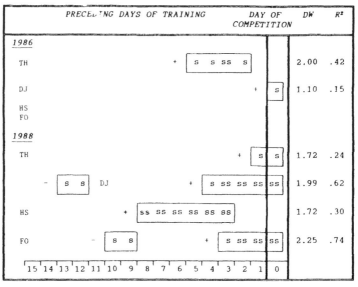

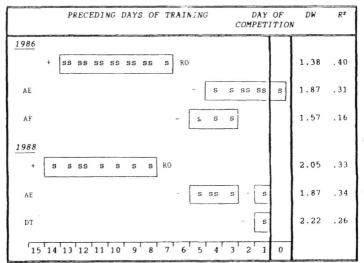

Fig. 3. Individual Delayed Training Effects (DTE) of (a) four water polo national players with early and (b) four players with late adaptations following high-volume endurance training in the course of preparation for the 1986 World Championships and the 1988 Olympic Games.

4 Conclusion

This study is based on the control, documentation and statistical
analysis of two training processes of the West German water polo
national team. In summary, the findings verify that for a two-year
time period the stability of the individual timescale for training
adaptations in dependence of the time period and the volume of the
swimming endurance training in the course of training processes.
Thus, the need for individualizing the contents, volumes and
temporal structure of endurance training for water polo is
emphasized. One can hypothesize that similar findings may occur in
other team and individual sports.

5 References

Hohmann, A. (1985) **Zur Struktur der komplexen Sportspielleistung.**
    Czwalina Verlag, Ahrensburg.
Hohmann, A. (1988) Zur Analyse zeitlich verzögerter Trainings-
    effekte im Sportspiel. **Leistungssport,** 5, 32-37.
Pindyck, R.S. and Rubinfeld, D.L. (1986) Econometric Models and
    Economic Forecasts. McGraw-Hill Inc., Singapore.
Werchozhanskij, J.W. (1988) **Effektiv trainieren.** Sportverlag,
    Berlin (Ost).

FORCE AND VELOCITY CHARACTERISTICS OF LAND TRAINING DEVICES IN SWIMMING

J. KLAUCK and K. DANIEL
Deutsche Sporthochschule, Köln, Germany

Abstract
The specific objectives of this study are the presentation and
discussion of mechanical parameters – force, velocity and mechanical
power – measured during land training of swimmers performing imitated
armstrokes (breaststroke or dolphin). The training devices used were
stretch cords, an isokinetic mini-gym, and a latissimus machine.
Force measurements were made by the means of a strain gauge cell
fixed between the traction rope and the hand of the swimmer. The
velocity-time curve of the hand was measured by using an ultra-sound
Doppler-system. The mechanical power was obtained by analogue
multiplication of force and velocity data. The forces measured
reached maximal values of 200-300 N, the peak "stroke" velocity of
the hand varied between 1 and 4 m/s. Maximum values of the
mechanical power up to 500 W were obtained. It is shown that an
imitation of arm strokes in swimming cannot be performed in the
force, velocity and time domain simultaneously. Furthermore, the
mechanical characteristics of the training devices used yield
different time distributions of force and/or velocity and/or
mechanical power within the armstroke cycle.
Keywords: Swimming Training, Training Devices, Armstroke, Traction
Rope, Isokinetic, Latissimus Machine, Force, Velocity, Mechanical
Power.

1 Introduction

The training devices to be discussed here can be characterised by the
possibility of executing cyclic arm or leg movements in order to
allow more or less perfect imitations of the arm or leg activities
in the water during swimming. This is valid especially for the
movements of the arms, which are important in the achievement of good
swimming performance. Special aspects of the comparison: swimming
movement/land training movement are given by the physical parameters:
kinematics of the hand, forces exerted and their dependence on time,
and the mechanical power generated.

2 Methods

Two test subjects (male and female) were involved in the experiments
using traction ropes, mini-gym and a latissimus machine. Both

individuals - swimmers - were familiar with the training devices and performed several tests under different conditions. A schematic view of the experiment set-up such as for the traction rope measurements is given in Fig. 1.

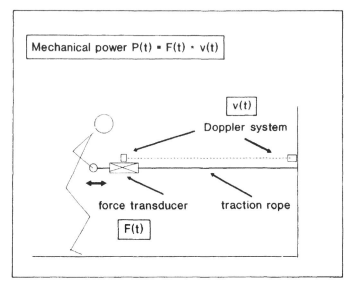

Fig. 1.   Measurement of pulling force F(t) and velocity v(t) during armstroke training by means of a traction rope.

Force measurements were made by means of a strain gauge load cell fixed between traction rope and the hand grip. The velocity was measured using a Doppler-velocimeter. The direction of force and velocity measurements is in every case given by the orientation of the traction rope. The mechanical power was obtained by analogue multiplication of force and velocity with each other. All measured parameters were stored by a multichannel tape recording.

3 Results

3.1 Traction rope measurements

According to the elastic properties of the traction rope the maximal force is developed at the end of the armstroke when maximal elongation of the rope occurs. An example of measured time curves of force and velocity combined with the mechanical power is given in Fig. 2.

The velocity curve corresponds to the derivative of the force curve as claimed by elasticity theory. Furthermore, the absolute value of the forces applied depends on the initial length of the rope, and the maximal force must be developed at the end of the armstroke when the elongation of the rope is maximal. The close connection between elongation of the rope and the force reduces the possibilities of training with respect to the force domain, while the kinematics of the arm movement can be chosen freely according to the

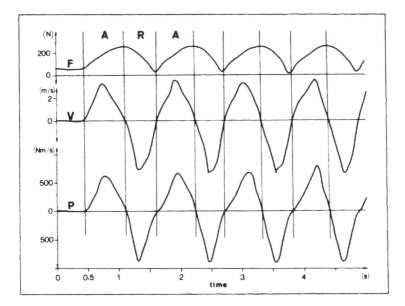

Fig. 2. Force (F), velocity (v) and mechanical power (P) in
armstroke land training by means of a traction rope.

special training aims. The maximal mechanical power is delivered in
the middle of the armstroke, possibly favourable for muscular
training. A further advantage is given by the fact that in the arm-
stroke/recovery-cycle a change of muscular work takes place from
concentric to eccentric mode, but it must be kept in mind that there
are no rest intervals in the cycle. For this reason, endurance
training using a traction rope seems not to be advisable. As the
quantitative parameters of the training are strongly influenced by
the elastic properties of the rope, it is useful to check them now
and then. A result of this is given in Fig. 3. Here we find the
force-length curves for two ropes of the same original quality, but
of different usage time.

It can be seen that the worn rope shows not only lesser starting
force values (length 2.5 m) but additionally the "spring constant" D
has changed to lower values, too. So, an athlete using such a device
would perform training in a lower force interval than possibly
intended, and the training effect of his exercise may be very low.

3.2 Isokinetic training device - mini-gym
The use of "isokinetic" training devices in swimming is based on the
imitation of the force-velocity relation found for the movements of
the extremities in the water. It is intended to generate great
constant forces at a constant angular velocity. In this case, a
regulation process between ·athlete and machine takes place. A
typical example as a result of the necessary adaptation is shown in
Fig. 4. The diagrams show relatively constant values for both parameters combined with minima in the middle of the armstroke, possibly
caused by the transition from pulling to pushing phase, suggesting a

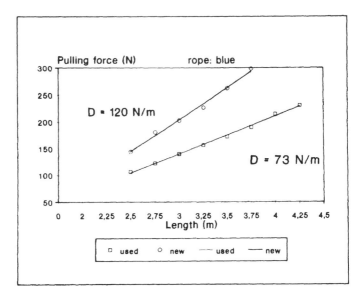

Fig. 3.   Length-dependent pulling forces of two traction ropes of
          different conditions.   D denotes the spring-constant.

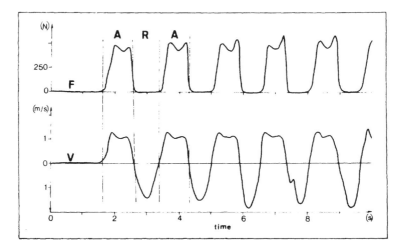

Fig. 4.   Force (F) and velocity (v)/time curves of imitated swimming
          movements using a mini gym.
          A: armstroke, R: recovery

lack of continuity in force development. The maximal value of the
velocity of the hand does not exceed 1.5 m/s (depending on the
setting of the machine) - the imitation of the swimming motion is not
perfect in the velocity domain. Additionally, the recovery time is
determined by the device and not by the swimmer, limiting the

possibility of choosing the duration and the rate of the armstroke during the training process.

3.4 Latissimus machine
This device uses the gravity forces of masses and the athlete is required to move up and down. The parameters to be defined are the starting and the final positions of the hands and the masses to be moved. With respect to the kinematics of the movement there exist unlimited possibilities to perform the imitated swimming arm motion – demanding a quantitative control of the armstroke kinematics. This can be done most effectively by measuring the acceleration of the masses moved, giving information about the kinematic parameters as well as about the inertial forces to be exerted, often being neglected by coaches and athletes. Here, nearly all parameters in the time, velocity and force domain can be chosen depending on the special objectives of the training phase.

4 Conclusions

The physical character of land training devices in swimming such as traction ropes, isokinetic mini-gyms or latissimus machines is decisive for the forces, the velocity and their distribution in the imitated armstroke and leg kick. Therefore, a knowledge of the physical properties is of great importance in order to grant a correct application of the devices in the training process, demanding the definition of training objectives using quantitative physical parameters, but also offering a training control on the basis of measurements performed.

PART SIX

LACTATE METABOLISM

A STUDY OF BLOOD LACTATE PROFILES ACROSS DIFFERENT SWIM STROKES

M. KELLY[*], G. GIBNEY[*], J. MULLINS[**], T. WARD[*], B. DONNE[**] and M. O'BRIEN[*]
[*]Trinity College, Dublin; [**]Newpark Sport Centre, Newpark, Co.
Dublin, Eire.

Abstract
Freestyle swims of varying frequency and intensity are recommended
for the determination of specific training programmes for competitive
swimmers. This study compared lactate and heart rate responses to
swims of the same relative intensity in all four basic swimming
strokes. Eleven swimmers (five females, six males) took part in the
study. Individual speeds, blood lactates and heart rates were
monitored during 4 × 200 m swims performed at four different
intensities between 80% and maximum in each of the four basic strokes
and in the medley. Multiple correlation analysis showed the
existence of significant correlation between speeds at the onset of
blood lactate accumulation for all strokes ($P < 0.01$). Significant
correlations were also found for maximum speeds across strokes ($P < 0.01$). The interstroke speed conversion ratio was constant at both
the onset of blood lactate accumulation and maximum effort in all
strokes. Lactate levels were more variable across strokes at
different swimming intensities. Heart rates also showed great
variability. The results of this study show that the most
significant stroke correlations are found using speed rather than
lactate or heart rate comparisons.
Keywords: Blood Lactate, Interstroke Speed Conversion, Heart Rate.

1 Introduction

Blood lactate responses to freestyle swims of various distances are
widely used to devise suitable training schedules. Recommended tests
include the Zwei-Streken-Test developed in 1975, which requires 2 ×
200 m freestyle swims, one at a lactate level of 4 mM and the other
at maximum effort. The two speed freestyle test was also recommended
by Madsen et al. (1984) and by Howat et al. (1990). Test sets
consisting of two or three 400 m freestyle swims are also commonly
used. Keskinen et al. (1989) recommended a combination of tests by
performing an incremental set with several steady state loadings
(aerobic) and one or two 100 m swims (anaerobic) in one test session.
Knowledge of a swimmer's lactate pattern enables the coach to
introduce specific swim speeds in training which will result in
fastest aerobic and anaerobic improvement and reduce the amount of
training time required. Race pace can be predicted and race strategy
altered to suit the capacity of the swimmer. Overtraining can be
identified early and prevented. Levels of blood lactate rise as a

result of imbalance between lactic acid production by exercising
muscles and rates of lactate removal by oxidation and/or reconversion
to glycogen. The size and location of the muscle mass involved in
the exercise will therefore have a very important effect on blood
lactate patterns. Each of the four different strokes – freestyle,
butterfly, breast and back – involve different groups of exercising
muscles. This study was designed to evaluate the similarities to,
and differences in, lactate profiles and heart rate responses in all
four basic strokes and in an individual medley swim.

2 Methods

Eleven swimmers volunteered for the study. They included six males
and five females of mean age 17.7 ($\pm$ 2.7) years. Characteristics of
performance are included in Table 1. It was a basic requirement of
the study that all swimmers were competent at individual medley swims
and the entire study was completed in a period of seven days to
obviate the effects of changes in training, climate, environment and
anthropometry. The tests were performed in a 25 m indoor, heated
swimming pool in randomised order. Each swimmer was tested for
resting blood lactate levels and then requested to swim four 200 m
swims at 85, 90, 95 and 100% of his/her personal best (PB) speed for
each particualr stroke. Swimming split times were monitored by stop-
watch from the poolside. At the end of each 200 m swim, heart rate
and blood lactate were measured and the swimmer did not commence the
next swim until blood lactate returned to resting levels. Heart
rates were measured by carotid palpation immediately the swim fini-
shed and before leaving the pool. Blood samples were taken from
either fingertip or ear lobe and were processed immediately in a
Yellow Spring lactate analyser (model 27). Because of constraint of
pool and subject availability, blood samples were taken 10 minutes
after swim completion, in each test; this means that all lactate
values stated were circa 1 mM below peak lactate values.
   Comparison of mean data for males and females was carried out
using a two-tailed Student's t test. Comparison of results across
strokes was performed using a two tailed paired student t test.
Investigation of relationships between strokes was performed using
linear regression analysis (least squares fit method) with statistical analysis of correlation coefficients.

3 Results

The swimming intensities requested were 85, 90, 95 and 100% of PB
times for 200 m in each stroke. The actual intensities achieved
varied between 83 and 97.5% (Table 2). Since PB times were invaria-
bly achieved in competition it would be unreasonable to expect
swimmers to achieve these times without tapering and the motivation
associated with competition. The percentages shown indicated
reasonable progression of effort and acceptable uniformity across all
strokes.
   Determination of speed at the onset of blood lactate accumulation
(V-OBLA) was based on each swimmer's lactate profile for the four
swims in each stroke (Figure 1). Two slopes were identified. In

Table 1. Characteristics of subjects. Best performance in metres per second.

Males			Females		
Stroke	Irish record	Personal best	Stroke	Irish record	Personal best
Breast	1.52	1.32 ± 0.15	Breast	1.29	1.17 ± 0.05
Back	1.66	1.37 ± 0.09	Back	1.47	1.25 ± 0.04
Butterfly	1.61	1.43 ± 0.14	Butterfly	1.45	1.32 ± 0.07
Free	1.79	1.66 ± 0.10	Free	1.61	1.49 ± 0.05
IM	1.64	1.50 ± 0.12	IM	1.42	1.33 ± 0.05

Table 2. 200 m sets as a % of personal best times ± SD

Stroke		Swim 1	Swim 2	Swim 3	Swim 4
Breast	M	86.74 ± 2.77	89.58 ± 2.16	92.41 ± 2.98	95.36 ± 2.61
	F	86.99 ± 1.14	90.01 ± 1.24	92.34 ± 1.43	95.01 ± 1.65
Back	M	87.71 ± 2.35	92.08 ± 2.20	94.75 ± 1.24	97.08 ± 2.29
	F	87.06 ± 1.62	90.22 ± 0.89	93.06 ± 2.01	96.07 ± 2.52
B'Fly	M	87.04 ± 4.20	90.35 ± 3.96	93.77 ± 3.10	95.58 ± 3.70
	F	85.25 ± 2.49	89.56 ± 3.53	91.57 ± 2.85	94.67 ± 3.43
Free	M	83.43 ± 3.21	88.39 ± 1.80	91.67 ± 1.55	95.08 ± 1.99
	F	85.56 ± 1.45	88.08 ± 2.53	90.35 ± 2.08	92.99 ± 1.04
IM	M	83.33 ± 2.18	87.75 ± 2.27	91.32 ± 1.67	94.17 ± 0.86
	F	85.51 ± 3.02	89.83 ± 1.81	90.74 ± 1.78	93.25 ± 1.01

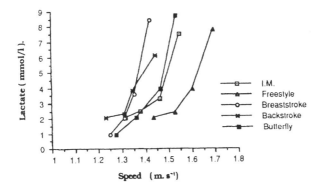

Fig. 1. An individual's lactate profile across all strokes.

each case a line was drawn through the two points obtained from Swim 3 and Swim 4 and continued downwards to its points of intersection with a slope incorporating at least two of the three lower points i.e. resting. Swim 1 and Swim 2 lactates. Both lactate in mM and speed in m/s were obtained from this point of intersection.

Comparing speed at V-OBLA in m/s across all strokes (see Figure 2)

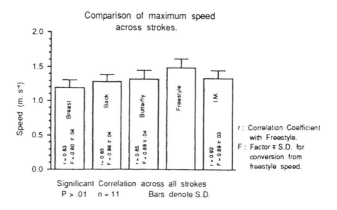

Fig. 2. Comparison of speed at V-OBLA across strokes.

it was apparent that the highest speed at V-OBLA occurred in
freestyle. When the speeds at V-OBLA for all other strokes were
compared to freestyle, correlation coefficients of r = 0.75, 0.76,
0.77 and 0.86 were obtained for breast, back, butterfly and IM
respectively and all were significant (P < 0.01).   Further
correlations across the strokes are shown in Table 3.

Table 3.   Correlation coefficients for speed at V-OBLA (m s^{-1}) for
all strokes

	IM	Fly	Back	Breast
Free	0.86	0.77	0.76	0.75
Breast	0.91	0.82	0.66	–
Back	0.86	0.83	–	–
Fly	0.93	–	–	–
IM	–	–	–	–

At V-OBLA the speed ratio for conversion from free to breast,
back, butterfly and IM are 0.81, 0.86, 0.89 and 0.90 respectively.
On comparing maximum speeds across strokes (Figure 3),
significantcorrelations were found for all strokes with r values
ranging from 0.83-0.96 (P < 0.01). The speed ratio for conversion
from freestyle was breast 0.80, back 0.86, butterlfy 0.89 and IM
0.89.
Standard t tests showed significant differences in speed at V-OBLA
and maximum between males and females for all strokes (P < 0.05),
except for V-OBLA during breaststroke where no significant
differences was found.
Analysis of lactate levels at OBLA and at maximum showed that
there was a significant differences between males and females in all
cases except butterfly. The level of significance varied in the
other four strokes (Figures 4 and 5). Correlation coefficients for
lactate concentrations at V-OBLA for the different strokes showed an
acceptable, though less significant correlation, than is seen with
speed. The V-OBLA lactate r values varied from 0.66-0.69 (P < 0.05),

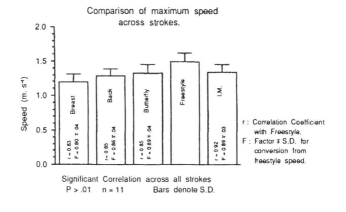

Fig. 3. Comparison of maximum speed across strokes.

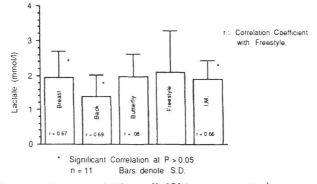

Fig. 4. Lactate (mM) at V-OBLA across strokes.

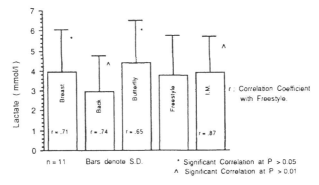

Fig. 5. Maximum lactate levels across strokes.

except for freestyle-butterfly where no correlation was seen.

The correlation of lactate values at maximum between freestyle and all other strokes was also somewhat variable. The r values varied from 0.65 for fly (P < 0.05), 0.71 for breast (P < 0.05), 0.74 for back (P < 0.01) and 0.87 for IM (P < 0.01).

Table 4. Comparison of blood lactate levels between males and females at V-OBLA and maximum

	Males		Females	
	Lactate (mM)		Lactate (mM)	
	OBLA	Max	OBLA	Max
Breast	2.38 ± 0.63	5.11 ± 1.43	1.40 ± 0.40*	2.05 ± 1.05*
Back	1.82 ± 0.56	4.06 ± 1.75	0.90 ± 0.06*	1.68 ± 0.53*
Fly	2.21 ± 0.65	5.43 ± 2.38	1.68 ± 0.50	3.12 ± 0.67
Free	2.85 ± 1.11	5.13 ± 1.33	1.18 ± 0.38**	2.18 ± 1.03**
IM	2.22 ± 0.44	5.01 ± 1.49	1.50 ± 0.39**	2.46 ± 0.68**

*indicates significant difference between males and females at
 P < 0.05
**indicates significant differences between males and females at
 P < 0.01

Table 5. Heart rates after each swim

Stroke		Swim 1	Swim 2	Swim 3	Swim 4
Breast	M	158 ± 11	171 ± 10	180 ± 7	189 ± 6
	F	152 ± 26	171 ± 17	182 ± 15	200 ± 16
Back	M	153 ± 20	162 ± 15	164 ± 0	180 ± 18
	F	138 ± 12	143 ± 13	153 ± 16	170 ± 15
Fly	M	173 ± 14	175 ± 11	179 ± 15	179 ± 8
	F	174 ± 18	172 ± 11	173 ± 10	173 ± 8
Free	M	149 ± 19	171 ± 11	178 ± 11	185 ± 5
	F	155 ± 11	166 ± 13	180 ± 7	190 ± 12
IM	M	148 ± 11	164 ± 7	180 ± 3	188 ± 9
	F	150 ± 12	169 ± 11	184 ± 11	189 ± 13

4 Discussion

A requirement of the study was to explore speed, lactate and heart rate patterns in a group of competitive swimmers. In Table 1 performance characteristics are shown in relation to current Irish record times and it can be seen that the group was capable of achieving times above 85% of the Irish record for all strokes except the backstroke where the level fell to 82.5% in males and 85% in females. During the study, however, performance nearest to 100% of PB was achieved in the backstroke (97.8% of PB in males and 96.7% in females). A further feature of the backstroke performance of the group which is difficult to interpret, is that both heart rate and lactate values were lower in the backstroke sets than in any other stroke. It would be reasonable to assume that the least efficient performance would result in highest lactates and heart rates and not the lowest as in this study.

The high correlation between speeds at OBLA has important practical implications for lactate testing and cross reference from one stroke to another. The indications from this study are that, provided the swimmers have a reasonable level of competence, suitable training speeds for aerobic improvement can be predicted for all strokes by testing in any one stroke, and then applying the relevant conversion factor for each individual stroke (the one exception being breast/back ratio). The high correlation for maximum speeds across strokes is important but has less practical significance since maximum performance should not normally be used in training prescription and cannot be used for reliable performance prediction since it will be affected by numerous factors not related to physical capacity alone. Comparing all strokes to freestyle, this study shows that the speed conversion factors for each of the other strokes at both OBLA and maximum speed are almost identical. This study also highlights the wide variations in lactate levels which occur. As expected the female group showed significantly lower blood lactate levels than the males ($P < 0.05$) for all strokes at both maximum and OBLA speeds except for the butterfly. In the total group mean, lactate levels 10 min post-exercise were below 2 mM in all strokers except freestyle where the level was 2.09 mM. Mean maximum lactate values ranged from 4.4 mM in butterfly to 2.98 mM in backstroke. The wide variability of lactate values at both speeds highlights the problems associated with the practice of using fixed lactate values such as V-4 mM or V-2 mM as reference points.

Heart rate values show wide variation and difficulty of measurement and interpretation at the two highest intensities.

5 Conclusions

(a) It is possible to predict accurately the specific speed at which the onset of blood lactate accumulation will occur in every stroke by using an incremental test protocol of 4 × 200 m swims in any one stroke and correcting by a fixed ratio. This statement applies to both sexes provided that swimmers are practised at each stroke.

(b) Isolated lactate values are less reliable than speeds determined from lactate profiles.

(c) Heart rates are difficult to measure accurately especially at above 90% of personal best speeds and also show wide variability.

(d) Further studies are necessary to confirm these findings and to explore relationships in younger swimmers and in those who limit training exclusively to one stroke.

6 References

Howat, R.C.L. and Robson, H. (1990) Training with times established from the modified two speed test. **The Swimming Times,** May 1990, 17-18.

Keskinen, K.L., Komi, P.V. and Rusko, H. (1989) A comparative study of blood lactate tests in swimming. **Int. J. Sports Med.**, 10, 197-201.

Madsen, P., Olbrecht, J., Mader, A., Liesen, H. and Hollman, W. (1983) **Specifics of Aerobic Training**. Institut fur Kreblau Fforschung und Sportmedizin, Deutsche Sporthochschule, Koln.

HEART RATE AND LACTATE RESPONSES TO SWIMMING

M.C. PEYREBRUNE and C.A. HARDY
Department of Physical Education, Sports Science and Recreation
Management, Loughborough University, England

Abstract
The purpose of the study was to determine a relationship between
heart rate (HR) and blood lactate (La) levels in swimmers using
swimming velocity as the dependent variable. Eleven male competitive
swimmers carried out two tests on separate days to establish this
relationship. The first test involved a 500 yard incremental swim;
lap times were recorded manually, and HR determined from a micro-
computer strapped below the chest. The second test involved five
successively faster 200 yard repeats with fifteen minuts rest between
each. Again lap times were recorded manually, and blood lactate
concentrations determined from a finger-prick sample after each
stage. Heart rate and La deflection velocities were then identified
from graphs obtained in the respective tests.
    Deflection (d) velocities in the HR test were recorded in eight
subjects while no deflection point was observed in the remaining
three. Retest results with five of the subjects obtained deflection
velocities in two subjects, but none in the three others. Blood
lactate deflection velocities were gained in all subjects, and the
2 mM and 4 mM speeds extrapolated from the graphs. Mean ($\pm$ SD)
velocities (m/s) for HR d, La d, 2 mM and 4 mM were 1.334 ($\pm$ 0.084)
m/s, 1.257 ($\pm$ 0.078) m/s, 1.291 ($\pm$ 0.113) m/s and 1.419 ($\pm$ 0.126) m/s
respectively. The HR deflection velocity was significantly higher
($P < 0.001$) than La d velocity and 2 mM velocity, but significantly
lower ($P < 0.01$) than 4 mM/l velocity. Blood lactate deflection
velocity was not significantly different from the 2 mM velocity.
    The time differences calculated from these speeds for 200 m and
500 m ranged from 4.2 to 18.2 s, and from 10.5 to 45.4 s respectively. The extent of these differences led the researchers to
conclude that although HR measurements are valuable when more
accurate methods are not available, there can still be a large margin
of error. This index may be unacceptable for the monitoring of
training intensity in international class swimmers.
Keywords: Heart Rate, Blood Lactate Concentration, Swimming Speed,
Training Intensity.

1 Introduction

The ability to evaluate even the slightest responses to the training
of élite swimmers has benefits in helping to explain the reasons for
competition performance. Researchers have used measures such as

HR (Treffene et al., 1980), oxygen consumption (Holmer, 1974; Troup, 1986) and La concentrations (Madsen, 1982; Maglischo et al., 1982, Madsen and Lohberg, 1987; Howat and Robson, 1990) to measure endurance capacity, one of the contributing factors to performance success in most swimming races.

The measurement of HR provides the coach or swimmer with an easy method of approximating intensity of effort, although errors may be obtained from manual palpation of the pulse, and also the influence of environmental factors on HR (e.g. the 'fight or flight' response). Many recent publications have focused on La measurements as a more valid and accurate indicator of endurance capacity, and the introduction of lactate analysers has made the testing easier to administer (Jacobs, 1986).

Many La values and responses to swimming intensity have been used to evaluate endurance capacity and performance, with attempts being made to associate these values with an 'anaerobic threshold' (McLellan, 1987). There has been some confusion over the interpretation of these results owing to the inconsistency of the La indicators used, the variations in test protocols and the lack of standardisation of terminology. A further complication has arisen with certain studies attempting to relate various definitions of the 'anaerobic threshold' to HR measurements (Treffene et al., 1980; Conconi et al., 1982; Cellini et al., 1986; Arabas et al., 1987; Pyne and Telford, 1988). It has been suggested that the point at which HR departs from linearity as endurance swimming approaches maximum, and which has been defined as the HR deflection or breakpoint velocity (Vd), is also the 'anaerobic threshold'. Blood lactate concentrations at this point have been reported as either very consistent (Conconi et al., 1982; Ribeiro et al., 1985; Cellini et al., 1986) or very inconsistent (Treffene et al., 1989, 1980; Tomakidis and Leger, 1988) amongst subjects.

The purpose of this study was to evaluate the non-invasive field test reported by Cellini et al. (1986), to determine the relationship betwween HR and several blood lactate indices in swimmers and analyse the appropriateness of each physiological measure in monitoring training intensity amongst swimmers of varying standards.

2 Methods

Eleven male competitive swimmers volunteered to participate in this study. All the tests were carried out in a 25 yard pool with the average water temperature being 29°C. The three tests were completed within two weeks, and each swimmer was tested individually. To ensure an even, calm water, one 'anti-wave' lane rope was used to isolate the swimmer from the rest of the pool. The subjects performed a fifteen minute warm-up of their own choice before each test. Times in tests were recorded manually from the poolside, converted to metres and speeds were calculated for each section.

The HR-speed (V) relationship was determined from subjects performing a 500 yard continuous swim on front crawl using kick turns with the HR monitoring equipment attached. The equipment consisted of a telemetric HR monitor strapped around the trunk just below the chest. Heart rate (in beats per minute) was recorded every 15 s and plotted against speed after the test. Instructions given to the

A.

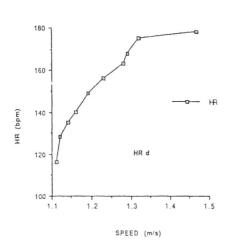

B.

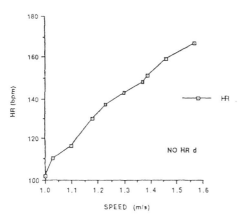

Fig. 1.   Example plots of subjects who did (A) and who did not (B)
          demonstrate a deflection point in the HR-V test.

(c) The significant difference found between the two variables Vd
and La d contrast with the close relationship found by Cellini et al.
(1986).

Heart rate data obtained in the present study showed a wide range
amongst subjects. A large inter-swimmer variation in HR and Vd was
also observed. This leads the researchers to believe that the HR
response to swimming is individually exclusive as well as inconsistent over repeated tests.

subjects were to increase their speed every 50 yards, beginning the
swim at a 'very steady' intensity and finishing at maximum effort
over the last 50 yard swim.

Determination of the La-V relationship was obtained from a further
test carried out by each of the 11 subjects one week after the HR-V
test. This interval type test involved five swims of 200 yards, each
at a successively faster pace. Each interval was separated by 15
minuts, and blood samples were taken after five minutes rest - post
exercise. Blood samples were analysed enzymatically for lactic acid
content at a later date using procedures suggested by Olsen (1971).

In order to determine significant differences between HR measures
and various lactate indices, a Wilcoxon matched pair test was
administered. This non-parametric test was chosen as small sample
sizes were used in the present study (n < 11), and some groups were
of uneven sample size. Mean (± SD) speeds for each physiological
variable were calculated and converted to 200 and 500 m (the test
distances) times for comparison.

3 Results

In the HR-V test, eight out of eleven subjects displayed a definite
breakpoint (Vd); the remaining three showed no clear breakpoint (Fig.
1). Mean (± SD) values for HR and V at this point (Vd) were 171.25
(± 9.896) beats per minute and 1.334 (± 0.084) m/s respectively.

HR-V retest results produced a breakpoint in the graph of three
out of five subjects. Inconsistency in obtaining a breakpoint was
observed between subjects and also within subjects (Fig. 2).

All eleven subjects in the La-V test demonstrated typical lactate
'profile' curves, and a breakpoint was obtained for each (Fig. 3).
The mean (± SD) lactate value at this point was 2.107 (± 0.755) mM,
with the corresponding mean (± SD) speed at the deflection being
1.257 (± 0.078) m/s).

Significant differences between the speeds at Vd and La d, Vd and
2 mM and Vd and 4 mM were found. There was no significant difference
between La d and the 2 mM speed in the La V test.

Absolute differences of 9.2 s between HR d and La d, 5.0 s between
HR d and 2 mM speed and 9.0 s between HR d and 4 mM speed were found
when the speeds were corrected back to time over 200 m. Similarly,
over 500 m, the time differences become 23.0, 12.5 and 22.4 s
respectively (Fig. 4).

4 Conclusions

The findings obtained in the present study did not support the
results reported by Cellini et al. (1986):

(a) The almost perfect straight line relationships found between
HR and V were not observed in any of the subjects in this study.

(b) Not all the subjects demonstrated a distinguishable deflection
point in their HR-V graphs, and inconsistencies were observed within
subjects after repeated measures. High post exercise blood lactate
levels and peak HR values suggested that effort was close to maximum,
and that the lack of Vd was not due to poor motivation.

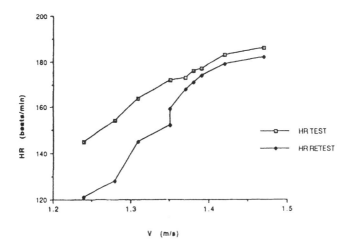

Fig. 2. Superimposed plots for the HR-V test and re-test showing inconsistency within subjects.

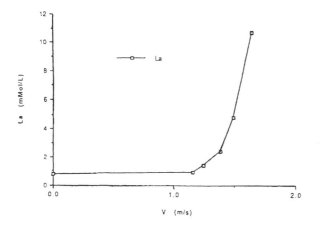

Fig. 3. A typical lactate-swimming speed relationship.

Problems in relating the current data collected to other studies ı the literature suggest that clearer definition of terms is needed ıd that more objective techniques for determination of breakpoints : deflections are necessary. Standardisation of test protocols and :ocedures would also help to avoid confusion over conflicting ısults.

Despite the value of HR as a useful monitor of intensity in rimming training, the time differences obtained when compared with .ood lactate indices, the inconsistency of the measurement and the .de individual variation indicate that its use may be limited in ıking some of the more accurate judgements in constructing the :aining programmes for international class swimmers.

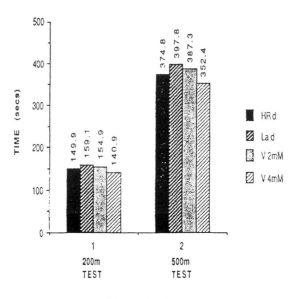

(Mean values).

Fig. 4.   200 and 500 m times converted from lactate deflection and
         heart rate deflection speeds.

5 References

Arabas, C., Mayhew, J.L., Hudgins, P.M. and Bond, G.H. (1987)
   Relationships among work rates, heart rates, and blood lactate
   levels in female swimmers. **J. Sports Med. Phys. Fit.**, 27,
   291–295.
Cellini, M., Vitiello, P., Nagliati, A. Ziglio, P.G., Martinelli, S.,
   Ballarin, E. and Conconi, F. (1986) Noninvasive determination of
   the anaerobic threshold in swimming. **Int. J. Sports Med.**, 7,
   347–351.
Conconi, F., Merrari, M., Ziglio, P.G., Droghetti, P. and Codeca, L.
   (1982) Determination of the anaerobic threshold by a noninvasive
   field test in runners. **J. Appl. Physiol.**, 52, 869–873.
Holmer, I. (1974) Energy cost of arm stroke, leg kick and the whole
   stroke in competitive swimming styles. **Eur. J. Appl. Physiol.**,
   33, 105–118.
Howat, R.C.L. and Robson, M. (1990) Established training times from
   blood lactate testing. **Swimming Times,** 67, 21.
Jacobs, I. (1986) Blood lactate: Implications for training and sports
   performance. **Sports Med.**, 3, 10–25.
McLellan, T.M. (1987) The anaerobic threshold: concept and

controversy. **Austral. J. Sci. Med. Sport,** 10, 3-8.

ladsen, O. (1982) Aerobic training: not so fast there. **Swimming Technique,** 19, 13-23.

ladsen, O. and Lohberg, M. (1987) The lowdown on lactates. **Swimming Technique,** 24, 21-26.

laglischo, E. (1982) **Swimming Faster.** Mayfield Publishing Company, California.

laglischo, E., Maglischo, C. and Bishop, R. (1982) Lactate testing for training pace. **Swimming Technique,** 19, 31-27.

)lsen, C. (1971) An enzymatic fluorimetric micromethod for the determination of acetoacetate, β-hydroxybutyrate, pyruvate and lactate. **Clin. Chim. Acta,** 33, 293-300.

?yne, D.B. and Telford, R.D. (1988) Classification of swimming training sessions by blood lactate and heart rate responses. **EXCEL,** 5, 7-9.

Ribeiro, J.P., Fielding, R.A., Hughes, V., Black, A., Bochese, M.A. and Knuttgen, H.G. (1985) Heart rate breakpoint may coincide with the anaerobic and not the aerobic threshold. **Int. J. Sports Medicine,** 6, 220-224.

Tomakadis, S.P. and Leger, L.A. (1988) External validity of Conconi's heart rate anaerobic threshold as compared to lactate threshold. **Exercise Physiology: Current Selected Research,** 60, 1523-1548.

Treffene, R.J., Craven, C., Hobbs, K. and Wade, C. (1979) Heart rates and plasma lactate study. **The International Swimmer,** 15, 19-21.

Treffene, R.J., Dickson, R., Craven, C., Osborne, C., Woodhead, K. and Hobbs, K. (1980) Lactic acid accumulation during constant speed swimming at controlled relative intensities. **J. Sports Med. Phys. Fit.,** 20, 244-253.

Troup, J. (1986) Setting up a season using scientific training. **Swimming Technique,** 23, 8-16.

THE IMPORTANCE OF A CALCULATION SCHEME TO SUPPORT THE INTERPRETATION OF LACTATE TESTS

J. OLBRECHT, A. MADER, H. HECK and W. HOLLMAN
German University of Sport Sciences, Cologne, Germany

Abstract
Blood lactate (BLa) response to exercise has become routine to determine the aerobic and anaerobic capacity of athletes and to monitor
training individually. For the interpretation of BLa as a parameter
of metabolic activity, there is no fundamental concept. This
contributes to multiple and debatable presentations of BLa thresholds
and leads to controversial conclusions and divergent applications of
BLa tests. The purpose of this study was to present some results of
a swim-specific calculation scheme (SCS) which depicts BLa in the
context of the whole metabolic process. The SCS is based on a mathematical approach to aerobic and anaerobic metabolism regulation and
describes BLa as a result of oxidative BLa elimination and BLa production (BLaP) rates related to the maximal capacity of BLaP and
oxygen uptake ($\dot{V}O_2$). The scheme also needs a speed-energy expenditure relation (SER). The study was performed on 778 male swimmers
using two-speed tests, competition or training series at constant
speed (TRS).
Keywords: Lactate Tests, Glycolysis, Metabolism.

1 Introduction

Blood lactate (BLa) measures are nowadays commonly used in the
assessment of metabolic performance. Despite the fact that BLa
concentrations were measured as early as 1923 by Hill and Lupton and
further elaborated upon by Jervell (1929) and Owles (1930), a clear
link between the measured BLa and the metabolic processes has not
been established. The purpose of this study was to use the swim
specific calculation scheme (SCS) reported by Mader and Heck (1986)
based on BLa, swimming time and speed, quantification of glycolytic
rate (LaP), as well as estimates of maximal aerobic power ($\dot{V}O_2$max)
and maximal glycolytic capacity (LaP_{max}).

2 Methods

Blood lactate was measured in 778 male swimmers during a two-speed
swim test of 200 m and of 400 m, as well as after competition and
steady state maximal swimming. Maximum oxygen uptake ($\dot{V}O_2$max) was
also measured in these swimmers. A combination of the BLa and $\dot{V}O_2$max
data allowed for a number of calculations to be made.

An increase of BLa above the resting level depends on the increase
of the lactate formation (dLa/dt gross) due to activation of glycolysis. During exercise lactate is also oxidised (dLa/dt el) according to the "Steady state $\dot{V}O_2$ ($\dot{V}O_2$ss)". Blood lactate (BLa) is the
result of "net lactate formation (dLa/dt net)" which is always lower
than the actual rate of glycolysis. In order to quantify the real
rate of glycolysis (dLa/dt gross) the definition of Mader and Heck
(1986) can be used for exercises between 80 and 600 s (Figure 1).

$$\frac{dLa}{dt} \text{ net} = \frac{dLa}{dt} \text{ gross} - \frac{dLa}{dt} \text{ el}$$

$$= \frac{60 \cdot \frac{dLa}{dt} \text{ max}}{1 + \frac{K''s}{\left(\frac{K's \cdot \dot{V}O_2 ss}{\overline{V}O_2 \text{max} - \overline{V}O_2 ss}\right)^{2/3}}} - \frac{\frac{0.01576}{Vol.rel.} \cdot \dot{V}O_2 ss}{1 + \frac{Kel}{(Class)^2}} \quad (1)$$

As $\dot{V}O_2$ss is a function of $\dot{V}O_2$max, dLa/dt net as well as La are
determined by dLa/dt max and $\dot{V}O_2$max. By increasing $\dot{V}O_2$ss from the
rest level towards $\dot{V}O_2$max, the "net" as well as the "gross" lactate
formation can be calculated for a given dLa/dt max (Figure 1).

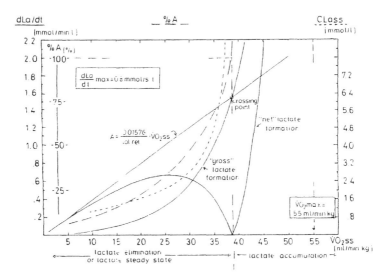

Fig. 1. Lactate elimination, "gross" and "net" lactate formation
         (mmol/lmin) as well as the steady state concentration of
         lactate (class; mmol/l) as a function of $\dot{V}O_2$ss (ml/kg/min)
         according to Equation 1.

If dLa/dt gross < dLa/dt el, the gross lactate formation falls
below the possible oxidation rate. It is assumed that in case of a
low blood and muscle pyruvate concentration the lack of pyruvate is

due to fatty acid oxidation.

If dLa/dt gross > dLa/dt el the gross lactate concentration exceeds the elimination and an accumulation of La occurs.

If dLa/dt gross = dLa/dt el (crossing point) lactate formation and elimination are balanced. A "maximal steady state of La (MaxLass)" may be established during endurance exercise.

The glycolytic rate can be converted into $\dot{V}O_2$-equivalents. Based on the $\dot{V}O_2$ and La-data of Holmer et al. (1988), Eriksson et al. (1978) Madsen (1982) and of Van Handel et al. (1988), the total energy supply in terms of $\dot{V}O_2$-equivalents ($\dot{V}O_2$tot; ml/min/kg) was calculated (Olbrechts, 1990, Fig. 2). The fitting of speed (v) to $\dot{V}O_2$tot has then been corrected for swimming in accordance with the data of Toussaint (1988) and can be used to estimate $\dot{V}O_2$tot related to speed (Equation 2).

$$\dot{V}O_2 tot = 34.88 . v^{1.647} \qquad\qquad (r = 0.979, n = 21) \qquad\qquad (2)$$

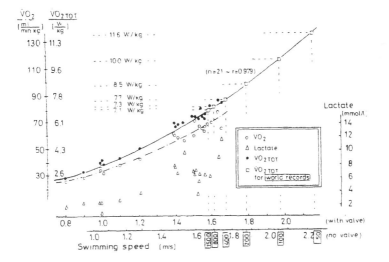

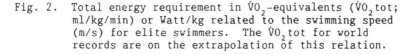

Fig. 2. Total energy requirement in $\dot{V}O_2$-equivalents ($\dot{V}O_2$tot; ml/kg/min) or Watt/kg related to the swimming speed (m/s) for elite swimmers. The $\dot{V}O_2$tot for world records are on the extrapolation of this relation.

3 Results

The mean "anaerobic threshold" (AT) values from 2-speed tests on 2 × 200 and 2 × 400 m were calculated (Table 1) for swimmers who partici-pated in regional (B), national (N), European (E) and world champion-ships (W). Aerobic threshold increased significantly with the impor-tance of the competition. The SCS reveals that in order to attain 4 mM a higher dLa/dt gross and a higher $\dot{V}O_2$ss are involved when anaerobic threshold (AT) improves (Figure 3). On 200 and 400 m swims, dLa/dt gross increased between B and W by 21.7% and 22.8% whilst $\dot{V}O_2$ss improved by 30.3% and 27.2%.

Table 1. Mean ($\bar{x}$) and standard deviation (s) of AT (m/s) for 2 × 200 and 2 × 400 m 2-speed tests for swimmers who participated in regional (B), national (N), European (E) and world championships (W)

2 speed test		Anaerobic threshold (m/s)			
		B	N	E	W
2 × 200 m	$\bar{x}$	1.348	1.424	1.461	1.576
	s	0.088***	0.071**	0.078**	0.044
	n	123	64	20	16
2 × 400 m	$\bar{x}$	1.320	1.409	1.449	1.524
	s	0.083***	0.056**	0.080**	0.077
	n	396	159	51	22

***$P < 0.001$; **$P < 0.01$; *$P < 0.05$

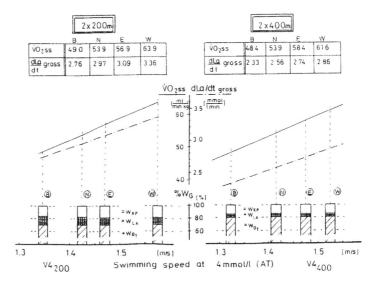

Fig. 3. Calculated $\dot{V}O_2$ss (ml/min/kg) and dLa/dt gross (mmol/l.min) related to the mean AT (m/s) on 200 and 400 m for B, N, E and W-swimmers (Table 1) and the corresponding % of the total energy (%W_G) delivered by phosphocreatine breakdown (W_{KP}), glycolysis (W_{LA}) and oxidation (W_{O2}).

From Olbrecht's (1990) study BLa and swimming speed for competitive distances from 50 to 1500 m for B, N, E and W-swimmers were used to calculate the data in Table 2. The dLa/dt gross decreases with the longer the distance but is always highest for the fastest swimmers.

The $\dot{V}O_2$max and dLa/dt max determine BLa (Figure 1). Each curve of Figure 4 (left) depicts various combinations of $\dot{V}O_2$max and dLa/dt max recorded experimentally for each test distance of the 2 × 200 and 2 × 400 m two 2-speed test, for a world class sprint middle- (SM) and a

Table 2. dLa/dt gross (mM/l/min) calculated on the basis of man La and swimming speed in competition for B, N, E and W swimmers

Distance (m)	B dLa/dt gross	n	N dLa/dt gross	n	E dLa/dt gross	n	W dLa/dt gross	n	G dLa/dt gross	n
50			24.71	3	(32.08		5)		29.31	8
200	6.79	11	8.73	33	9.54	5	9.50	11	8.24	60
400	4.40	16	4.54	13	4.98	13	5.13	8	4.54	50
800									3.51	6
1500									2.78	7

long- (L) distance swimmer.
    For each swimmer the concurrence of the curves depicts $\dot{V}O_2$max and dLa/dt max which can be used to reproduce (Eq.(1)) the La-speed-curves experimentally defined (Figure 4, right). Anaerobic threshold determined from both the two-speed tests and the SCS, $\dot{V}O_2$ss, dLa/dt gross, $\dot{V}O_2$max, and dLa/dt max are denoted here for SM and L in Table 3.
    The Maxlass speed (speed accorded to the "crossing point"; Figure 1) was 1.444 and 1.529 m/s for SM and L and closely approached the average speed of a 30 min steady state swim at maximal but constant intensity (SM: 1.446 and L: 1.517 m/s).

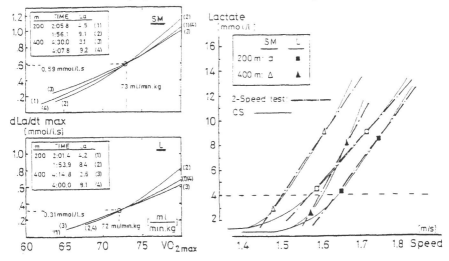

Fig. 4.   Pairs of $\dot{V}O_2$max and dLa/dt max determining La and speed recorded for each test distance of a 2 × 200 and 2 × 400 m 2-speed test for a world class spring - middle (SM) and long (L) distance swimmer (left). Lactate-speed-curves of the 2-speed tests can be reproduced after defining $\dot{V}O_2$max and dLa/dt max (concurrence of curves). The higher AT of L is due to his lower glycolytic and not to a higher aerobic capacity.

Table 3. The $\dot{V}O_2$max, $\dot{V}O_2$ss (ml/min.kg), dLa/dt max and dLa/dt gross (mmol/1.s) and AT (m/s) defined by CS for two elite swimmers. Anaerobic threshold fixed by the 2-speed tests (exp) is compared to AT calculated by CS (CS).

$\dot{V}O_2$max (ml/kg/min)	dLa/ dt max (mM/s)	Distance (m)	AT (m/s)		$\dot{V}O_2$ss (ml/kg/min)	dLa/ dt gross (mM/s)
			exp	CS		
SM 73	0.59	200	1.576	1.565	58.79	0.0604
		400	1.501	1.508	55.56	0.0467
L 72	0.31	200	1.641	1.639	62.65	0.0656
		400	1.595	1.593	61.16	0.0531

Maximal aerobic capacity ($\dot{V}O_2$max) did not differ between SM and L (Table 3). Differences of AT cannot therefore be related to the aerobic capacity ($\dot{V}O_2$max) but to the lower glycolytic capacity (dLa/dt max) of L. If both athletes swim at AT, SM will swim 200 and 400 m at 87.0% and 85.0% of $\dot{V}O_2$max, and 21.2% and 17.12% of dLa/dt max. SM however reaches the same 4 mmol/l speed at 80.5% and 76.1% of $\dot{V}O_2$max and 10.2% and 8.1% of dLa/dt max.

4 Discussion

The swim specific calculation scheme revealed that a higher AT did not always imply a better aerobic capacity ($\dot{V}O_2$max). A decrease of the glycolytic capacity (dLa/dt max) improved AT even when $\dot{V}O_2$max remained the same. In this case the glycolytic rate according to AT increased and amounted to a higher percentage of dLa/dt max. This may explain the coaches' experiences that distance swimmers get midrange BLa with greater difficulties than sprinters.

Anaerobic threshold correlated significantly with swimming speed in competition (r = 0.85 to 0.96; Olbrecht 1990). It seems however to be a determining factor for good performances in competition to possess not only a high AT but also a high dLa/dt max, particularly for the shorter competitive distances. A lower dLa/dt max for distance swimmers compared to sprinters (Olbrecht, 1990) may explain why in sprint events long distance swimmers with a better AT for 100 m do not swim as fast as sprinters with a lower 100 m AT.

The swim-specific calculation scheme enabled the glycolytic rate for exercises between 80 and 600 s to be quantified and to estimate the aerobic and glycolytic capacity. This is important not only to detail the different aspects of the metabolic performance capacity of a swimmer but also to be able to differentiate the load of training exercises. The swim-specific calculation needs a speed-energy equation (Eq.2). The technical ability of the swimmer may affect this equation and thereby the results of SCS. Due to the error on La measurements a shift of $\dot{V}O_2$max-dLa/dt max curves (Fig. 4, left) may occur. The concurrence of the curves can then be somewhat diffuse so that a range of $\dot{V}O_2$max or dLa/dt max and not a single value must be defined. The swim-specific calculation scheme is a first step to link La with whole metabolic activity and there is still room for improvement.

5 References

Eriksson, B.O., Holmer, I. and Lundin, A. 91978) Physiological effects of training in elite swimmers, in **Swimming Medicine IV** (eds B. Eriksson and B. Furberg), University Park Press, Baltimore, pp. 177-187.

Hill, A.V. and Lupton, H. (1923) Muscular exercise, lactic acid and the supply and utilization of oxygen. **Quart. J. Med.**, 16, 135-170.

Holmer, I., Lundin, A. and Eriksson, B.O. (1974) Maximum oxygen uptake during swimming and running by elite swimmers. **J. Appl. Physiol.**, 36, 711-714.

Jervell, O. (1929) Investigation of the concentration of lactic acid in blood and urine. **Acta Med. Scand.**, Suppl. 24.

Margaria, R. (1976) **Biomechanics and energetics of muscular exercise.** Clarendon Press, Oxford.

Mader, A. (1984) **Eine Theorie zur Berechnung der Dynamik und des steady state von Phosphorylierungszustand und Stoffwechselaktivität der Musckelzelle als Folge des Energiebedarfs.** Habil. DSHS, Cologne.

Mader, A. and Heck, H. (1986) A theory of the metabolic origin of "anaerobic threshold". **Int. J. Sports Med.**, 7, 45-65.

Madsen, Ö (19872) Untersuchungen über Einflussgrössen auf Parameter des Energiestoffwechsels beim freien Kraulschwimmen. Diss. DSHS, Cologne.

Olbrecht, J. (1990) Metabolische Beanspruchung bei Wettkampfschwimmern unterschielicher Leistungsfähigkeit. Diss. DSHS, Cologne.

Owles, J. (1930) Alternations in lactic acid content of the blood as a result of light exercise and associated changes in the CO_2-combining power of the blood and in the alveolar CO_2 pressure. **J. Physiol.**, 69, 214-237.

Toussaint, H.M. (1988) **Mechanics and energetics of swimming.** Rodopi, Amsterdam.

Van Handel, P.J., Katz, A., Morrow, J.R., Troup, J.P., Daniels, J.T. and Bradley, P.W. (1988) Aerobic economy and competitive performance of US elite swimmers, in **Swimming Science V** (eds B. Ungerechts, W. Wilke and K. Reischle), Human Kinetics Books, Champaign, Ill, pp. 219-227.

EFFECT OF LEG ACTION ON STROKE PERFORMANCE IN SWIMMING

K.L. KESKINEN and P.V. KOMI
Department of Biology of Physical Activity, University of Jyväskylä,
Jyväskylä, Finland

Abstract
The present study was designed to make comparisons among biomechanical parameters between normal crawl (CN) and crawl arm swimming (CA).
These parameters included mean velocity (V), stroke rate (SR) and
distance per stroke (d/S). The comparisons were complemented with
the simultaneous recording of blood lactate (BLa) responses. Eight
well conditioned competitive male swimmers carried out two sets of 15
times 100 m swims in both ways. In the comparisons of BLa vs V
diagrams, CN and CA demonstrated different ($P < 0.05$) V values at 0.5
mM increase in BLa (anaerobic threshold, AT). The d/S was longest
around aerobic-anaerobic transition. The values of d/S were higher
($P < 0.05$) in the CN curve when BLa increased by 0.5 mM above basal
level and at V above AT. In CA swimming the SR curve became
different ($P < 0.05$) from that of the CN at higher levels of V and
BLa. However, at maximum pace SR values were equally high (0.76 Hz)
in both swimming conditions. It is concluded that the support of leg
kick could be seen in d/S values at V around AT and above, as well as
in SR values at higher intensity levels.
Keywords: Swimming Velocity, Blood Lactate, Distance per Stroke,
Stroke Rate.

1 Introduction

In the training of competitive swimmers, arm stroke swimming
especially in crawl style ("Crawl Arms", CA), has become an important
part of normal daily practice. Evidently, this training mode
improves both competitive performance and physical fitness of a crawl
swimmer. Several studies have reported that the arms contribute more
to propulsion than the legs in different swimming styles (e.g. Adrian
et al., 1966; Alley, 1952; Magel, 1970; Hollander et al., 1988).
    As was reported by Holmer (1974a) the efficiency of CA at a
constant submaximal velocity is higher than in normal crawl swimming
("Crawl Normal", CN) or in leg kicking. These results were in good
agreement with those obtained by Rennie et al. (1973). On the other
hand, when CN and CA swimming have been compared with respect to
oxygen consumption (Holmer, 1974b), CN was noted to have higher $\dot{V}O_2$
values at all velocities.
    In training CN seems to allow maintenance of higher velocities,
heart rates and lactate concentrations, and lower pH-values as
compared to CA swims (Huber et al., 1978). In addition, the

comparison of maximum velocity between CN, CA and leg kicking has
shown that kicking is the most inefficient part of the swimming
movements, while swimming that includes both arms and legs produces
the highest performances and best competition results (Karpovich,
1935; Bucher, 1974). No reported data exist regarding the
differences in the technical performance between CN and CA swimming.

The present study was designed to make comparisons among the
biomechanical parameters between the CN and CA swimming. These
comparisons were complemented with the simultaneous recording of
blood lactate responses.

2 Methods

Eight well conditioned, competitive male swimmers volunteered to
serve as subjects (Table 1). An indoor, 50 m long swimming pool with
standard water temperature of 26-27°C was used. The subjects carried
out two sets of 15 times 100 m swims, by normal crawl swimming (CN)
and by crawl stroke with arms only (CA). In CA swimming pull-buoys
with ankle ties were used to inactivate the legs in a conventional
way. The two sets were conducted on separate days, one rest day in-
between. The order of the performance was randomized so that four
subjects carried out CN before CA and vice versa.

Biomechanical parameters included mean velocity (V), stroke rate
(SR) and distance per stroke (d/S). Time was measured for each of
the swims (no dive in starting) to obtain V (m/s). The SR was
obtained so that in each length of the pool the time for ten stroke
cycles was measured and SR was calculated in cycles/s. The d/S was
calculated by V/SR (m/cycle). Blood samples were drawn from
hyperemisized ear lobes to analyze blood lactate concentration (BLa)
before and after the 100 m swims.

The subjects were allowed to warm up by very slow, steady paced
swimming for about 10 minutes preceding the trials. Additionally,
just before starting, each of the swimmers performed 2-3 times 100 m
swims at the first target time (2 min) to make sure they would start
with the correct pacing and also to lower the BLa values down to the

Table 1. Individual data for age, height, weight, personal best time
on 100 m freestyle (50 m pool) and arm span.

Subject (number)	Age (yr)	Height (cm)	Weight (kg)	Time (s)	Arm Span (cm)
1.	22.3	180.0	73.0	56.4	188.5
2.	26.0	178.0	74.0	58.8	187.5
3.	18.2	188.6	72.0	59.6	192.0
4.	20.0	186.5	89.5	57.7	195.0
5.	19.1	188.0	81.5	54.9	196.0
6.	21.4	187.5	77.5	55.4	192.0
7.	20.2	182.0	75.5	55.8	191.5
8.	20.4	183.5	75.0	57.8	199.0
Mean	21.0	184.3	77.3	57.1	192.7
S.D.	2.4	4.0	5.8	1.7	3.9

initial level. Thereafter, swimmers were asked to swim at an even pace and to improve time by 5 s in each successive 100 m effort.

The data were handled so that BLa values were plotted against V values and individual diagrams between BLa and V were drawn. At first the lowest level in BLa during the exercises was defined and the highest V at initial BLa level (I) was chosen as a common reference point to observe the changes in BLa (dBLa). Then the parameters (V, SR, d/S) were averaged according to dBLa in individual diagrams in both CN and CA experiments separately. The V axis, from the start to the I point, was used to average the parameters when dBLa was around zero. For data analysis t-tests with paired observations were used to test the statistical significance of the difference between the parameters in the two modes of exercise at different dBLa levels.

3 Results

The comparison between BLa and V diagrams (Fig. 1) for CN and CA experiments revealed that the two curves were almost identical in low intensity swims until the anaerobic threshold (AT; Gullstrand and Holmer, 1980; Keskinen et al., 1989). The curves became different ($P < 0.05$) in V at 0.5 mM dBLa and this difference stayed significant thereafter at each dBLa level tested up to maximum effort.

The examination of V, SR and d/S showed that SR and V were positively interrelated through all tested conditions, while d/S and V demonstrated a more complex relationship. The comparison between d/S and V (Fig. 2) as well as d/S and dBLa (Fig. 3) showed that d/S was longest around the area of the aerobic-anaerobic transition. The d/S values were higher ($P < 0.05$) in the CN curve at dBLa levels above 0.5 mM and at V levels above AT. In CA swimming the SR curve became different ($P < 0.05$) from that of the CN at higher levels of V and BLa (Figs. 4 and 5). However, at maximum pace, SR values were equally high (0.76 Hz) in both swimming conditions.

4 Discussion

The present data demonstrated considerable effect of leg action especially by d/S (Figs. 2 and 3). At around the AT level, the difference was about 11 cm (4.5%) in favour of CN and even larger at V above AT. Although the difference was nearly the same between CN and CA in low pace swims, it was not statistically significant. This may be partly due to a large variation in individual d/S values in this phase of exercise. It seems evident that CA was a very economical way of swimming just before the increase in BLa started. After the AT was reached the lack of support from the legs could be seen from the lowered d/S values as compared to the CN in swimming. These findings agree with those of Holmer (1974b). He noticed that CA swimming demanded lower $\dot{V}O_2$ at a given submaximal V than the CN swimming.

On the other hand, SR was very similar between the sets at V less than 1.3 m/s (Figs. 4 and 5). This suggests that SR is strongly dependent on V at submaximal exercise level, while d/S depends also on such factors as muscle force of the upper extremities and on the support of the leg action during swimming (Craig and Pendergast,

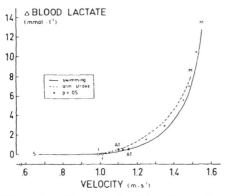

Fig. 1. Change in Blood Lactate vs Velocity. Symbols:
S=Start, I=Initial Level of Blood Lactate, AT=Anaerobic
Threshold, M=Maximum Velocity.

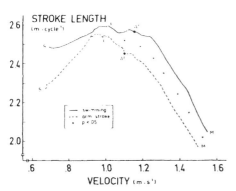

Fig. 2. Relationship between
Stroke Length and Velocity.

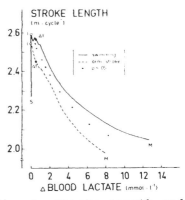

Fig. 3. Stroke Length and
Change in Blood Lactate.

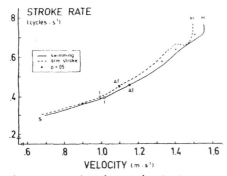

Fig. 4. Relationship between
Stroke Rate and Velocity.

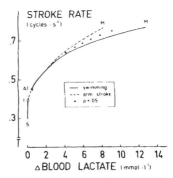

Fig. 5. Stroke Rate and
Change in Blood Lactate.-

1979; Keskinen and Komi, 1988). An interesting observation can be made from inspection of Fig. 4. The CA curve became nearly identical to the CN curve at V of 1.46 m/s. It occurred in almost every subject during the second/third to the last effort. This may be the result of a dolphin kick when the subjects were trying really hard. The very last effort was then so exhaustive that the CA curve again became different in V from that of CN.

Thus, it is suggested that if one wants to improve swimming economy, CA swimming should be practised at around the aerobic-anaerobic transition with high d/S and low SR. Kicking under these conditions would be compensated by pull-buoys to keep the body in a streamlined position. However, the exercises at race pace should include the leg kicking to obtain competition-like coordination between upper and lower extremities.

5 References

Adrian, M.J., Singh, M. and Karpovich, P.V. (1966) Energy cost of leg kick, arm stroke, and whole crawl stroke. **J. Appl. Physiol.**, 21, 1763-1766.

Alley, L.E. (1952) An analysis of water resistance and propulsion in swimming the crawl stroke. **Res. Quart.**, 23, 257-270.

Bucher, W. (1974) The influence of the leg kick and the arm stroke on the total speed during the crawl stroke, in **Swimming II** (eds J.P. Clarys and L. Lewillie), University Park Press, Baltimore, pp. 180-187.

Craig, A.B. Jr. and Pendergast, D.R. (1979) Relationships of stroke rate, distance per stroke and velocity in competitive swimming. **Med. Sci. Sports Exerc.**, 11, 278-283.

Gullstrand, L. and Holmer, I. (1980) Fysiologiska tester av landslagssimmare: Anaerob energileveransmätningen av blod mjölksyra. **Simsport**, 3, 13-17.

Hollander, A.P., Groot, G. de, Ingen Schenau, G.J. van, Kahman, R. and Toussaint, H.M. (1988) Contribution of the legs to propulsion in front crawl swimming, in **Swimming Science V** (eds B.E. Ungerechts, K. Wilke and K. Reischle), Human Kinetics Books, Champaign, Ill., pp. 39-43.

Holmer, I. (1974a) Propulsive efficiency of breaststroke and freestyle swimming. **Eur. J. Appl. Physiol.**, 33, 95-103.

Holmer, I. (1974b) Energy cost of armstroke, leg kick, and the whole stroke in competitive swimming styles. **Eur. J. Appl. Physiol.**, 33, 105-118.

Huber, G., Keul, J., Kinderman, W. and Stoklasa, L. (1978) Herzfrequenzen, Lactaspiegel und pH-Wert bei verschiedenen Trainingsform im Kraulschwimmen. **Dtsch. Z. Sportmed.**, 29, 282-291.

Karpovich, P.V. (1935) Analysis of the propelling force in the crawl stroke. **Res. Quart.**, 6, 49-58.

Keskinen, K.L. and Komi, P.V. (1988) Interaction between aerobic/ anaerobic loading and biomechanical performance in freestyle swimming, in **Swimming Science V** (eds B.E. Ungerechts, K. Wilke and K. Reischle), Human Kinetics Books, Champaign, Ill., pp. 285-293.

Keskinen, K.L., Komi, P.V. and Rusko, H. (1989) A comparative study of blood lactate tests in swimming. **Int. J. Sports Med.**, 10,

197–201.

Magel, J.R. (1970) Propelling force measured during tethered swimming in the four competitive swimming styles. **Res. Quart.**, 41, 68–74.

Rennie, D.W., Prampero, P. di, Wilson, D.R. and Pendergast, D.R (1973) Energetics of swimming the crawl. **Fed. Proc.**, 32, 1125 (abs.).

POST-COMPETITION BLOOD LACTATE IN DISABLED SWIMMERS

G.S. ROI and C. CERIZZA
Dipartimento di Scienze e Tecnologie Biomediche, Cattedra di
Fisiologia, Universitá di Milano, Instituto Scientifico San Raffaele,
Milano, Italy

Abstract
The time taken to cover 50 m in freestyle swimming and the post-
competition blood lactate levels were measured in healthy and
disabled swimmers. The results of this study show that disabled
swimmers take more time and accumulate a lower lactate per unity of
time than healthy subjects. These differences can be due to the
lower muscular mass utilized by disabled swimmers and to the
particular technique they employ according to their handicap.
Furthermore the high values of lactate found at the end of the race
indicate that the contribution of the anaerobic energetic sources is
important in disabled athletes too.
Keywords: Disabled Athletes, Lactate, Metabolism.

1 Introduction

Swimming is a very agreeable sporting activity for the disabled
because, in many cases, it allows them to get out of their wheel-
chairs. Technical and biomechanical aspects of the disableds' water
locomotion have been and are the topic of many scientific studies,
while metabolic aspects have not been investigated enough.
    Particularly the simple measurement of post-competition blood
lactate concentration indicates the involvement of anaerobic
energetic sources. Several data can confirm an increase in post-
competition blood lactate in healthy swimmers (Mader et al., 1976;
Sawka et al., 1979; Telford et al., 1988; Chatard et al., 1988). On
the contrary measurements of blood lactate in disabled athletes are
unknown.
    The purpose of this study was to compare post-competition blood
lactate concentration in disabled athletes and healthy swimmers.

2 Methods

We examined nine top disabled swimmers (paraplegic and polio with
different handicap levels) participating in a national competition of
50 m freestyle swimming. Seventeen top level healthy swimmers were
taken as control subjects.
    Lactate concentration was determined by microsamples of capillary
blood taken from a preheated ear lobe and analyzed by Lactate
Analyzer (Kontron 640). Each sample was taken 5 min after the end of

the competition for disabled and after a simulated competition for healthy athletes. Both groups were tested after swimming in a 25 m pool. The differences between the two groups were tested by Student's t-test.

3 Results

The results of this study are shown in Table 1.

Table 1. Performances of the swimmers in a 50 m freestyle competition. PCL: Post-competition blood lactate concentration.

Subjects	Handicap	Time (s)	Velocity (m/s)	PCL (mM)	PCL/time (mM/min)
1	Polio	77.00	0.65	7.03	5.48
2	Polio	84.32	0.59	7.94	5.42
3	Polio	40.32	1.24	10.05	14.94
4	Polio	55.10	0.91	6.22	6.78
5	Para	47.50	1.05	8.17	10.32
6	Para	51.40	0.97	9.12	10.62
7	Para	54.80	0.91	7.47	8.16
8	Para	75.44	0.66	9.38	7.44
9	Para	65.70	0.76	5.84	5.33
Mean		61.29	0.86	7.91	8.31
± SD		15.02	0.12	1.43	3.17
Mean	Controls	26.66	1.90	8.97	20.27
± SD	(n = 17)	1.77	0.11	1.61	4.47

Disabled athletes take 40"32 to 84"32 to cover 50 m in freestyle swimming. Mean (± SD) speed was significantly lower than that of healthy athletes (P < 0.001). The difference in post-competition blood lactate between healthy and disabled swimmers was not significant (P > 0.05).

The ratio between blood lactate and mean time employed to cover 50 m freestyle was significantly higher in top healthy swimmers (P < 0.001).

4 Discussion

The disabled athletes examined in this study could not utilize their lower limbs for water locomotion, in spite of the different levels of spinal cord injury. It is well known that in top healthy freestyle swimmers the arm stroke has a more decisive importance than leg kicks (Holmer, 1974, 1974a) and that the trunk muscles are involved in maintaining the right position. In polio and paraplegic swimmers the position of the body in the water is affected by the level of spinal cord lesion and by the occurrence of muscle spasma as confirmed by EMG studies (De Witte et al., 1988). Therefore, the upper limbs are involved in progression and also in correcting continuously the body position in the water. In this situation the disabled take more time to cover 50 m in freestyle swimming and accumulate a lower lactate per unity of time, than healthy swimmers. These differences can be due to the lower muscular mass utilized by disabled swimmers and to the particular technique they employ according to their own handicap. These facts can also explain the wide time-ranges to swim 50 m.

Lactate values found at the end of the 50 m race are higher than the value of 4 mM that is commonly indicated as "anaerobic threshold" (Heck et al., 1985). This means that anaerobic sources are involved in delivering the required energy in disabled swimming competitions. This fact should be considered when programming a 50 m freestyle training for disabled athletes.

5 References

Chatard, J.C., Paulin, M. and Lacour, J.R. (1988) Post-competition blood lactate measurements and swimming performance: illustrated by data from a 400 m Olympic record holder, in **Swimming Science V** (eds B.E. Ungerechts, K. Wilke and K. Reischle), Human Kinetics Books, Champaign, Ill., pp. 311-316.

De Witte, B., Loyens, R., Robeaux, R. and Clarys, J.P. (1988) The activity of trunk muscles in paraplegic patients after breast-stroke initiation, in **Swimming Science V** (eds B.E. Ungerechts, K. Wilke and K. Reischle), Human Kinetics Books, Champaign, Ill., pp. 319-331.

Heck, H., Mader, A., Hess, G., Mucke, S., Muller, R. and Hollman, W. (1985) Justification of the 4-mmol/l lactate threshold. **Int. J. Sports Med.**, 6, 117-130.

Holmér, I. (1974) Propulsive efficiency of breaststroke and freestyle swimming. **Europ. J. Appl. Physiol.**, 33, 95-103.

Holmér, I. (1974a) Energy cost of arm stroke, leg kick and the whole stroke in competitive swimming styles. **Europ. J. Appl. Physiol.**, 33, 105-118.

Mader, A., Heck, H. and Hollmann, W. (1978) Evaluation of lactic acid anaerobic energy contribution by determinatio of post-exercise lactic acid concentration of ear capillary blood in middle distance runners and swimmers. **Exerc. Physiol.**, 4, 187.

Sawka, M.N., Knowlton, R.G., Miles, D.S. and Critz, J.B. (1979) Post competition blood lactate concentrations in collegiate swimmers. **Eur. J. Appl. Physiol.**, 41, 93-99.

Telford, R.D., Hahn, A.G., Catchpole, E.C., Parker, A.R. and Sweetenham, W.F. (1988) Post-competition blood lactate concentration in highly ranked Australian swimmers, in **Swimming Science V** (eds. B.E. Ungerechts, K. Wilke and K. Reischle), Human Kinetics Books, Champaign, Ill., pp. 277-283.

PART SEVEN

PERFORMANCE AND PHYSIOLOGY

ADJUSTMENT TO MAXIMAL WORK INTENSITY DURING INTERVAL SWIMMING USING VARIOUS WORK:REST RATIOS

J.P. TROUP, A. BARZDUKAS and S. TRAPPE
U.S. Swimming, International Center for Aquatic Research, Colorado Springs, Colorado, USA

Abstract
While the duration of work will affect the relative energy contributions during work of an interval type, little is known of the role of the rest duration during interval work. The purpose of this study was to determine what effect varying the work:rest ratio has on the energy contributions when the work duration and intensity are kept constant. Well trained swimmers participated in a series of interval work sets of 12 × 100 m freestyle swims at each of the following work:rest ratios, 1:2, 1:1 and 1:1/2. All tests were conducted on separate days. During each swim, accumulated O_2 uptake was measured to describe the percent aerobic contributions. Additionally, accumulated O_2 deficit was calculated in order to describe the anaerobic profile of each swimming set. From the accumulated O_2 uptake data, the rate of adjustment to 25% of total energy demand was determined for each workout set interval. Blood lactate and base excess for all work repeats were also measured. The data suggest that (1) the rate of adjustment is faster when the work:rest ratio is shorter, (2) at a given distance, a short rest interval results in a higher aerobic contribution and (3) longer rates of adjustment reflect a greater anaerobic contribution.
Keywords: Aerobic:Anaerobic Energy, Rate of Adjustment, O_2 Kinetics, Lactate, Base Excess, Interval Training.

1 Introduction

The effects of interval training are primarily determined by two components, (i) the duration of the workbout and (ii) the duration of the rest interval. Recent studies have shown that, in spite of swimming at the same intensity, the length of the rest interval determines the net energy cost of the workout set (Troup, 1989). In general the workout will have a more anaerobic emphasis if the rest periods are longer. This may be related to the ability to adjust to the energy demand required by each interval swim. To this end the level of adjustment to total energy demand will be greater for interval training using longer rest periods (Åstrand and Rodahl, 1974). If this is true, it should be possible to measure differences in the time course of adjustment in the accumulated O_2 uptake of each work interval. The purpose of this project, therefore, was to determine the rate of adjustment to total energy demand for all work periods in an interval training set. This approach should, in turn,

explain the differences in energy utilization of workout sets caused
by varying the rest interval.

2 Methods

2.1 Subjects
After signing informed consent, eight highly trained swimmers
participated in this project. All swimmers were involved in year
round training programmes and had participated in previous testing
sessions. All tests were administered in a swimming treadmill
(Richardson et al., 1990) for greater control of swimming velocity.
Performance time trials were also conducted to determine each
swimmer's best time and achievable work duration.

2.2 Calculation of energy demands
Each swimmer participated in a series of four submaximal and one
maximal effort swim for description of the swimming economy profile
(Troup, 1986). Each of the submaximal swims was completed at a
progressively faster speed with the last swim not exceeding a heart
rate above 160 beats/min. During all swims, expired air samples were
collected on line with O_2 and CO_2 levels measured with Applied
Electrochemistry analyzers. The steady state $\dot{V}O_2$ values at each of
the swims were determined via direct computer analysis. From the
resulting linear relationship of O_2 uptake vs velocity cubed
(Hollander, 1990) the total energy demand for the test intensities
and each interval duration was determined. The O_2 demand was taken
as the product of the energy cost at 120% of $\dot{V}O_2$max (Troup, 1989) and
the duration of the swim for 100 m. Since the total time for the
interval training was set the same for all interval sets (see 2.3),
the O_2 demand was the same for all test conditions.

   Following each swim, heart rate was determined. A finger prick
blood sample was collected post-swim for determination of lactate
concentration using a YSI-L23 automated analyser.

2.3 Interval training set design
The desired work intensity for examination was selected specific to
200 m race pace which has been shown to correspond to 120% of $\dot{V}O_2$max
(Troup, 1989). One repeat distance was used to examine three
different work:rest ratios. These sets are typically used by
swimming coaches (Counsilman, 1978) and included sets of 12 × 100 m
swims. For all tested swimming sets the swimming velocity was the
same and averaged 1.66 ± 0.02 m/s for the group. For each workout
set, the total work duration was 12.20 ± 0.2 min. All swims were
done using the freestyle stroke.

   The effect of the rest interval was measured by using three
different work:rest ratios for each of the above listed workout sets.
These work:rest ratios included 1:2, 1:1 and 1:1/2. All interval set
design conditions (a total of nine; three per work repeat type) were
completed by all subjects on separate days. Randomization of
assigned testing schedules was used in this study for all subjects.

2.4 Interval set energy cost analysis
During each repeat of all workout sets, expired air samples were
collected and the accumulated O_2 uptake was calculated at 10 sec

increments. Using the previously determined O_2 demand values, accumulated O_2 uptake values were subtracted and calculation of the O_2 deficit was made (Medbø et al., 1988). While the accumulated O_2 was used to describe the aerobic energy contributions, the O_2 deficit was used to express the anaerobic capacity (Hermansen and Medbø, 1984). For purposes of comparison, these values were expressed per entire interval set based on the group mean data for the individual repeat averages.

Finger stick blood lactate values were collected after each interval swim and analyzed for lactate concentration (YSI-L23). An additional sample was collected for blood gas analysis (Instrumentation Laboratory Blood Gas Analyzer 3033) and base excess measured to determine the extent of the metabolic challenge (West, 1980).

2.5 Rate of adjustment
The time to reach 25% (t1/4) of total energy demand for each repeat swim of all work:rest ratios was calculated. The calculation was based on the accumulated O_2 uptake response for interval set conditions (Hagberg et al., 1980). Based on the total O_2 demand for each repeat, 25% of that value was determined. From the accumulated O_2 uptake of each swim, the time to reach this 25% value was then determined. The mean value for all repeats of each interval work set was determined and the average value for the set expressed. A semi-log plot of accumulated O_2 uptake vs time was used to confirm the rate of adjustment for each swim (Hagberg et al., 1980).

2.6 Statistics
Analysis of variance with repeated measures (SPSS) was carried out for all test conditions. A level of $P < 0.05$ was selected for significance.

3 Results

The data are presented as group mean data for the entire interval set examined. Figure 1 presents the O_2 deficit data (anaerobic capacity) for each work:rest ratio. While the O_2 demand remained the same for all rest interval conditions, the O_2 deficit value fell with shorter rest periods. A significant difference between the 1:1/2 set and both 1:1 and 1:2 work:rest interval sets was observed ($P < 0.05$).

Similarly, the percent aerobic energy contributions increased while the work:rest ratio fell. To this end, the shorter the rest interval the more aerobic was the interval design. A significant difference between the 1:2 and 1:1 sets vs 1:1/2 was observed ($P < 0.05$).

Blood lactate and base excess data are presented in Table 1. While both lactate and base excess data fell with shorter rest duration, no significant difference in these levels was observed.

Figure 3 illustrates the difference in the rate of adjustment of each test set. As suggested by the percent aerobic data, the rate of adjustment to 25% of total energy demand was significantly faster with shorter rest intervals. The rates of adjustment were faster for 1:1/2 work:rest ratios compared to 1:1 and 1:2 sets as was the set of 1:1 vs 1:2 ($P < 0.05$).

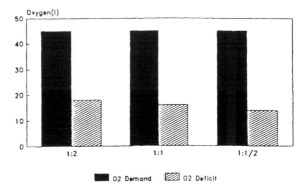

Fig. 1. The O_2 demand and O_2 deficit of interval training sets
using various work:rest ratios (1:2, 1:1 and 1:1/2).
*denotes differences between 1:2 and 1:1 vs 1:1//2
(P < 0.05).

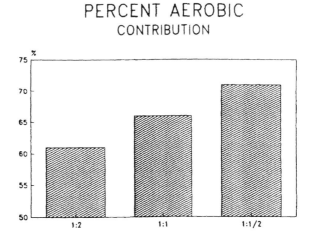

Fig. 2. Percent aerobic contribution during work:rest ratios of
of 1:2, 1:1 and 1:1/2 at common work intensity and
duration. *denotes a significant difference between
1:2, 1:1 vs 1:1/2.

Table 1.   Blood lactate and base excess response to interval training
          of work:rest ratios of 1:2, 1:1 and 1:1/2

	1:2	1:1	1:1/2
Blood lactate (mM)	9.5 ± 0.8	8.8 ± 0.9	8.3 ± 0.9
Base excess	-15.8 ± 0.7	-16.8 ± 0.6	-12.7 ± 0.8

RATE OF ADJUSTMENT

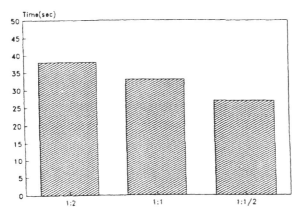

Fig. 3.   Rate of adjustment to 25% (t1/4) of total energy demand
         to interval training repeats of varying work:rest ratios.

4 Discussion

Interval training has been described by a number of investigators
over the years (Åstrand and Rodahl, 1974). Most studies have limited
their discussion to a description of what physiological changes take
place as a result of alternating work and rest periods (Åstrand and
Rodahl, 1974). While the benefits of interval training appear to be
in the swimmer's ability to swim at a greater percent of $\dot{V}O_2$max, the
design of interval training has never been well understood
(Counsilman, 1978). In fact, most interval training sets are
designed on the basis of being able to swim as fast as possible using
the shortest selected rest interval. Most coaches utilize this
specific approach in that it is commonly believed that the longer the
rest interval the less beneficial would be the adaptations to
training. The purpose of this study, therefore, was to determine
what differences exist as a result of varying the rest interval and
why.
     It is clear from the data presented that the shorter the rest
interval the more aerobic the training response becomes. This is
true regardless of the intensity of work selected. In other words,
even if the work selected is of a race specific type, by decreasing
the length of the rest interval, the net effect of the workload will

be aerobic in nature. Previous studies have revealed similar findings in that the oxygen uptake during intermittent exercise is greater when short rest periods are used (Åstrand and Rodahl, 1974). Why this is the case has essentially been speculative.

One possible way of explaining how the rest interval affects the aerobic or anaerobic contributions is to look at the rate of adjustment to energy demand. Hagberg et al. (1980) described differences in endurance trained athletes using this technique suggesting that these athletes are able to utilize energy at a faster rate than untrained athletes. It would seem that in interval training designs, the faster this rate of adjustment the closer will steady state exercise be reached. In this way the shorter rest interval allows for near maximum energy utilization for a given pace with less time spent in re-adjusting to the next work bout. The net effect of this type of exercise is aerobic since a greater amount of accumulated oxygen will be reached over the entire work period. In contrast to this, the more time required to adjust to an energy demand, the greater will be the need for anaerobic metabolism: as more time is needed the immediate energy demands will be met by the stored ATP and other anaerobic energy sources (Åstrand and Rodahl, 1974).

5 Conclusions

These data suggest that when the rest interval is short, the aerobic contribution significantly increases for the entire workout set. It is noteworthy that while lactate values decreased, this was not significant. This might suggest that the measurement of lactate alone during work intervals may not provide as accurate a picture of the energy demands of training as needed. In summary, it is important when designing the interval set to give attention to the length of the rest interval. Additionally, it is important to realize that more anaerobic type work can be achieved when the rest interval is longer in spite of the intensity of work.

6 References

Åstrand, P.O. and Rodahl, K. (1974) **Textbook of Work Physiology.** McGraw-Hill, New York.

Counsilman, J.E. (1978) **Science of Swimming.** University Park Press, Baltimore.

Hagberg, J.M., Mullin, J.P. and Nagle, F.J. (1980) Effect of work intensity and duration on recovery O_2. J. **Appl. Physiol: Respirat. Environ. Exercise Physiol.**, 48, 540-544.

Hermansen, L. and Medbo, J.I. (1984) The relative significance of aerobic and anerobic processes during maximal exercise of short duration. **Medicine, Sport and Science**, 17, 56-67.

Hollander, A.P. (1990) O_2 deficit and energy stores. Unpublished manuscript (Vrije Universiteit, Amsterdam).

Medbo, J.I., Mohn, A.C., Tabata, I., Bahr, R., Vaage, O. and Sejersted, O.M. (1988) Anaerobic capacity determined by maximal accumulated O_2 deficit. **J. Appl. Physiol.**, 64, 50-60.

Richardson, A.B., Troup, J.P. and D'Acquisto, L.J. (1990) Swimming treadmill: Validation of physiological and biomechanical aspects.

Communication to ACSM Conference.

Troup, J.P. (1986) Swimming economy - an overview. **J. Swimming Res.**, 1(2), 3-7.

Troup, J.P. (1989) Training intensities. **Proc. the VIIth FINA Conference on Medical and Scientific Aspects of Aquatic Sports, London.**

West, J.B. (1980) **Repiratory Physiology - The Essentials.** 2nd Ed. Williams and Wilkins, Baltimore.

PERFORMANCE RELATED DIFFERENCES IN THE ANAEROBIC CONTRIBUTION OF COMPETITIVE FREESTYLE SWIMMERS

J.P. TROUP, A.P. HOLLANDER, M. BONE, S. TRAPPE and A.P. BARZDUKAS
U.S. Swimming, International Center for Aquatic Research, Colorado
Springs, Colorado, USA

Abstract
The purpose of this project was to determine (1) how the anaerobic
energy contributions of competitive swimming distances may vary with
performance level, and (2) whether the adjustment in O_2 uptake to
maximal swimming intensities are different between high vs low
performance level swimmers. Based on 200 m freestyle performances,
well trained swimmers were divided into two groups, (a) low
performers (LP) (n = 30) 1.58 $\pm$ 0.02 m/s and (b) high performance
(HP) (n = 34) 1.69 $\pm$ 0.02 m/s. A swimming economy test was completed
by all swimmers from which the O_2 demand was determined corresponding
to 100, 200 and 400 m work intensities. Each swimmer returned to the
laboratory on separate days to complete swims at these prescribed
intensities. During the swims expired gases were collected continuously on line with accumulated O_2 uptake determined at 10 s increments. The O_2 deficit was calculated as the difference between the
O_2 demand and the accumulated O_2 uptake and used to describe the
anaerobic capacity and the percent anaerobic energy contribution.
Prior to the start and following each swim a mixed arterialized blood
sample was collected for analysis of base excess, pH, lactate and
buffer capacity. From the accumulated O_2 uptake curves, the time to
reach 25% of the total O_2 demand was determined. Analysis of variance with repeated measures was carried out to determine significance
at $P < 0.05$. Results suggest that at the same relative work intensity, (1) anaerobic capacity varies with performance level, (2)
anaerobic energy contributions differ with performance level and (3)
swimmers of higher performance levels adjust to work at faster rates.
Keywords: Anaerobic Capacity, Buffer Capacity, Aerobic:Anaerobic
Contribution, O_2 Kinetics, Lactate.

1 Introduction

Anaerobic energy contributions play a key role during high intensity,
short duration work bouts (Åstrand and Rodahl, 1974; Hermansen, 1969;
Gollnick, 1978). While previous studies (Troup, 1990; Hollander,
1990b) have described the energy contribution requirements of swimming specific events, little work has been available that describes
the relationship of energy systems to performance. Most studies that
have presented a link between performance level and physiological
capacity have limited their description to the aerobic demands
(Van Handel et al., 1988). However, with the recent subtantiation of

an anaerobic measurement test (Hermansen and Medbø, 1984), it becomes possible to evaluate the role that the anaerobic system plays in swimming performance.

Through the determination of O_2 demand (Hermansen, 1969), and the direct measurement of accumulated oxygen uptake, the anaerobic capacity of the exercising swimmer can be described by calculating the O_2 deficit (Medbø and Burgers, 1990; Medbø et al., 1988). While this technique has been useful in describing the role of the anaerobic energy contributions, only recently has it been used to determine the aerobic:anaerobic contributions of each swimming distance (Hollander, 1990b; Troup, 1990). It would seem possible, therefore, that a difference in the anaerobic capacity of athletes would exist that could better describe the energy demand relationship to swimming performances.

The purpose of this project was, for swimmers of different performance levels, to (1) determine whether or not a difference in the anaerobic capacity exists, (2) to describe how the adjustment in O_2 uptake at maximal swimming intensities may differ and (3) to describe the anaerobic characteristics when swimming at 100, 200 and 400 m race paces.

2 Methods

2.1 Subjects and performance characteristics
Highly trained swimmers who are involved in competitive training programmes year-round participated in this project. All subjects were male swimmers specializing in the freestyle events. These swimmers were divided into two testing groups based on their 200 m freestyle times, including (i) low performers (n = 30) with an average performance time of 1.58 ± 0.02 m/s, and (ii) high performers (n = 34) with an average performance time of 1.69 ± 0.1 m/s. Prior to the start of the study, all swimmers participated in a time trial competition in order to determine their current best performances in the 100, 200 and 400 m freestyle.

2.2 Energy demand measurements
During the first week of the project, all subjects completed a series of four submaximal swims lasting 5 min each. Each swim was progressively faster than the previous effort with the last effort having a heart rate below 160 beats/min. All swims and tests were conducted in a swimming treadmill which allowed for the accurate control of all test speeds (Troup, 1989). During each swim, expired air samples were collected on line at 10 s increments. Applied Electrochemistry analyzers were used to determine the concentrations of O_2 and CO_2. A specialized computer software program determined oxygen consumption values during the course of each swim. Following the series of submaximal effort swims, a progressive maximal effort swim to exhaustion was administered to determine the maximal oxygen uptake values.

After each swim, a finger stick blood sample was collected for determination of lactate (YSI L-23), and blood gases were analysed (Instrumentation Laboratories model 3033) for determination of base excess.

2.3 Oxygen demand and O_2 deficit

From the resulting linear relationship of O_2 uptake vs velocity cubed an extrapolation to 140, 127 and 108% of $\dot{V}O_2$max was made as described by Hollander (1990a). These intensities were selected as they have previously been shown (Troup, 1986) to describe the energy costs of 100, 200 and 400 m freestyle swimming, respectively. The O_2 demand was then calculated as the product of O_2 cost and the duration of each swim (Hermansen and Medbø, 1984). The duration was taken as the time actually achieved by each swimmer at each distance during a time trial swim in a 25 yard pool. The accumulated O_2 deficit can then be calculated as the difference between the accumulated O_2 uptake during the workout and the estimated O_2 demand for a selected work intensity (Hermansen and Medbø, 1984).

2.4 Test swims and accumulated O_2 uptake

Each swimmer, by randomized selection, returned to the test facili- ties during the second week of the project to complete swims at each of the three distances selected. All individual swims were completed on different days and all swimmers swam at speeds selected from their specific energy demand cost curves for 100, 200 and 400 m work bouts.

During each swim, expired air samples were collected continuously on-line via computer interface. Accumulated O_2 uptake values were determined at 10 s increments using the same equipment as described under section 2.2. This accumulated oxygen uptake was then used to determine the accumulated O_2 deficit values as described above. The determined values for O_2 deficit were used to describe the anaerobic capacity (Hermansen and Medbø, 1984). Accumulated values for the entire swim are presented in the Results section.

Prior to the start and immediately after each swim, a mixed arterialized blood sample was collected from the finger-tip. These samples were used to determine lactate concentration (YSI L-23) and blood gases (Instrumentation Laboratories) for calculation of buffer capacity (Sahlin, 1985).

2.5 Rate of adjustment

During each swim test at all distances the accumulated O_2 uptake value at 10 s increments was determined. These data were then graphically expressed for use in determining the time to reach 25% (t1/4) of the estimated O_2 demand for each swimmer and group. A semi-log plot of accumulated O_2 uptake was plotted vs time as described by Hagberg et al. (1980). The O_2 demand was used as the point of comparison since this value represents the actual energy contributions of both energy systems. Time of 25% of total O_2 demand was selected as it represented a common time increment for all subjects.

2.6 Statistics

Analysis of variance with repeated measures (SPSS) was used to identify differences between test swims and performance levels. Correlation analysis was also carried out to examine the relation- ships between performance time and the anaerobic capacity (i.e. O_2 deficit). Finally, linear regression analysis of the adjustment in O_2 vs time of each swim was completed. In all cases significance was determined at the $P < 0.05$ level.

3 Results

The results presented below suggest that swimmers of higher performance levels also have greater energy reserves. It is possible to
compare athletes of different ability levels by measuring the energy
contributions of each group at the same relative intensities. This
was done by having all swimmers complete three swims on separate days
at race specific intensities. The group means for each swim were
(expressed as a percent of $\dot{V}O_2$max) 100 m: 144 $\pm$ 4 (HP), 140 $\pm$ 5 (LP);
200 m: 127 $\pm$ 5 (HP), 126 $\pm$ 2 (LP); 400 m: 105 $\pm$ 5 (HP), 107 $\pm$ 5 (LP).
   The accumulated O_2 deficit was used to express the anaerobic
contribution at each swim. The highest value, attained after swims
lasting longer than 2 min, was used to express the maximal anaerobic
capacity. Figure 1 illustrates the findings that the anaerobic
capacity at each distance was greater in the high performer group.
While the anaerobic capacity at the 200 and 100 m swims was higher in
the better trained group (P < 0.05), a significant difference in
maximal anaerobic capacity was seen between groups.

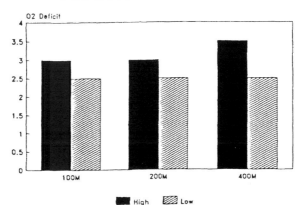

Fig. 1. Anaerobic capacity of high vs low performance groups.
Measured as O_2 deficit (1).

It is interesting to note that in spite of the larger anaerobic
capacity a difference between groups as well as between swim intensities exists in the percent anaerobic contribution. In this case, the
better trained swimmers had a lower percent energy contribution from
the anaerobic sources when compared to the lower performance group.
   The enhanced anaerobic capacity is further illustrated by looking
at the lactate, base excess and calculated buffer capacity values.
These results, described in Table 1, reveal that the better trained
swimmers can produce higher lactate values at each swim, have lower
base excess and have a better buffering capacity (B) than the less
well trained, low performer, group.
   The rate of total energy outlay is presented in Table 2 and shows
that the better trained swimmers also can adjust to the energy
demands of the swimming intensity faster than the less well trained
swimmers.

PERCENT ANAEROBIC
CONTRIBUTION

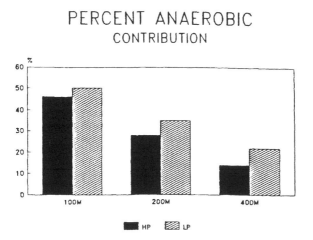

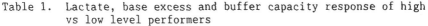

Fig. 2. Percent anaerobic energy contribution for each swimming
distance.

Table 1. Lactate, base excess and buffer capacity response of high
vs low level performers

	100 m	200 m	400 m
Lactate (mM):			
HP	10.5 ± 0.2	10.2 ± 0.2	9.5 ± 0.3
LP	7.9 ± 0.3	9.8 ± 0.3	11.7 ± 0.3
Base excess:			
HP	$-12.6 \pm 0.2^*$	-12.5 ± 0.3	$-13.5 \pm 0.5^*$
LP	-7.8 ± 0.3	$-12.4 \pm 0.1^+$	$-16.0 \pm 0.1^+$
Buffer capacity:			
HP	$89.0 \pm 1.5^*$	$121.6 \pm 12.0^{*+}$	$52.0 \pm 4.0^{*+}$
LP	$46.5 \pm 1.0^*$	$63.4 \pm 5.0^+$	$44.0 \pm 2.0^+$

*Group difference; $^+$Difference between swims (P < 0.05)

Table 2. Time of adjustment of 25% of total energy demand (s)

	100 m	200 m	400 m
t 1/4			
HP	$33.0 \pm 1.5^*$	$53.0 \pm 1.0^*$	$235 \pm 5^{*+}$
LP	43.0 ± 1.0	$61.0 \pm 2.0^+$	$295 \pm 10^+$

*Group difference; $^+$difference between swims (P < 0.05

4 Discussion

The results of this study suggest that the better, well trained
swimmer has a larger source of energy and can adjust to the use of
energy at a faster rate than the less well trained. Furthermore, it
appears that the swimmer who is of a higher performance level also
utilizes a greater percent of energy from the more efficient aerobic

energy sources.

These data are supported by previous studies which have described similar data but independently of each component. Medbø et al. (1988) showed that sprint athletes have a higher anaerobic capacity while trained athletes also show a similar elevated capacity when compared to the untrained athlete. This study is significant in that the data suggest that even in athletes who are highly trained, the anaerobic capacity will be higher than those of a lower talent level. Toward this end, correlation analysis revealed a rather high relationship between anaerobic capacity (i.e. O_2 deficit) and 100 m freestyle performances ($r = 0.77$, $P < 0.05$). These data are significant in that anaerobic capacity can be used to determine levels of performance – something previously limited to endurance profiles of athletes as described in the literature (Åstrand and Rodahl, 1974; Brooks and Fahey, 1984).

While few studies have measured the percent of aerobic:anaerobic contributions in swimming, studies described by Åstrand and Rodahl (1974) have suggested that the more efficient energy source is the aerobic system. Similarly, this study also shows that in spite of a larger anaerobic capacity, a greater percent of energy is derived from the aerobic sources. Similarly, the rate of adjustment of energy utilization is also faster in the group of athletes more talented and likely better trained. This is also supported by previous studies (Hagberg et al., 1980) that revealed that endurance trained athletes have a faster rate of adjustment than untrained swimmers.

Blood data collected in these studies also confirm the characteristics described by the O_2 uptake data. In all test events, those athletes of a higher performance level were able to produce higher lactate levels as well as lower base excess values. To this end, calculations of the buffer capacity also revealed better buffering potential for the high performance levels. These data also support the many studies in the literature that described adaptations and distinguishing features of elite, world class swimmers (Troup, 1990).

5 Conclusions

In summary, even though highly trained athletes have high energy system profiles, differences between athletes can be described. This includes differences in both the aerobic and anaerobic energy systems. Furthermore, these data also support the use of the O_2 deficit measurement as a test describing anaerobic capacity and can therefore be used to describe differences between athletes of different talent and performance levels.

6 References

Åstrand, P.O. and Rodahl, K. (1974) **Textbook of Work Physiology.** McGraw-Hill, New York.

Brooks, G.A. and Fahey, T.D. (1984) **Exercise Physiology: Human Bioenergetics and its Application.** John Wiley and Sons Inc., New York, pp. 330-336.

Gollnick, P.D. (1978) Anerobic contributions. **Exercise and Sport**

Science Reviews, 1, 3-20, University Park Press.

Hagberg, J.M., Mullin, J.P. and Nagle, F.J. (1980) Effect of work intensity and duration on recovery O_2. J. Appl. Physiol: Respirat. Environ. Exercise Physiol., 48, 540-544.

Hermansen, L. (1969) Anaerobic energy release. Med. Sci. Sports Exerc., 1, 32-38.

Hermansen, L. and Medbø, J.I. (1984) The relative significance of aerobic and anaerobic processes during maximal exercise of short duration. Medicine, Sport and Science, 17, 56-67.

Hollander, A.P. (1990a) Economy regression lines and their meaning. Unpublished manuscript (Vrije Universiteit, Amsterdam).

Hollander, A.P. (1990b) O_2 deficit and energy stores. Unpublished manuscript (Vrije Universiteit, Amsterdam).

Medbø, J.I. and Burgers, S. (1990) Effect of training on the anaerobic capacity. Med. Sci. Sports Exerc., 22, 501-507.

Medbø, J.I., Mohn, A-C., Tabata, I., Bahr, R., Vaage, O. and Sejersted, O.M. (1988) Anaerobic capacity determined by maximal accumulated O_2 deficit. J. Appl. Physiol., 64, 50-60.

Sahlin, K. (1985) Buffer capacity of exercise trained cyclics. Acta Physiol. Scand., 124, 97-109.

Troup, J.P. (1986) Swimming economy - an overview. J. Swimming Res., 1, 3-7.

Troup, J.P. (1989) Training intensities. Proc. VIIth FINA Conference on Medical and Scientific Aspects of Water Sports, London.

Troup, J.P. (1990) International Center for Aquatic Research Annual, Colorado Springs.

Van Handel, P.J., Katz, A., Morrow, J.R., Troup, J.P., Daniels, J.T. and Bradley, P.W. (1988) Aerobic economy and competitive performance of US elite swimemrs, in Swimming Science V (eds B. Ungerechts, K. Wilke and K. Reischle), Human Kinetics Books, Champaign, Ill..

AEROBIC:ANAEROBIC CONTRIBUTIONS DURING VARIOUS DISTANCES AT COMMON
WORK:REST RATIOS

J.P. TROUP, S. TRAPPE, G. CRICKARD, L. D'ACQUISTO, A. BARZDUKAS
U.S. Swimming, International Center for Aquatic Research, Colorado
Springs, Colorado, USA

Abstract
Interval type training is widely used in the sport of swimming. This
type of training, however, is affected by the rest period selected.
The purpose of this project, therefore, was to determine how the
aerobic:anaerobic energy contribution at a selected work intensity is
altered with different interval distances at a common work:rest
ratio. A secondary objective was to determine which repeat distance
may be most specific to the energy demands of 200 m specific
training. Workout sets of the same swimming intensity with different
repeat distances and common work:rest ratios (1:2) were examined. On
separate days swimmers completed one of the following sets, 6 × 200,
12 × 100 and 24 × 50 m swims. During each swim of each set accumulated O_2 uptake was determined with the resulting percent aerobic:
anaerobic contributions calculated. Mixed arterialized blood samples
were taken after each repeat for analysis of lactate and base excess.
The results demonstrated that (1) the aerobic energy contribution
increased with shorter repeat distances, (2) the anaerobic contribution increases with shorter work duration and (3) the 100 m repeat
distance is most specific to 200 m pace specific swimming.
Keywords: Interval Training, Aerobic:Anaerobic Energy, O_2 Kinetics,
O_2 Demand.

1 Introduction

Interval training is commonly used for preparation of racing distances requiring high intensity short duration effoerts. Whenever
intermittent training is used, however, the energy contributions may
be altered as a result of the length of either the rest interval or
the selected work distance (Åstrand and Rodahl, 1974). Recent
studies (Hollander, 1990b) have described the energy continuum of
competitive swimming distances which should help establish the most
accurate interval training design for a specific event. Interval
training design is difficult since the selection of a repeat distance
and work:rest ratio will alter the energy contributions in spite of
working at the same relative intensities (Troup, 1990). The purpose
of this project, therefore, was to determine how the aerobic:
anaerobic energy contribution changes by altering work duration while
maintaining work intensity at a common work:rest ratio. A secondary
consideration was to establish which interval training distance is
the most specific to the energy demands of a 200 m freestyle race.

2 Methods

2.1 Methods and selection of work intensity

Highly trained male swimmers (n = 8) participated in this project after signing informed consent. All swimming specific testing was done in a swimming treadmill (Richardson et al., 1990) in order to control velocity at a steady state while collecting $\dot{V}O_2$ data. Each participant participated in year round training with data collected during the mid-season phase of training.

All subjects completed a series of four submaximal and one progressive maximal effort swim for determination of the swimming economy profile. During each submaximal effort, the swimming speed was progressively faster with the pace of the last submaximal effort not above a heart rate of 160 beats/min. During each swim, expired air samples were collected continuously on-line with analysis of O_2 and CO_2 with Applied Electrochemistry analyzers. A computer program was used to directly calculate $\dot{V}O_2$ at each effort (Costill and Wilmore, 1973). The resulting linear relationship of O_2 uptake vs velocity cubed (Hollander, 1990a) was used to determine the energy demand of 200 m freestyle swimming by extrapolation to 120% of $\dot{V}O_2$max (Troup, 1989). The resulting swimming velocity was then used for all subsequent testing.

2.2 Interval set design

Typical workout sets used in the sport of swimming were designed to evaluate the effect of repeat duration. All sets were designed to be of common work duration based on the swimming velocity and duration of each set. In all interval design sets, the total work period was 12.36 ± 0.1 min. The average swimming velocity was a pace of 1:01.8 per 100 m. Additionally, for all interval sets, a common work:rest ratio of 1:2 was used. Each of the following three interval sets was then completed by all swimmers on separate days by assignment in randomized order. The sets included 6 × 200, 12 × 100 and 24 × 50 m freestyle swims. Since the swimming treadmill was used for all tests, the duration of each repeat swim was selected on the basis of the actual time swum for each distance at the selected velocity.

2.3 O_2 demand and O_2 uptake

From the swimming economy profile, the energy demand or O_2 demand for each repeat and entire set duration was determined as the product of the energy cost and the duration of work. During each repeat swim, expired air samples were collected continuously on-line with the accumulated O_2 calculated at 10 s increments (Medbø et al., 1988). The calculated O_2 deficit (i.e. O_2 demand minus accumulated O_2 uptake (Medbø et al., 1988)) was used to describe the percent anaerobic contribution. Accumulated O_2 uptake was used to describe the percent aerobic contribution.

2.4 Blood analysis

Following each repeat swim of each interval set a mixed arterialized blood sample was taken from the finger tip. The samples were then analyzed for lactate concentration (YSI 23L) and base excess (Instrumentation Laboratory Blood Gas Analyzer 3033). For time comparative purposes, the data are presented as mean data for each interval set.

2.5 Statistics
Analysis of variance with repeated measures was used for statistical analysis (SPSS). Appropriate post-hoc tests were completed with the P < 0.05 level selected for significance.

3 Results

Figure 1 illustrates the differences between the accumulated O_2 uptake between each interval workout set. It is interesting to note that the calculated O_2 demand was the same (45.1 ± 3.0 l) for all interval sets since the work duration was the same in all cases. However, the accumulated O_2 uptake was significantly lower for both 100 and 50 m sets when compared to the 200 m sets, with the 50 m set different from the 100 m set (P < 0.05).

ACCUMULATED O2 UPTAKE

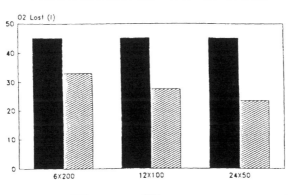

Figure 1. Accumulated O_2 uptake (l) and O_2 demand (l) for workout sets of 6 × 200, 12 × 100 and 24 × 50's each of the same work duration.

Just as the accumulated O_2 uptake fell with decreasing work distance, the percent aerobic contribution fell as the percent anaerobic contribution increased.

Results of blood analyses are presented in Table 1. Patterns

Table 1. Blood lactate and base excess response following interval work sets of 6 × 200, 12 × 100 and 24 × 50

	6 × 200	12 × 100	24 × 50
Blood lactate (mM)	11.10 ± 0.4	8.96 ± 0.8	5.60 ± 0.6 [*][+]
Base excess	-15.18 ± 0.3	-13.73 ± 0.2*	-10.37 ± 0.3 [*][+]
Intensity (% $\dot{V}O_2$max)	120	120	120

[*]difference between 200's vs 100's and 50's
[+]difference between 100's and 50's   (P < 0.05)

observed here are somewhat different than anticipated based on the percent anaerobic contribution observed. With decreasing work duration, in spite of the same work intensity, both the lactate and base excess values were observed to fall. These data appear to respond to a duration effect rather than strictly an intensity effect. Nevertheless, lactate values differed ($P < 0.05$) only between the 200, 100 m swims vs the 50 m set. Base excess differences were also apparent ($P < 0.05$) between the sets.

4 Discussion

These data describe the differences in the aerobic:anaerobic contributions of interval training sets. While the work intensity and the rest intervals were both controlled in this study, observed differences were due to the work duration differences.

The accumulated O_2 uptake values fell ($P < 0.05$) with decreasing work duration. This is due to the fact that the work was not long enough for an elevated energy demand (Åstrand and Rodahl, 1974). This suggests that, in spite of swimming at the same velocities, work duration will affect the category of work achievable. It would seem, therefore, that the speed must be increased at shorter distances in order to increase the aerobic contribution.

Previous studies (Troup, 1990) have described the aerobic: anaerobic contributions for each swimming distance. In the case of 200 m race specific training an aerobic:anaerobic contribution of 61-39% is required. Review of the percentages achieved in each of the work sets examined reveals that the 100 m set was most specific to this requirement, the 200 m sets being too high and the 50 m sets too low ($P < 0.05$). This suggests that the 100 m repeat work duration is most specific to the desired type of training.

In review of the blood data with decreasing duration of work, the lactate value at each repeat distance fell, a significant difference being observed in the 50 m sets ($P < 0.05$). This suggests that the production of lactate is also duration dependent. It would seem that caution must be used when performing lactate testing at a selected intensity while training at short work durations. This situation could be addressed by adjusting the repeat swims of the shorter duration efforts in such a way that the velocity is increased. This would have the net effect of increasing the energy cost as well as increasing the lactate values. Similarly, base excess values revealed similar changes to that of lactate. This further suggests that the 100 m efforts are more specific to 200 m race paces.

5 Conclusions

In summary, these data suggest (1) accumulated O_2 uptake decreased with shorter repeat distance thus reflecting a decrease in the aerobic contribution, (3) the anaerobic component increases as the work duration falls and (3) 100 m repeats appear to be more specific to 200 m race specific training.

6 References

Åstrand, P.O. and Rodahl, K. (1974). **Textbook of Work Physiology.** McGraw-Hill, New York.

Costill, D.L. and Wilmore, J. (1973) The semi-automated method for determination of exercising oxygen consumption. **Med. Sci. Sport Exercise**, 6, 25-30.

Hollander, A.P. (1990a) Economy regression lines and their meaning. Unpublished manuscript (Vrije Universiteit, Amsterdam).

Hollander, A.P. (1990b) O_2 deficit and energy stores. Unpublished manuscript (Vrije Universiteit, Amsterdam).

Medbø, J.I., Mohn, A.C., Tabata, I., Bahr, R., Vaage, O. and Sejersted, O.M. (1988) Anaerobic capacity determined by maximal accumulated O_2 deficit. **J. Appl. Physiol.**, 64, 50-60.

Richardson, A.B., Troup, J.P. and D'Acquisto, L.J. (1990) Swimming treadmill: validation of physiological and biomechanical aspects. **Communication to 1990 ACSM Conference.**

Troup, J.P. (1989) Training intensities. **Proc. VIIth FINA Conference on Medical and Scientific Aspects of Aquatic Sports, London.**

Troup, J.P. (1990) International Center for Aquatic Research Annual, Colorado Springs.

EVALUATION OF MAXIMAL AEROBIC VELOCITY AND PREDICTION OF PERFORMANCE
IN BACKSTROKE

S. SANO[1], J. BONGBÉLÉ[2] J.-C. CHATARD[3] and J.-M. LAVOIE[4], [1]INSEPS,
Dakar, Sénégal; [2]ISEPS, Brazzaville, Rep. Pop. du Congo, [3]Université
de Saint-Etienne, France; [4]Université de Montréal, Canada

Abstract
The functional and maximal aerobic power (FMAP) of approximately 200
swimmers (males and females) of different ages (11-12, 13-14, > 15
years) were evaluated using backstroke swimming according to a
maximal multistage swim test recently developed (Lavoie et al.,
1985). In addition, an estimate of the energy cost of swimming, the
arm stroke index (ASI), i.e. the ratio of the number of arm strokes
and swimming velocity, was measured. The results indicate a clear
progression of both these variables with age. Using the best
performance times produced by these swimmers, a regression equation
for the prediction of performance times was established, taking into
account the following variables: FMAP, ASI, age, sex and the swimming
distance. For the 100 and 200 m backstroke, the equation is: $y =
1.08 + (0.033 \text{ FMAP}) - (0.00044 \text{ ASI}) - (0.019 \text{ sex}) - (0.00082
\text{ distance})$, with a correlation coefficient of 0.8 and the standard
error of estimate of 5.2%. These data can be used as a tool to
partial out the swimming economy and energetic capacity in backstroke
swimming.
Keywords: Backstroke, Functional Maximal Aerobic Power, Arm Stroke
Index, Training.

1 Introduction

In recent years, field tests based on the measurement of functional
maximal aerobic power (FMAP) were introduced (Léger and Lambert,
1982). The FMAP is a combined index of maximal aerobic power and
mechanical efficiency, and corresponds to the velocity (running or
swimming) at which VO_2max is reached. The notion of FMAP has been
recently applied to front crawl and breaststroke swimming (Lavoie et
al., 1988; Bongbélé et al., 1989), in connection with the measurement
of an estimate of swimming economy: the arm stroke index (ASI). This
index of swimming economy consists simply of the number of arm
strokes for a given distance (125 m) divided by the swimming velocity
in m/s. The purpose of the present investigation was to evaluate the
FMAP and ASI of a large number of competitive swimmers using
backstroke swimming and to compare these values with those found
using front crawl and breaststroke swimming.

2 Methods

A large group of active swimmers (n = 206) volunteered to take part in this study. These swimmers, from both sexes, were classified in three groups according to their age: 11–12 (20 males, 38 females), 13–14 (32 males, 43 females) and 15+ years (35 males, 38 females). The swimmers had their FMAP and ASI evaluated in approximately the middle of the training season. The FMAP was evaluated through a maximal multistage swim test recently developed by Lavoie et al. (1985). Briefly, this test consists of swimming a series of continuous 2-min stages at a progressively increasing velocity until the swimmer is unable to keep up with the speed. In the present study, the test started at 0.7 m/s (stage 1) and the speed was increased by 0.05 m/s up to 1.15 m/s, and by 0.025 m/s thereafter. The subjects were paced by light pacers placed on the side of the pool. The ASI was also measured during the test. The number of arm strokes (averaged for 125 m) was divided by the swimming velocity in m/s. The ASI was calculated at the speed of 1.10, 0.95 or 0.8 m/s depending on the ability level of the swimmer.

During the course of these evaluations the best performances (100, 200 m) registered by these swimmers during the most recent swimming meet were recorded. To predict swimming performance, these performance times were multiple regressed with FMAP, ASI, swimming distance, sex and age. For statistical comparison, an analysis of variance non-repeated measures design was utilized.

3 Results

Averaged values for FMAP and ASI according to sex and age groups are presented in Table 1. A significant ($P < 0.005$) increase in FMAP and a significant decrease in ASI with age in both sexes was observed. There were, however, no significant differences between male and female swimmers for the three age groups.

Table 1. Comparisons of functional maximal aerobic power (FMAP) and arm stroke index (ASI) using front crawl (C), backstroke (BS) and breaststroke (BR) swimming (means $\pm$ SD).

Age	Sex	FMAP (m/s)			ASI	
		C	BS	BR	C	BS
11–12	M	1.09 ± 0.1	0.95 ± 0.1	0.95 ± 0.1	153 ± 28	135 ± 24
13–14	M	1.28 ± 0.1	1.05 ± 0.1	1.04 ± 0.1	113 ± 18	99 ± 12
15+	M	1.37 ± 0.1	1.15 ± 0.1	1.11 ± 0.1	97 ± 16	89 ± 11
11–12	F	1.10 ± 0.1	0.95 ± 0.1	0.93 ± 0.1	153 ± 22	127 ± 27
13–14	F	1.16 ± 0.1	1.05 ± 0.1	1.00 ± 0.01	131 ± 23	102 ± 12
15+	F	1.27 ± 0.1	1.15 ± 0.1	1.04 ± 0.06	110 ± 16	92 ± 13

A regression equation for the prediction of performance times was established, using FMAP (stage), ASI, age, sex and the swimming distance. For the 100 and 200 m swims, the equation is: $y = 1.08 + (0.033\ \text{FMAP}) + (0.00044\ \text{ASI}) - (0.019\ \text{sex}) - (0.0082\ \text{distance})$, with a correlation coefficient of 0.80 and a standard error of estimate of 5.21%. The age group in the regression equation corresponds to the number 11, 13 or 15, and the sex to the number 1 and 2 for males and females respectively. The predicted variable y is velocity in m/s.

Comparisons of FMAP and ASI values measured using backstroke swimming to values measured using front crawl and breaststroke swimming (Bongbélé et al., 1989) are presented in Table 1. As expected FMAP velocities were respectively faster in front crawl, backstroke and breaststroke swimming. Although the ASI in breaststroke swimming (using both arms simultaneously) cannot be compared to the two other strokes, it is interesting to observe that the ASI was lower in backstroke than in front crawl swimming in all of the six groups of swimmers.

4 Discussion

The improvement of FMAP and ASI with age using backstroke swimming confirms similar findings found previously using front crawl and breaststroke (Lavoie et al., 1988; Bongbélé et al., 1989). These results reinforce the notion that the improvement of performance times with age depends not only on improvements of energy production systems, but also on improvements of swimming economy. In all three styles, the FMAP was similar between the 11-12 years old male and female swimmers. This was not the case for the 13-14 and 15+ year groups in front crawl and breaststroke swimming. The absence of differences in FMAP between male and female swimmers (13-14 and 15+ years) using backstroke swimming is probably due to the fact that in our sample, females represented a group of relatively better backstroke swimmers than males. This contention is supported by the finding of comparable ASI in females and in males using backstroke swimming. On a practical point of view, these FMAP and ASI results using backstroke swimming can be used to get an unbiased evaluation of aerobic capacity and swimming economy.

The high correlation coefficient (0.8) and low standard error of estimate (5.21%) found for the present regression indicate an acceptable level of accuracy for predictive responses. The FMAP and ASI have previously been reported to be good predictors of swimming performances (Lavoie et al., 1988). This regression equation can be used to determine a target time that a swimmer should be able to realize according to his or her FMAP and ASI. An interesting finding of the present study is the observation that in all groups of swimmers the ASI is lower in backstroke than in front crawl swimming (Table 1). This might reflect a sampling problems in the quality of backstroke versus front crawl swimmers. Even though the available information on swimming economy of backstroke swimming is scarce (Smith et al., 1988), higher distances/stroke in backstroke compared to front crawl swimming have been previously reported (Craig and Pendergast, 1979). The better ASI in backstroke compared to front crawl swimming might also be the result of a greater mechanical efficiency or a greater contribution of the legs in backstroke swimming.

5 Acknowledgement

This study was supported by a grant from Sport Canada.

6 References

Bongbélé, J., Leone, M., Lafond, A. and Lavoie, J.-M. (1989) Etude normative de la puissance aérobie maximale et fonctionelle en crawl et en brasse. **Science et Motricité**, 7, 25-28.

Craig, A.B. and Pendergast, D.R. (1979) Relationships of stroke rate, distance per stroke, and velocity in competitive swimming. **Med. Sci. Sports**, 11, 278-283.

Lavoie, J.-M., Léger, L.A., Leone, M. and Provencher, P. (1985) A maximal multistage swim test to determine the functional and maximal aerobic power of competitive swimmers. **J. Swimming Res.**, 1, 17-22.

Lavoie,. J.-M., Leone, M. and Bongbélé, J. (1988) Functional maximal aerobic power and prediction of swimming performances. **J. Swimming Res.**, 4, 17-19.

Léger, L.A. and Lambert, J. (1982) A maximal multistage 20 m shuttle run test to predict VO_2max. **Eur. J. Appl. Physiol**, 49, 1-12.

Smith, H.K., Montpetit, R.R. and Perrault, H. (1988) The aerobic demand of backstroke swimming, and its relation to body size, stroke technique and performance. **Eur. J. Appl. Physiol.**, 58, 182-188.

DIFFERENCES IN THE ANAEROBIC POWER OF AGE GROUP SWIMMERS

S. TAKAHASHI, M. BONE, S. SPRY, S. TRAPPE and J.P. TROUP
U.S. Swimming, International Center for Aquatic Research, Colorado
Springs, Colorado, USA

Abstract
In order to determine (1) the anaerobic capacity and characteristics
of age group swimmers and (2) how the anaerobic energy contributions
change with age, 28 well trained swimmers were tested in the following age groups based on mean age, AG1 - 9.5 $\pm$ 0.5 years (n = 6), AG2
- 11.5 $\pm$ 0.5 years (n = 6), AG3 13.45 $\pm$ 0.6 years (n = 5), AG4 - 16.0
$\pm$ 0.4 years (n = 5), and AG5 18.0 $\pm$ 0.5 years (n = 5). All swimmers
first completed a series of four submaximal swims followed by a
maximal swim for determination of individual energy cost curves. The
resulting linear relationship ($\dot{V}O_2$ vs velocity^3) was extrapolated to
140% of $\dot{V}O_2$max for each swimmer. On a subsequent day, subjects
completed a single swim at the prescribed intensity - an O_2 deficit
swim. During the O_2 deficit swim, accumulated O_2 uptake was measured
continuously and the accumulated O_2 deficit calculated following the
swim. A blood sample was taken 2 min post-swim for analysis of
lactate. Girth measurements of the upper arm were taken for
determination of muscle area. A 45 s swim bench test was also
administered for determination of total muscular work. Peak muscle
power values were expressed as watts per muscle area. Regression
analysis of the economy profile revealed significant differences
between all ages in all submaximal swims. All data (velocity,
$\dot{V}O_2$max, O_2 deficit, lactate, muscle area, % anaerobic contribution,
power/muscle, total muscular work) showed a tendency to increase with
age. The O_2 deficit, lactate, muscle area, power/muscle, and total
muscular work showed the greatest increase between AG2 and AG3.
Correlation analysis revealed relationships (P < 0.05) between O_2
deficit, muscle area, velocity and total muscular work. The data
suggest that (1) prior to 13.4 years (AG4) the aerobic contribution
is greater than the anaerobic component, (2) improvement in anaerobic
capacity closely follows development of muscle area during growth,
(3) change in anaerobic characteristics affects swimming performance.
Keywords: Anaerobic, O_2 Deficit, Power, Age Group Swimmers, Muscle
Area.

1 Introduction

Physical and morphological changes in children during puberty are
well documented. Both aerobic and anaerobic capacity are improved
upon during adolescence. Koch and Fransson (1986) and Atomi et al.
(1986) reported that aerobic and anaerobic capacity in children

improved with training. The degree of improvement, however, is still lower than in adults. We observed that the anaerobic capacity of age group swimmers was improved following the development of muscle area. This may explain why children cannot produce power in high intensive exercise to the degree adults can.

The purpose of this study was (1) to describe the anaerobic capacity and characteristics of age group swimmers and the developmental changes that take place, and (2) to determine how the anaerobic energy contributions change with age.

2 Methods

2.1 Subjects
Twenty-eight well trained swimmers participated in this study. They were divided into the following groups based on mean age, AG1 - 9.1 $\pm$ 0.5 years (n = 6), AG2 - 11.5 $\pm$ 0.5 years (n = 6), AG3 - 13.4 $\pm$ 0.6 years (n = 6), AG4 - 16.0 $\pm$ 0.4 years (n = 5), AG5 - 18.0 $\pm$ 0.5 years (n = 5). Physical characteristics of subjects are shown in Table 1. All swimmers were fully informed of the experimental procedure and the risks associated with the experiment, and gave written consent.

Table 1. Subject characteristics: Mean $\pm$ SD

	AG1 (n = 6)	AG2 (n = 6)	AG3 (n = 6)	AG4 (n = 5)	AG5 (n = 5)
Age (yrs)	9.5 $\pm$ 0.5	11.5* $\pm$ 0.5	13.4* $\pm$ 0.6	16.0* $\pm$ 0.4	18.0* $\pm$ 0.5
Height (cm)	140.2 $\pm$ 6.0	152.9* $\pm$ 2.6	161.1* $\pm$ 7.4	172.6* $\pm$ 2.0	178.2* $\pm$ 6.9
Weight (kg)	32.8 $\pm$ 2.5	39.9* $\pm$ 4.67	51.7* $\pm$ 6.0	68.1* $\pm$ 6.5	72.1 $\pm$ 1.9
Body fat (%)	15.0 $\pm$ 3.76	13.8 $\pm$ 2.1	11.28* $\pm$ 0.8	11.6 $\pm$ 1.8	11.3 $\pm$ 1.2

*denotes significant difference (P < 0.05) as listed before.

2.2 Measurements

2.2.1 $\dot{V}O_2$ submaximal and maximal tests
All subjects completed a series of four submaximal swims followed by a maximal swim for determination of individual energy cost curves. The sub-maximal velocities were determined as 60%, 70%, 80% and 90% of 200 m freestyle best time. For the maximal swim test, the swimmers swam at the 4th sub-maximal velocity for 2 min, then it was increased by 0.5 m/s every 30 s to fatigue. During each test, expired gases were collected continously and analyzed by O_2 and CO_2 analyzers (Morgan & Co. Ltd.). Heart rate was measured immediately after each swim. Blood samples were taken immediately after each submaximal swim and 2 min after the maximal swim for determination of lactate. All tests were conducted on-line in a swimming treadmill.

2.2.2 O_2 deficit swim

The resulting linear relationship ($\dot{V}O_2$ vs velocity) was extrapolated to 140% of $\dot{V}O_2$max and a corresponding velocity was selected. The O_2 demand was calculated (Hermansen and Medbø, 1984). On a subsequent day subjects returned and completed a freestyle swim at the above pace. During this time, oxyten uptake was recorded continuously and analyzed. The accumulated O_2 uptake was determined at 10 s increments and accumulated O_2 deficit calculated following the swim (Hermansen and Medbø, 1984). The O_2 deficit measured in this way has previously been shown to be an accurate estimate of an individual's anaerobic power (Medbø et al., 1988). A blood sample was collected 2 min ppst-swim for determination of lactate.

2.2.3 Girth measurements

Skinfold thickness was measured at four sites using Lang Skinfold Calipers (Cambridge Scientific Industries Inc). Girth measurements of upper arm were taken for determination of muscle mass.

Muscle/bone area (MBA) was estimated from the formula (Malina, 1989, unpublished lecture):

Arm MBA = G - 0.157*(S bicep + S tricep)

2.2.4 Swim bench tests

The peak power test was measured using a Pacer 2A Biokinetics Swim Ergometer (Isokinetics Inc.). Each athlete completed a series of three double arm pulls through a full range of motion, while prone, at different settings (0, 3, 6, 9) on the swim ergometer. Then a 45 s muscle fatigue test was administered for determination of total muscular work. Peak muscle power values were expressed as watts per muscle area.

2.3 Statistics

MANOVA was used to determine differences at the 0.05 level of probability.

3 Results

Submaximal economy curves for each group are shown in Figure 1. Regression analysis of the economy profile revealed significant differences between all ages in all submaximal swims. All of the data from the O_2 deficit swim and the 45 s fatigue test are shown in Table 2.

The swim velocities were selected at 140% of $\dot{V}O_2$max pace from the economy profile and showed a tendency to increase with age with the greatest difference between AG3 and AG4. There were significant differences in $\dot{V}O_2$max between AG1 and AG2, and AG4 and AG5. The O_2 deficit values showed significant differences between AG2 and AG3 and AG4 and AG5. Muscle area measurements revealed significant differences between AG2, AG3 and AG5. Percent anaerobic contribution was significantly different between AG2, AG3 and AG4, and the value of the AG4 was highest in all ages but no significant difference between it and AG5. Peak power and 45 s muscular fatigue tests indicated significant differences between AG2 and AG3 respectively.

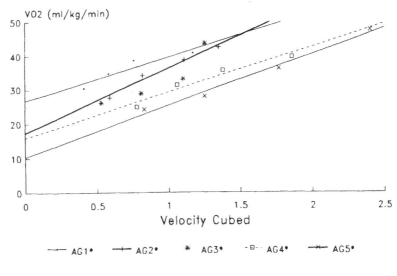

Fig. 1.   A comparison of elite age group swimming economies.

Table 2.   Selected physiological characteristics of elite age group
swimmers

	AG1	AG2	AG3	AG4	AG5
Swim velocity (m/s)	1.33 ± 0.09	1.44 ± 0.05	1.56 ± 0.01	1.70 ± 0.02	1.74 ± 0.02
$\dot{V}O_2$ max (ml/kg/min)	35.14 ± 1.20	47.49* ± 1.67	47.90 ± 1.50	47.90 ± 0.73	51.66* ± 0.89
O_2 deficit (watts)	700.0 ± 5.4	742.0 ± 7.5*	983.0* ± 9.3*	1032.0 ± 11.4	1225.0* ± 13.5
Lactate (mM)	5.43 ± 0.40	7.50* ± 0.45	9.30* ± 0.26	11.40 ± 0.85	13.50 ± 1.00
Muscle area (cm²)	16.64 ± 0.26	18.29 ± 0.38	22.25* ± 0.50	24.50* ± 1.20	26.11 ± 1.00
% Anaerobic contribution	37.00	40.00	45.00*	55.00*	52.00
Power/muscle (watts/cm²)	21.63 ± 0.69	23.74 ± 0.09	28.21* ± 2.10	31.00 ± 2.50	33.00 ± 2.10
45 s muscular work (kpm)	153.0 ± 10.0	252.0 ± 5.9	389.0* ± 22.0	392.2 ± 30.0	450.0 ± 30.0

*denotes significant difference (P < 0.05) from the groups listed
previously

All data revealed a tendency to increase with age. The greatest increases in the measured parameters occurred between groups AG2 and AG3.

4 Discussion

The influence of training on physical development is well documented. Nomura (1983) has reported that swim training during growth accelerated the development of body height and aerobic capacity. Vos et al. (1986) reported that maximal aerobic power was affected by age, training, sex and genetic endowment. Gunter and Lief (1987) suggested that increased oxygen uptake in children was correlated with increasing ventilatory development and cardiac output associated with normal growth and training. The results of the present study support these findings. The data also suggest that improvement in $\dot{V}O_2$max in children is related to increases in swimming velocity. It is, moreover, suggested that age correlates with improvement of stroke length and stroke frequency (Table 1), and improvement of swimming technique by training, and improvement of technical efficiency in swimming energy. When we observed the relationship between muscle area, muscle strength and performance in age group swimmers aged from 13 to 17 years, we found that the swimming performance and muscle strength significantly improved following the development of muscle area between pre- and post-puberty. Clausen and Lassen (1971) and Nordenfeld (1974) observed that after the age of 15 years, when muscle mass had remarkably increased in all the subjects, relative muscle blood flow tended to be lower than in young men with normal physical activity and fitness. In this study, a similar observation of developmental muscle area was observed, and at the transition from 13 to 14 years of age, a significantly larger development in anaerobic factors was correlated with a significant development of muscle area. Observations in our study, moreover, suggest that the maximum accumulated O_2 deficit is strongly related to improved 100 m performance following the development of muscle area between pre- and post-puberty. Additionally, Atomi et al. (1986) suggested that lactate threshold and $\dot{V}O_2$max of trained boys were higher than in untrained ones. Thus it was expected that the swimmers in this study have had a large influence of training in the development of anaerobic capacity.

5 Conclusions

In conclusion, these data suggested that (1) prior to 13.4 years (AG3) at the same relative work intensity the aerobic energy contribution is greater than the anaerobic component, (2) improvement in anaerobic capacity closely follows improvement in muscle mass taking place during growth, (3) the changes in anaerobic characteristics of age group swimmers affects the capacity for improvement in performance.

6 References

Atomi, Y., Fukunaga, T., Yamamoto, Y. and Hatta, H. (1986) Lactate threshold and $\dot{V}O_2$max of trained and untrained boys relative to muscle mass and composition, in **Children and Exercise XII** (eds J. Rutenfranz, R. Mocellin and F. Klimt), Human Kinetics Publishers, Champaign, Ill., pp. 53-65.

Clausen, J.P. and Lassen, N.A. (1971) Muscle blood flow during exercise in normal man studied by the 133-Xenon clearance method. **Cardiovascular Res.,** 5, 245-250.

Hermansen, L. and Medbø, J.I. (1984) The relative significance of aerobic and anaerobic processes during maximal exercise of short duration. **Medicine, Sport and Science,** 17, 56-67.

Kich, G. and Fransson, L. (1986) Essential cardiovascular and respiratory determinants of physical performance at age 12 to 17 years during intensive physical training, in **Children and Exercise XII** (eds J. Rutenfranz, R. Mocellin and F. Klimt), Human Kinetics Publishers, Champaign, Ill., pp. 275-292.

Medbø, J.I., Mohn, A.C., Tabata, I., Bahr, R., Vaage, O. and Sejersted, O.M. (1988) Anaerobic capacity determined by maximal accumulated O_2 deficit. **J. Appl. Physiol.,** 64, 50-60.

Nomura, T. (1983) The influence of training and age on $\dot{V}O_2$max during swimming in Japanese elite age group and Olympic swimming, in **Biomechanics and Medicine in Swimming** (eds A.P. Hollander, P.A. Huijing and G. de Groot), Human Kinetics Publishers, Champaign, Ill., pp. 251-257.

Nordenfeld, I. (1974) Bloodflow of working muscles during autonomic blockade of the heart. **Cardiovascular Res.,** 8, 1227-1231.

Vos, J.A., Geurts, W., Brandon, T. and Binkhorst, A.R. (1986) A longitudinal study of muscular strength and cardiorespiratory fitness in girls (13 to 18 years), in **Children and Exercise XII** (eds J. Rutenfranz, R. Mocellin and F. Klimt), Human Kinetics Publishers, Champaign, Ill., pp. 233-243.

LEG EXTENSION POWER OF ELITE SWIMMERS

M. MIYASHITA, S. TAKAHASHI[*], J.P. TROUP[*] and K. WAKAYOSHI[**]
University of Tokyo, Tokyo, Japan; [*]International Centre for Aquatic
Research, Colorado Springs, USA; [**]Osaka University, Osaka, Japan

Abstract
The maximal leg extension power of elite swimmers was determined
using an electric measuring device. There was a positive
relationship between starting performance and leg extension power. A
large sex difference was found in the maximal power event though
expressed relative to body weight. Age group swimmers were inferior
to the national swimmers in absolute power, but when compared in
values relative to body weight, the difference decreased, especially
in female swimmers. No racial difference existed in the maximal
power between American swimmers and Japanese swimmers.
Keywords: Swimming, Starting, Turning, Leg Extension Power.

1 Introduction

Most swimmers understand the significance of starting and turning to
their overall race time. Counsilman (1968) described, "the three
qualities needed to be a good starter are good reaction time, power,
and good mechanics". The reaction time is hardly shortened with
practice, while the mechanics, in other words, technique is appreciably improved during the early stage of training as a competitive
swimmer. Power is developed naturally with physical growth, and
consciously by resistance training.

In general, however, swimmers who have acquired the basic techniques of start and turn tend to fail in positive workouts on improving
those two movements. As was described already, greater muscular
power is primarily important to shorten the time spent in starting
and turning. Many investigations have been conducted on the starting
and turning. In most cases, however, the performances are discussed
biomechanically, while few investigations exist concerning the
swimmer's ability to produce the necessary power (Counsilman et al.,
1988).

The present study was designed to propose a method to determine
the maximal power of leg extension, and to discuss the data obtained
from elite swimmers.

2 Methods

Forward speed in starting and turning is developed mainly by the
contractions of extensor muscles of hip, knee and ankle joints during

295

the take-off or push-off phase. Therefore, the maximal power generated by combined extension of hip, knee and ankle joints under a certain condition should be determined to evaluate the swimmer's potential. A leg extension power meter (Leg Power B type, Takei & Company Ltd., Tokyo) was used, which consisted of a reclining seat and a footplate (Furuya et al., 1986). The force applied to the footplate was detected by a strain gauge type load cell. The swimmer sits fully back on a seat with hip, knee and ankle joints bent and feet fastened to the footplate. Instantly after a starting voice, the swimmer pushes his feet as much as possible against the foot-plate, which moves away in a straight direction at a constant speed. The reason why a speed of 0.8 m/s is adopted is as follows. The distance of the plate from the starting point to the end point varies from 0.35 to 0.46 m according to the individual leg length. The time spent in extension ranges from 0.44 to 0.56 s, which is a little shorter than the block-time, the elapsed time from start to take-off (0.78 to 0.88 s reported by Miller et al., 1984), when taking the reaction time into account. Also, mean duration of push-off was reported to be 0.42 s in a flip turn (Takahashi et al., 1983).

Mean power is obtained as the products of the force applied to the footplate by the speed. Since an unfamiliar swimmer cannot push against the moving plate with his best power, the test was repeated four or five times. The maximal value was chosen for the results and discussion.

The subjects tested were American national selected swimmers and age group swimmers, Japanese swimmers of the 1988 Olympic team, and female swimmers of the Colorado College swim team. Moreover, in order to ascertain the relationship between starting performance and leg extension power, Japanese elite and ordinary competitive swimmers were tested. In this case, each swimmer was asked to start and swim 25 m in the same manner as in the actual race, and the distance from the starting block to the point where the swimmer's fingers entered the water and the elapsed time from the starting signal to the moment when the swimmer's head reached the 5 m line were determined by using a high speed video camera. All subjects were fully informed of the purpose and procedure of the present measurements, and positively participated in the test.

3 Results

There was a statistically significant relationship between diving distance and leg extension power in 69 swimmers using freestyle, butterfly and breaststroke ($r = 0.760$, $P < 0.01$). Furthermore, a statistically significant relationship was found between swimming time to the 5 m line and leg extension power in 57 swimmers using freestyle and butterfly ($r = -0.675$, $P < 0.01$).

There was a large sex difference in power even though expressed per kg body weight. Female swimmers had only 50% of the absolute value and 70% of the relative value per kg body weight of the maximal power of male swimmers.

Age group swimmers were inferior to national swimmers in absolute power. When compared in relative values per kg body weight, the difference decreased, especially in female swimmers.

No racial difference existed in the maximal power between American

Table 1. Mean values of maximal power of leg extension and starting performance

	Maximal power (W)	Maximal power (W/kg)	Distance (m)	Time (s)
Male:				
Freestyle (20)	1032 (123)	14.3 (1.3)	342.6 (15.1)	1.68 (0.09)
Butterfly (13)	952 (95)	13.8 (1.1)	340.7 (26.5)	1.71 (0.06)
Breaststroke (8)	1061 (107)	15.7 (1.3)	350.3 (18.8)	1.69 (0.05)
Female:				
Freestyle (17)	584 (122)	10.5 (1.7)	295.5 (21.5)	1.89 (0.14)
Butterfly (7)	578 (71)	10.7 (1.0)	278.3 (9.4)	1.85 (0.06)
Breaststroke (4)	578 (61)	10.2 (0.4)	290.7 (4.1)	1.96 (0.12)

national swimmers and Japanese Olympic swimmers, except in absolute power between American and Japanese male swimmers. Also there was no difference in the maximal power between elite female swimmers and the ordinary competitive female swimmers.

When the maximal values of American national swimmers were examined individually, the sprinters were found to have a larger power than the distance swimmers; males, 1793 W (18.1 W/kg) and 1697 (19.4 W/kg) and female, 1084 W (13.8 W/kg). These values are 20 to 44% more than the respective mean value for each group as a whole.

Table 2. Mean values and (SDs) of the maximal power of leg extension

	Age (yr)	Maximal power (W)	Maximal power (W/kg)
Male:			
National Selected	18.6	1240	14.9
Swimmers (N = 7)	(1.5)	(347)	(2.8)
Selected Age-Group	14.0	912	13.8
Swimmers (N = 23)	(0.2)	(144)	(1.3)
Japanese Olympic	20.2	1033	14.5
Swimmers (N = 11)	(2.9)	(204)	(2.7)
Female:			
National Selected	17.6	662	10.9
Swimmers (N = 10)	(3.6)	(179)	(1.4)
Selected Age-Group	12.9	514	10.1
Swimmers (N = 24)	(0.3)	(106)	(1.7)
Japanese Olympic	17.1	605	11.2
Swimmers (N = 11)	(2.8)	(87)	(1.2)
College Swimmers	19.3	615	10.1
(N = 19)	(1.2)	(97)	(1.3)

4 Discussion

The results obtained in the present measurements are almost as expected; males, matured swimmers and sprinters have large power, because males and mature individuals have larger muscle mass than females and immature individuals, respectively. Also sprinters are thought to have a greater percentage of fast twitch fibres in the leg muscles than long distance swimmers.

On the other hand, these results imply that most swimmers tested have not performed the training necessary to develop the explosive force of lower extremities in their daily workouts. This implication might be partially supported by the facts that there was no significant difference in the maximal power between the elite swimmers and the college swimmers, and that there was no distinct difference in relative power per kg body weight between age group swimmers and national swimmers.

The lactic acid and the oxygen energy systems are mainly involved in 200 m and 400 m swim (Fox, 1979). Thus, in most daily workouts swimmers swim at submaximal speeds around the "anaerobic threshold". Human muscles consist of three major different fibres, i.e. slow oxidative (SO) fibres, fast oxidative-glycolytic (FOG) fibres and fast glycolytic (FG) fibres (McArdle et al., 1986). These muscles fibres are recruited in the order of SO, FOG, FG fibres, as the exercise intensity increases (Sale, 1987). Therefore, it is inferred that swimmers exert the propulsive force mostly through the contractions of SO and FOG fibres utilizing both the lactic acid and the oxygen energy systems. In other words, swimmers hardly recruit their FG fibres during swimming workouts.

Some coaches claim that swimmers perform the maximal push-off against the wall at each start on intermittent training and/or turning. This might be true. However, the problem is how intensively they perform each push-off. If a swimmer wants to train the fastest motor units, he must work against high loads, because only high loads guarantee maximal voluntary contraction (Schmidtbleicher, 1988). Water resistance and body mass might not be sufficient to activate all of FG fibres. Therefore, special resistance exercise must be arranged for improving the start and turn so that swimmers can work against high loads as fast as possible.

In the present paper, the authors would like to suggest that the swimmer should perform the following exercise. Stand with light weights in his hands or on shoulders at the back of the neck. Bend the knees as deeply as is adopted in an actual race, raising the heels slightly off the floor. Jump straight up as high as possible. Repeat 5 to 8 times a day.

5 Acknowledgements

The authors would like thank Takei & Company Limited, who donated the Leg Power Apparatus, to US Swimming Inc.

6 References

Counsilman, J.E. (1968) **The Science of Swimming.** Prentice-Hall, New Jersey.

Counsilman, J.E., Counsilman, B.E., Nomura, T. and Endo, M. (1988) Three types of grab starts for competitive swimming, in **Swimming Science V** (eds B.E. Ungerechts, K. Wilke and K. Reischle), Human

Kinetics Books, Champaign, Ill., pp. 81-91.

Fox, E.L. (1979) **Sports Physiology.** W.B. Saunders, Philadelphia.

Furuya, K., Funato, K., Takatoh, S., Mutoh, Y. and Miyashita, M. (1986) A new isokinetic dynamometer for measuring human leg extension power. **Jpn. J. Sports Sci.,** 5, 669-675.

MacArdle, J.A., Katch, F.I. and Katch, V.L. (1986) **Exercise Physiology.** Lea & Febiger, Philadelphia.

Miller, J.A., Hay, J.G. and Wilson, B.D. (1984) Starting techniques of elite swimmers. **J. Sports Sci.,** 2, 213-223.

Sale, D.G. (1987) Influence of exercise and training on motor unit activation, in **Exercise and Sports Science Reviews Vol. 15** (ed K.B. Pandolf), Macmillan, New York, pp. 95-151.

Schmidtbleicher, D. (1988) Muscular mechanics and neuromuscular control, in **Swimming Science V** (eds B.E. Ungerechts, K. Wilke and K. Reischle), Human Kinetics Books, Champaign, Ill., pp. 131-148.

Takahashi, G., Yoshida, A., Tsubakimoto, S. and Miyashita, M. (1983) Propulsive force generated by swimmers during a turning motion, in **Biomechanics and Medicine in Swimming** (eds A.P. Hollander, P.A. Huijing and G. de Groot), Human Kinetics Publishers, Champaign, Ill., pp. 192-198.

VALIDATION OF A DRYLAND SWIMMING SPECIFIC MEASUREMENT OF ANAEROBIC POWER

S. TAKAHASHI, M. BONE, J.M. CAPPAERT, A. BARZDUKAS, L. D'ACQUISTO,
A.P. HOLLANDER and J.P. TROUP
U.S. Swimming, International Center for Aquatic Research, Colorado
Springs, Colorado, USA

Abstract
The purpose of this study was to develop a simple dryland test that
could be used to measure the anaerobic power of competitive swimmers.
Sixteen well trained swimmers (17 ± 1 years) completed a series of
four submaximal and one maximal effort swims for determination of
swimming economy. A linear relationship (VO_2 vs velocity^3) was
extrapolated to 110% of $\dot{V}O_2$max for each swimmer. Within seven days
swimmers completed a freestyle swim at this pace for an average of
3.36 ± 0.20 min. During this time, oxygen uptake was measured continuously, accumulated O_2 uptake was determined at 10 s increments and
O_2 deficit (anaerobic capacity) calculated (Hermansen and Medbø,
1984). A blood sample was taken 2 min post-swim for analysis of
lactate. A 45 s maximal effort test was also administered using an
isokinetic swim bench for determination of total muscular work,
average power and force (last 5 s of the bout), and a fatigue ratio
(percent decline in power from the first to last 5 s increment). The
data revealed significant correlations between the O_2 deficit swim
and the swim bench test. It is suggested that a 45 s maximal effort
test on the swim bench can be used as an accurate way of measuring
and predicting a swimmer's anaerobic profile.
Keywords: Anaerobic Capacity, Blood Lactate, Swim Bench.

1 Introduction

Anaerobic capacity influences performances in swimming, especially in
the short events. Anaerobic capacity (maximal anaerobic power and
anaerobic stamina) can be defined as the aptitude to exert short-term
maximum work loads under oxygen deficit conditions (Hermansen and
Medbø, 1984; Medbø et al., 1988). This is influenced by physical
qualities (speed, strength and coordination), morphological factors
(muscle mass and percentage of fast twitch fibres), functional
factors (impulse transmission speed, the influence of the biofeedback
of proprioreceptors, and the utilization of elastic energy), and
metabolic factors (alactacid energy reserves, glycolytic rate, and
acidosis tolerance). These factors are trainable to different
degrees (Szogy, 1988). It is, however, difficult to evaluate the
anaerobic capacity during swimming.
    The purpose of this study, therefore, was to develop a simple dry-
land test that could be used to measure the anaerobic profile of
competitive swimmers.

2 Methods

2.1 Subjects
Sixteen well trained swimmers participated in this study. Physical characteristics of subjects are shown in Table 1. All swimmers were fully informed of the experimental procedure and the risks associated with the experiment, and gave written consent.

Table 1. Subject characteristics. Mean $\pm$ SD

Age (yrs)	Height (cm)	Weight (kg)	Body fat (%)
17.53 ± 1.25	174.4 ± 4.1	70.0 ± 3.99	11.7 ± 2.1

2.2 Measurements

2.2.1 Swimming economy
All subjects first completed a series of four submaximal swims followed by a maximal effort for determination of individual energy cost curves (i.e. swimming economy profile). The sub-maximal velocities were prescribed as 60%, 70%, 80% and 90% of 200 m best time individually in submaximal swim. For the maximal swim test, the swimmers swam at the fourth sub-maximal pace for 2 min, after which velocity was increased by 0.5 m/s for every 30 s to fatigue. During each test, respiratory gases were collected continuously and analyzed by O_2 and CO_2 analyzers (Morgan & Company Ltd.). Heart rate was measured immediately after swims by palpation of the carotid artery. Blood samples were taken immediately after each submaximal swim and 2 min after the maximal swim for determination of lactate. All tests were performed on-line in a swimming treadmill (flume).

2.2.2 O_2 deficit swim
The resulting linear relationship ($\dot{V}O_2$ vs velocity[3]) was extrapolated to 100% of $\dot{V}O_2$max and a corresponding velocity selected. The O_2 demand was calculated (Hermansen and Medbø, 1984) and within seven days swimmers returned to the facility and completed a single swim at the prescribed intensity for an average of 3.36 ± 0.20 min. During this swim, oxygen uptake was measured continuously and analyzed. The accumulated O_2 uptake was determined at 10 s increments and the accumulated O_2 deficit calculated following the swim (Hermansen and Medbø, 1984). The O_2 deficit measured in this way has previously been shown to be through accurate estimate of an individual's anaerobic power (Medbø, 1985). A blood sample was collected 2 min post-swim for determination of lactate.

2.2.3 Swim bench test
Following complete recovery of the test swim, a swim bench test was administered consisting of: (1) a single double arm pull to determine peak power, (2) a 45 s maximal effort double arm pull. A computer program interfaced to the swim bench determined the total work (kpm) during the 45 s bout, average power and force during the last 5 s of the bout, and a fatigue ratio expressed as percent decline in power

from first to last 5 s increment. A bench test blood sample was
collected 2 min post-swim for determination of lactate.

2.3 Statistics
A MANOVA was used to determine the total work, average power, fatigue
rate, average force and maximal lactate differences between tests at
a probability level of 0.05. The Pearson-product moment correlation
coefficient was calculated to determine the strength of the
relationship between these variables.

3 Results

For the O_2 deficit swim, velocity at 110% $\dot{V}O_2$max and the fatigue time
were 1.58 m/s and 3.36 $\pm$ 0.20 min, respectively. The values of
$\dot{V}O_2$max, HR_{max} and LA_{max} for both the O_2 deficit swim and maximal $\dot{V}O_2$
test are shown in Table 2.

Table 2. The maximal values in $\dot{V}O_2$max test and O_2 deficit swim

	$\dot{V}O_2$max (1/min)	HR_{max} (beats/min)	Peak lactate (mM)
$\dot{V}O_2$max test	4.25 $\pm$ 0.53	185.0 $\pm$ 9.62	11.60 $\pm$ 0.49
O_2 deficit	4.16 $\pm$ 0.49	181.8 $\pm$ 6.80	12.33 $\pm$ 2.58

The O_2 demand was calculated as described by Hermansen and Medbø
(1984) and the O_2 uptake determined at 10 s increments. Correlation
analysis was carried out between O_2 deficit (1064 $\pm$ 75 watts) and the
variables listed in Table 3.

Table 3. Correlation (r, P < 0.05) values between accumulated O_2
deficit and selected dry-land power variables

Total work (kpm)	508.0 $\pm$ 4.4	0.83*	
Average power (final 5 s) (watts)	370.29 $\pm$ 30	0.83*	
Fatigue rate (%)	39.0 $\pm$ 6	0.80*	
Average force (final 5 s) (Newtons)	162.75 $\pm$ 4.4	0.79*	
Maximal lactate (mM)	10.0 $\pm$ 0.8	0.28*	

*denotes significance at P < 0.05)

A significant relationship (total work load, average power,
average force and fatigue rate) between swim bench variables and O_2
deficit was revealed. There was no significant relationship between
maximum peak lactate and O_2 deficit.

4 Discussion

Several researchers have attempted to determine anaerobic capacity in various sports. These previous tests were performed by using a bicycle ergometer (Gollnick et al., 1974), running treadmill (Fujitsuka et al., 1982; Ohkuwa et al., 1984), and by step up (Margaria, 1976). Szogy (1988) observed that no significant relationship exists between anaerobic capacity (maximum anaerobic power and anaerobic stamina) and free swimming, hand grip ergometer and a universal ergometer. It is likely that, in these studies, different muscle groups had led to different work load levels. The anaerobic capacity in top swimmers, however, showed a significant correlation between free swimming and hand grip ergometry, with no significant relation to performance on the bicycle ergometer. This is reasonable, for the swimmer has trained these muscle groups and corresponding anaerobic energy delivery from them. Therefore, it was concluded that the muscle masses participating in swimming and bicycling are quite different because of the different form of exercise.

To improve swimming performance, swimmers train with weights and surgical tubing on dry land as well as in the pool. In 1988, Strass reported strength training caused greater improvement in maximal explosive force production than in the maximal force and also in the sprint swimming performance. Similar observations were reported by Costill et al. (1980). However, in reference to swimming specific strength training, several authors (Costill et al., 1980; Pipes and Wilmore, 1976; Sharp et al., 1982) demonstrated a clear superiority of isokinetic training procedures over isotonic or isometric procedures. The isokinetic apparatus is motion specific and allows the simulation of the swimming movement, and therefore improvements in muscle strength may affect the arms' underwater movement.

For these reasons, we examined the use of the swim bench which is widely utilized in training on dry land for comparison of the anaerobic capacity. As the results indicate, there were significant correlations between anaerobic capacity and the swim bench measurements. These findings are supported by Szogy's (1988) opinion. In other words, it is suggested that testing on the swim bench is similar to swimming, so that similar body parts and similar number of muscle fibres bear the work load in both tests. It was observed, however, that there was no significant relationship between O_2 deficit and peak maximal lactate level. In the past, blood lactate measurements have been used to evaluate the anaerobic profile of the swimmer. This test has been used and interpreted to suggest that peak lactate values are descriptive of the anaerobic capacity of the athletes (Haper, 1972). These data suggest that this previous interpretation is not accurate.

5 Conclusions

In conclusion, these data suggest that (1) post swim blood lactate is a poor determinant of an individual's anaerobic capacity, and (2) a 45 s fatigue test on the swim bench can be used as an accurate means of measuring and predicting a swimmer's anaerobic power.

6 References

Costill, D.L., Sharp, R. and Troup, J.P. (1980) Muscle strength: contribution to sprint swimming. **Swimming World**, 21, 29-34.

Fujitsuka, N. et al. (1983 Peak blood lactate after short periods of maximal treadmill running. **Europ. J. Appl. Physiol.**, 48, 289-296.

Gollnick, P.D., Piehl, K. and Saltin, B. (1974) Selective glycogen depletion pattern in human muscle fibre after exercise of varying intensity and various pedalling rates. **J. Physiol.**, London, 241, 45-57.

Hermansen, L. and Medbø, J.I. (1984) The relative significance of aerobic and anaerobic processes during maximal exercise of short duration. **Medicine, Sport and Science**, 17, 56-67.

Margaria, R. (1976) **Biomechanics and Energetics of Muscular Exercise.** Clarendon Press, Oxford.

Medbø, J.I., Mohn, A.C., Tabata, I., Bahr, R., Vaage, O. and Sjersted, O.M. (1988) Anaerobic capacity determined by maximal accumulated O_2 deficit. **J. Appl. Physiol.**, 64, 50-60.

Ohkuwa, T. et al. (1984) Blood lactate and glycerol after 400 m and 3000 m runs in spring and long distance runner. **Europ. J. Appl. Physiol.**, 53, 213-218.

Pipes, T.V. and Wilmore, J.H. (1976) Muscular strength through isotonic and isokinetic resistance training. **Athletic J.**, 57, 42-45.

Sharp, R.L., Troup, J.P. and Costill, D.L. (1982) Relationship between power and spring freestyle swimming. **Med. Sci. Sports Exerc.**, 14, 53-56.

Szögy, A. (1988) Assessment of anaerobic capacity in swimmers by a two-phase laboratory and field test, in **Swimming Science V** (eds B.E. Ungerechts, K. Wilke and K. Reischle), Human Kinetics Books, Champaign, Ill., pp. 305-310.

RELATION BETWEEN METABOLIC PERFORMANCE CAPACITY AND TEST RESULTS ON ISOKINETIC MOVEMENTS BY FIN SWIMMERS

J. OLBRECHT[*], B. UNGERECHTS[**], B. ROBBEN[+], A. MADER[*] and W. HOLLMANN[*]
[*]German University of Sports Sciences, Cologne, Germnay; [**]Olympic Training Center, Hannover, [+]Coach of the German National Team

Abstract
In fin swimming the leg muscles are dominant during propulsion. It was felt that tests using isokinetic movements (Cybex) might provide some insight into the physical ability of the athletes' muscles. The purpose of this study was to compare performance and blood lactate response (BLa) to exercises in water with isokinetic measures. Fin swimmers (six male and eight female) of the German national team had their BLa and anaerobic thresholds (AT) assessed for 100 m and 400 m ($V\text{-}4mM_{100}$ and $V\text{-}4mM_{400}$) swims using the 2 × 100 and 2 × 400 m two-speed tests (BLa_{100}max = BLa after 100 m sprint). Five maximal isokinetic extensions, peak torque (PKT) and average power (AP) of the repetition with the highest total work (TW) as well as BLa (BLa_{60}), total work (TW_{60}) and decrease of work (ΔSW) for 60 maximal repetitions were measured for each leg and the different speeds. Blood lactate increased significantly after each test. Peak torque, AP, TW and TW_{60} correlated with the 100 m sprint time, $V\text{-}4mM_{100}$ and BLa_{100}max but not with $V\text{-}4mM_{100}$. Despite a strong relation between ΔSW and both BLa_{100}max and BLa60, BLa60 did not correlate with BLa_{100}max. An increase of both $V\text{-}4mM_{400}$ and BLa_{100}max improved PKT (multiple r = 0.87) but caused a greater ΔSW. It can be concluded that PKT, AP, TW and TW_{60} reflect the sprint performance capacity of fin swimmers. The Cybex results are related to the swim specific aerobic and anaerobic performance capacities. After the prolonged maximal test on land BLa_{60} was not related to BLa_{100}max in water.
Keywords: Leg Strength, Fin Swimming Performance, Lactate, Isokinetic Test.

1 Introduction

The world records for 50 m and 100 m fin swimming are 15.48 s and 36.80 s respectively. Only the leg muscles are used for propulsion. Since the surface of a fin is approximately 0.3 m^2 (Kerll, 1989a) and as the best sprinter's kick up to 2.80 Hz on 50 m (Kerll, 1989b), it is obvious that great muscle forces have to be involved.

Therefore we tested elite fin swimmers for leg extension on a Cybex isokinetic device to determine the physical ability of these muscle groups. The relevance of the tests for the performance capacity of the fin swimmers was checked by comparing the Cybex results with the current individual 100 m sprint best time. Based on blood lactate levels (BLa), the metabolic response to the tests on the Cybex was compared to that of fin swimming specific tests in the water.

2 Methods

Six male and eight female fin swimmers from the German national team swam a 2 × 100 and a 2 × 400 m speed test (Mader et al., 1980; Olbrecht et al., 1988) to provide blood lactate (BLa) values after the fastest 100 m (BLa_{100}max) and anaerobic thresholds (AT) for 100 ($V-4mM_{100}$) and 400 m ($V-4mM_{400}$).

Measurements of peak torque (PKT) and the average power (AP) of the repetition with the highest work (TW) were measured on a Cybex 340 during five maximal extensions of each leg at 1.04, 2.08 and 3.14 rad/s (TSH). Furthermore two sets of 30 maximal extensions at 3.14 rad/s with 7 s rest between each set were performed with the left (Test II) and right leg (Test III). The total work for 60 repetitions (TW_{60}) as well as the decrease in work (ΔSW) between the first (SW1, SW3) and last six (SW2, SW4) reps of each set were recorded. A 30 min rest was given between each test. The amplitude of knee extension was restricted to the range during fin swimming. A blood sample was taken from the earlobe to determine lactate concentration before and 1, 3 and 5 min after each test on the Cybex equipment.

3 Results

The males presented significantly higher $V-4mM_{100}$ and $V-4mM_{400}$ than the females although no significance was found for sex differences of BLa_{100}max (Table 1). For the Cybex test, a small but significant increase of BLa after Test I and an increase after Tests II and III were found for both sexes.

Tests II and III lasted 54.69 $\pm$ 1.67 s and 56.42 $\pm$ 1.07 s for the females and 54.79 $\pm$ 1.90 s and 56.23 $\pm$ 1.46 s for males. The highest isokinetic strength values were obtained for the left leg in all tests whereas in Test I the right leg scores were higher (Figure 1). The differences between the two legs, however, were not significant. Peak torque, AP, TW and TW_{60} for both legs were significantly higher for the males (Figures 1 and 2). About 60 to 63% of TW_{60} was delivered in the first set. For both sexes SW2 and SW4 decreased by about 37 and 62% compared to SW1 (Figure 2).

Table 2 presents the data correlating Cybex test results with performance criteria. The highest correlations (r = -0.63 to -0.84) were found between the 100 m sprint time (t_{100}: m 43.93 $\pm$ 2.18 s, f 50.48 $\pm$ 1.25 s) and PKT, Ap, TW and TW_{60}. The strength parameters also correlated with $V4mM_{100}$ (r = 0.61 to 0.75) and BLa_{100}max. Both ΔSW12 and ΔSW14 improved significantly with PKT at 3.14 rad/s in Test II (r = 0.81 and 0.92) and Test III (r = 0.83 and 0.96). An increase of both $V-4mM_{400}$ and BLa_{100}max improved PKT (multiple R = 0.87) but caused also a greater ΔSW14.

Table 1. Mean ($\bar{x}$) and standard deviation (SD) of BLa before (RBlaI, RBLaII, RBLaIII) and after (BLaI, BLaII, BLaIII) the test on the Cybex machine (a) and before (RBLa) and after (BLa_{100}max) the 100 m sprint in water (b). Anaerobic threshold on 100 ($V-4mM_{100}$) and 400 m ($V-4mM_{400}$) for male (m) and female (f) elite fin swimmers are determined by a 2 × 100 and a 2 × 400 m 2-speed test.

(a) Cybex tests

		RBLaI (mM)	BLaI (mM)	RBLaII (mM)	BLaII (mM)	RBLaIII (mM)	BLaIII (mM)
f	$\bar{x}$	1.23	1.76	1.71	5.16	1.76	5.65
	SD	0.18	0.45	0.18	0.99	0.45	1.72
m	$\bar{x}$	1.08	2.02	1.82	7.12	1.80	7.33
	SD	0.16	0.45	0.42	1.40	0.35	1.61

(b) Swim tests

		RBLa (mM)	BLA_{100}max (mM)	$V-4mM_{100}$ (m/s)	$V-4mM_{400}$ (m/s)
f	$\bar{x}$	1.12	9.58	1.754	1.518
	SD	0.15	1.34	0.053	0.033
m	$\bar{x}$	1.17	10.70	1.883	1.619
	SD	0.21	2.11	0.060	0.042

Table 2. Correlations between Cybex results and performance in water as well as BLa response to a maximal exercise in water and on land

	$V-4mM_{10}$	$V-4mM_{100}$		t_{100}		BLa_{100}max		BLaII or BLaIII	
		from	to	from	to	from	to	from	to
PKT'	NS	0.69	0.75	-0.63	-0.82	0.56	0.68	0.60	0.74
AP'	NS	0.61	0.66	-0.68	-0.84	0.57	0.68	0.54	0.69
TW'	NS	0.65	0.72	-0.75	-0.83	0.56	0.71	0.54	0.73
TW_{60}'	NS	0.62	0.67	-0.76	-0.80	0.53	0.59	0.50	0.64
SW1-SW2'	NS	NS		-0.65	-0.67	NS		0.54	0.82
SW1-SW4'	NS	NS		-0.66	-0.80	0.57	0.81	0.62	0.69

4 Discussion

It has been demonstrated that higher PKT, AP, TW and TW_{60} improve 100 m sprint time. A previous study (Olbrecht, 1990) also showed high correlations between the specific endurance capacity, measured at $V-4mM_{100}$ (r = 0.96) or $V-4mM_{400}$ (r = 0.74) and the 100 m sprint time for fin swimmers in competition. It can then be expected that Cybex test results and specific endurance capacity of fin swimmers should statistically be related. This actually happens for $V-4mM_{100}$ but not for $V-4mM_{100}$.

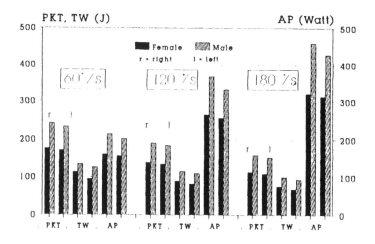

Fig. 1. Mean peak torque (PKT), average power (AP) and highest total work (TW) for a single repetition during five maximal extensions for the right (r) and left (l) leg by female and male fin swimmers at 1.04, 2.08 and 3.14 rad/s.

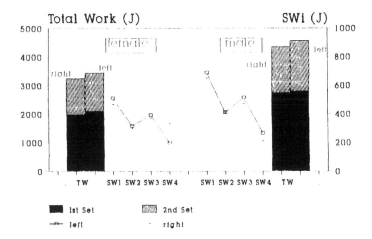

Fig. 2. Mean total work (TW) of two sets of 30 maximal extensions with right and left leg by female and male fin swimmers at 3.14 rad/s. A decrease of the mean total work between the first (SW1, SW3) and last six (SW2, SW4) repetitions of each set is also depicted for each leg.

It is also worthy of note that the faster the swimmer (over 100 m) the more pronounced the decrease of work (ΔSW) during the prolonged Cybex test. The reason for this may be that the fastest swimmers have the higher PKT and that PKT correlates with BLa. It is assumed that the relation between PKT and BLa reflects the glycolytic capacity of the muscle group. As FT-fibres are characterized by a high glycolytic capacity and a high power output, the high PKT of the fastest sprinters may partly be explained by the quantity or activity of the FT-fibres. The decrease of work during successive muscle contractions could then result in accumulation of muscle lactate and of a decrease of pH due to the high glycolytic activity. A lower BLa may reflect a greater aerobic capacity (ST-fibres) of the muscles.

According to swim training, more endurance trained swimmers show a smaller decrease of AT by increasing the distance (Olbrecht, 1989) which may be due to a smaller decrease of work during prolonged exercises.

A multiple regression analysis shows that an increase of both $V-4mM_{100}$ and BLa_{100}max is related to an improvement of PKT. This demonstrates the close relation between the metabolic and physical capacity of the muscle. It should then be obvious that training in water has to be combined with power training on land. Furthermore, as BLa after a 100 m sprint did not correlate with BLa after a maximal test on land, lasting for about the same time, it is clear that the anaerobic capacity should be improved by swimming.

5 References

Kerll, H. (1989a) **Fin Swimming Manual.** Stephanie Naglschmid, Stuttgart.

Kerll, H. (1989b) **Die Entwicklung des Tauchens zum Mono-Flossenschwimmen als Hochleistungssport** (The development from diving to mono fin swimming in competition). University Munster.

Mader, A., Madsen, O. and Hollman, W. (1980) Zur Beurteilung der laktaziden Energiebereitstellung für Trainings- und Wettkampfleistungen im Schwimmen (The evaluation of the anaerobic energy supply with regard to the performances in training and competition in swimming). **Leistungssport,** 10, 263-279, 408-418.

Olbrecht, J. (1989) Metabolische Beanspruchung bei Wettkampfschwimmern unterschiedlicher Leistungsfähigkeit (Metabolic response of competition swimmers with different qualifications). Dissertation, DSHS, Cologne.

Olbrecht, J. (1990) **Trainingssteuerung im Flossenchwimmen** (Training monitoring in fin swimming). Stephanie Naglschmid, Stuttgart (in press).

Olbrecht, J., Mader, A., Madsen, Ö, Liesen, H. and Hollman, W. (1988) The relationship of lactic acid to long distance swimming and the 2 x 400 m 2-speed test and the implications for adjusting training intensities, in **Swimming Science V** (eds B.E. Ungerechts, K. Wilke and K. Reischle), Human Kinetics Books, Champaign, Ill., pp. 261-267.

ANALYSIS OF SWIMMING SPEED AND ENERGY METABOLISM IN COMPETITIVE WATER POLO GAMES

A. HOHMANN and R. FRASE
Universität Stuttgart, Germany

Abstract
This study investigated the individual swimming profiles of 24 elite
water polo players in a competitive situation i.e. during games at
the 11th European Championships in Bonn, 1989. After an analysis of
the individual maximum swimming speed (V_{max}) and the speeds corresponding to the aerobic threshold of 2 mM ($\dot{V}$-2mM), the anaerobic
threshold of 4 mM (V-4mM) and the limit of the super aerobic training
zone of 6 mM (V-6mM), all movements of the players during the games
were recorded using a time-lapse video recorder and evaluated by
computer. The findings indicated that water polo necessitates an
energy release which mainly results from high energy phosphates (ATP
and CP) and aerobic metabolism.
Keywords: Water Polo, Swimming Profiles, Aerobic Threshold, Anaerobic
Threshold, Super Aerobic Training Zone, Video Analysis.

1 Introduction

In order to devise appropriate training regimens and indeed to
monitor correctly any improvements as a consequence of water polo
training, it is necessary to understand the demands of the game and
the energy requirements in competition. Consequently this study
examined the swimming profiles of centre forwards, wing and back
players, and compared the playing involvement of those players who
played a full match with those who played for one quarter only.

2 Methods

During water polo games the movements of selected players (Table 1)
were recorded by a video camera combined with a time lapse recorder
(VHS), which took single shots every second. The actual positions of
the players were tagged with a trackball and the coordinates were
defined in a grid of 720 × 540 lines using a video-position-analyzer.
A processor "analysis" then calculated, on an XT-personal computer,
the actual swimming speeds at every second of the game. The set-up
of the equipment is shown in Figure 1.
Prior to the tournament most of the players participated in a 30 m
sprint test to measure the individual maximum swimming capability
(V_{max} test). The German players additionally performed a 2 × 400 m
"2-speed test" (Mader et al., 1980). From these data (Table 2) the

Table 1. List of the 24 players and their positions

	Whole game	One quarter
Centre forwards	FE (IRA)	GO (ESP)
	PO (TCH)	MI (YUG)
	HO (TCH)	
	ST (FRG)	
Wing players	PE (HUN)	FP (ITA)
	SA (ESP())	SC (FRG)
	BU (YUG)	ST (FRG())
	RE (FRG)	
Back players	ES (ESP)	NA (URS)
	CA (ITA)	KO (URS)
	OT (FRG)	AP (URA)
	TH (FRG)	OS (FRG)
		HU (FRG)
		EH (FRG)
		TO (FRG)

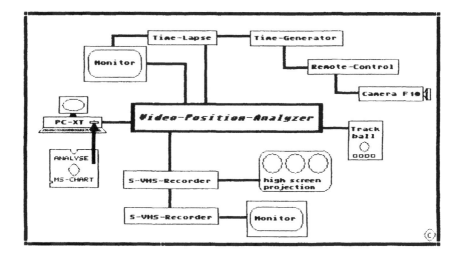

Fig. 1. Diagram of the equipment used.

individual speeds at the aerobic threshold of 2 mM (V-2mM), the anaerobic threshold of 4 mM (V-4mM) and the limit of the super aerobic training zone of 6 mM (V-6mM) (Maglischo, 1988) were estimated. The four speed data were used to estimate the players' energy requirements during the game.

3 Results and discussion

The structure of the individual swimming speed of player ST is illustrated in Figure 2. It is interesting to note the number of sprint swims of greater than V-6mM which led to horizontal jump move

Table 2. Test report on the performance capacity of a male swimmer
(Olbrecht et al., 1988)

Distance test – 2 × 400 m FS

	1st swim	2nd swim
Time (s)	5:06.00	4:36.00
Velocity (m/s)	1.307	1.449
Peak lactate (mM)	1.74	5.78

Diagnosis about the tested distance – 400 m

Lactate	Linear		Exponential	
	Speed	Time	Speed	Time
2 mM	1.316	5:03:87	1.319	5:03.17
4 mM	1.386	4:48.23	1.395	4:46:69
6 mM	1.457	4:34.53	1.455	4:34.83
8 mM	1.527	4:21.89	1.507	4:25.29

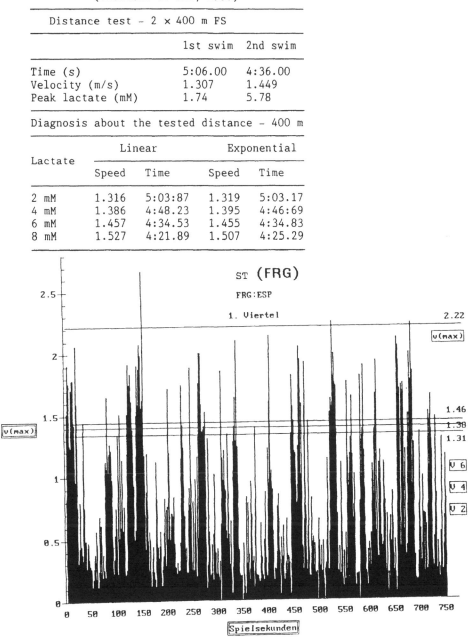

Fig. 2. Swimming speed of subject ST during the 1st quarter of the
game FRG vs ESP.

ments. Only three sprints lasted longer than 10 s. This indicates a reliance on anaerobic energy release mainly from the high energy phosphates (ATP and CP) and to a lesser extent on the breakdown of glycogen to lactic acid. On the basis of these data a high accumulation of lactic acid is unlikely. Thereby the player can avoid severe fatigue and significant loss in swimming speed.

The observations in general demonstrate varying intensities during actual playing time of t_{total} = 2881 $\pm$ 129 s. Players with an uninterrupted playing time of four quarters have a total swimming distance of 1_{total} = 1776 $\pm$ 114 m.

Table 3 shows great differences in the total distance swum by the centre forwards depending on the time of uninterrupted play. Thus the 2 m men, who only play one quarter and then get a rest, swim greater distances in these quarters than those who play the full match without a break. The difference of the total swimming distance between the two groups was significant (t = 3.14; P < 0.05). The reason was that the recovered players were more likely to 'drive in' or go into the 'hole' position.

With regard to the three different game positions, there was no evidence of any difference in the total swimming distance between the groups. This is because all the players of a team must participate in a counter-attack as soon as their own team gains ball possession. With the counter-attack, all players reach a narrow semi-circle zone of offence close to the opposite goal either until the team scores or loses the ball. In this case all players have to withdraw immediately to the zone of defence.

There were no significant differences in the swimming intensity, that is the mean swimming velocity (V/V_{max} test in %), between the game positions or between long- and short-playing fielders.

The contributions of the different sources of energy release are not equivalent. The most important form of energy supply in water polo appears to be the anaerobic alactic breakdown of adenosine triphosphate (ATP) and its continual replacement by creatine phosphate (CP). These two high energy phosphates provide most of the energy for the large number of sudden high speed jump movements and sprints (n_y > 2.0 m/s) required in water polo. The German players swam 10.8 $\pm$ 2.2% of their total playing time at sprint speed i.e. between V~6mM and the maximum swimming speed in the game (V_{max} game), which is sometimes even higher than the tested maximum swimming speed (V_{max} test). As only very few sprints last longer than 10 s, anaerobic metabolism, or the breakdown of glycogen to lactic acid, does not appear to be of the same importance for energy release in water polo.

Swimming velocities close to the anaerobic threshold (i.e. between V2 and V6) are rare. The German players swam at this speed only 3.6 $\pm$ 0.8% of their total playing time.

The aerobic metabolism, however, is of very great importance in water polo. This source of energy release results from the breakdown of glycogen to carbon dioxide and water, and later from fatty acid oxidation. Of the total playing time, 85.6 $\pm$ 2.8% (of the German players) was concerned with steady state swimming below the aerobic threshold or with resting. Thus the most economical energy source plays a dominant role for ATP replacement between the repeatedly occurring high speed movements in the course of the game.

Table 3. Individual data of swimming load of (a) centre forward, (b) wing and (c) back national players in competition water polo games

(a) Centre forwards

Name; game	$<V_2$ (%)	<0.5 (m/s) %	$V_2\text{-}4$ (%)	0.5-1.4 (m/s %)	$V_4\text{-}6$ (%)	>1.4 (m/s) %	$>V_6$ (%)	S tot (m)	V (m/s)	V_{max} (m/s)	n > 2.0 (m/s)	V_{max} test	$\dfrac{V}{V_{max}}$ test (%)
ST; FRG:ESP	85.8	53.8	2.26	38.0	2.31	8.2	9.6	1971	0.66	2.67	30	2.22	29.7
FE; ITA:YUG		73.4		7.0		19.2		1846	0.66	2.31	26	2.11	31.3
HO; CSFR:POL								1744	0.64	2.35	9		
PO; CSFR:FRG								1511	0.62	2.24	7		
GO; ESP:FRG		51.6		40.0		8.4		504	0.57	2.37	3	2.03	28.3
MF; YUG:URS		51.7		36.0		12.3		585	0.67	2.24	2	2.01	33.3
KO; URS:FRG		55.0		31.0		14.0		506	0.62	1.98	0		
URS:JUG		49.0		35.0		16.0		399	0.68	2.22	7		

(b) Wing players

Name; game	$<V_2$ (%)	<0.5 (m/s) %	$V_2\text{-}4$ (%)	0.5-1.4 (m/s %)	$V_4\text{-}6$ (%)	>1.4 (m/s) %	$>V_6$ (%)	S tot (m)	V (m/s)	V_{max} (m/s)	n > 2.0 (m/s)	V_{max} test	$\dfrac{V}{V_{max}}$ test (%)
RE; FRG:CSFR	83.4		1.94		1.57		15.1	1816	0.66	2.28	14	2.09	31.6
PE; HUN:FRG								1829	0.66	2.43	13		
SA; ESP:CSFR								1767	0.68	2.51	15	2.23	30.5
BU; JUG:ITA		75.0		8.0		17.0		1789	0.64	2.53	16	2.31	25.3
PO; ITA:FRG		48.0		42.0		10.0		436	0.65	1.95	0	1.85	35.1
SC; FRG:JUG	82.5		1.62		1.35		14.5	467	0.63	2.28	8	2.22	28.4
ST; FRG:CSFR	79.3		2.46		2.60		15.6	461	0.67	2.06	2	2.25	29.8
NA; URS:FRG		47.0		41.0		12.0		553	0.68	2.90	4		
URS:ROM		51.4		39.0		9.6		436	0.62	2.35	4		

Table 3 (continued).

(c) Back players

Name; game	< V2 (%)	< 0.5 (m/s %)	V2-4 (%)	0.5-1.4 (m/s %)	V4-6 (%)	> 1.4 (m/s %)	> V6 (%)	S tot (m)	V (m/s)	V_{max} (m/s)	n > 2.0 (m/s)	V_{max} test	$\frac{V}{V_{max}}$ (%) test
TH; FRG:URS	84.0	55.9	1.69	34.0	1.94	10.1	12.3	1774	0.62	2.35	12	2.21	28.1
OT; FRG:JUG	89.0		1.36		1.35		8.3	1693	0.61	2.25	10	2.19	27.9
CA; ITA:FRG		52.6		36.0		11.4		1693	0.62	2.54	13	2.20	28.2
ES; ESP:ROM								1882	0.67	2.42	39	2.24	29.9
OS; FRG:JUG	88.9		0.43		0.86		9.8	390	0.56	2.39	4	2.26	24.8
EH; FRG:CSFR	83.6		2.01		2.73		11.8	434	0.63	2.07	2	2.03	31.0
TO; FRG:JUG	87.1		0.40		1.07		10.4	437	0.62	2.29	3	2.37	26.2
HU; FRG:JUG	83.5		2.01		2.73		11.8	434	0.63	2.07	2	2.03	31.0
AP: URS:FRG		52.3		35.0		12.7		519	0.64	2.43	11		
URS:ITA		53.0		36.0		11.0		485	0.67	2.43	5		

4 Conclusions

The implications of these findings are that elite water polo players should use conditioning programmes that prepare the players for the expected maximum swimming load in a very specific way. This means that for speed training a total of 40 resisted sprints is recommended. For the development of endurance training we suggest a training load of double the total swimming distance in a game, i.e. 4000 m. For overload endurance training a distance of 2000 m seems optimal. For specific endurance training the players should use fartlek training with about 20% of the time swimming at sprint speed and 80% at low speed. The slow speed swimming should be interrupted frequently by series of scissor kicks or eggbeater kicks.

5 References

Mader, A., Madsen, O. and Hollmann, W. (1980) Zur Beurteilung der laktaziden Energiebereitstellung für Trainings- und Wettkampf-leistungwen im Schwimmen. **Leistungssport,** & (Suppl.), 63–79.

Maglischo, E.W. (1988) The application of energy metabolism to swimming training, in **Swimming Science V** (eds B.E. Ungerechts, K. Wilke and K. Reischle), Human Kinetics Books, Champaign, Ill., pp. 209–218.

Olbrecht, J., Mader, A., Madsen, O., Liesen, H. and Hollmann, W. (1988) The relationship of lactic acid to long-distance swimming and the 2 × 400 m "2-speed test" and the implications for adjusting training intensities, in **Swimming Science V** (eds B.E. Ungerechts, K. Wilke and K. Reischle), Human Kinetics Books, Champaign, Ill., pp. 261–267.

PHYSIOLOGICAL AND BIOMECHANICAL LOAD PARAMETERS IN LIFE-SAVING

K. DANIEL and J. KLAUCK
Deutsche Sporthochschule Köln, Germany

Abstract
To determine a profile of load during life-saving heart rate, lactic
acid concentration and dynamic forces were measured as parameters of
load during the event "50 m saving a dummy". Lactic acid determinations were made during rest and then at four intervals in the
recovery phase after a maximum effort. The mean values of lactate
accumulation for the total group (testpersons: n = 17 m/f) showed an
increased concentration from the first to the second sample for all
testpersons and a significant decrease from the second to the fourth
measurement ($P < 0.05$). The curve patterns of all test persons were
similar to those of competitive swimmers over sprint distances.
Heart rate was recorded and stored during swimming and recovery every
5 seconds. The mean heart rate showed a pattern, which highlighted
the influence of the diving reflex ($P < 0.01$). Dynamic forces were
measured using a strain gauge load cell fixed between the traction
rope and a gondola driving above the surface of a 50 m indoor pool.
During tethered swimming drag forces increased because of added loads
for about 10 to 19% depending on the kind of load (v = 1.2 m/s
const.).
Keywords: life-saving, Lactic Acid, Heart Rate, Drag Forces.

1 Introduction

Life-saving societies are organized in a dual system of swim
education and life-saving, in which water safety competitions are
integrated with national and international programmes and fixed
technical regulations. Because of the combinations of different
life-saving techniques most life-saving training and competitive
events are endurance-predominant. To determine work intensities
involved in life-saving it is necessary to measure parameters such as
heart rate, blood lactic acid concentration (BLa) and drag forces (to
measure biomechanical factors).

Lactate accumulation during intense swimming is usually above the
anaerobic threshold. In life-saving events, the results of lactic
acid determinations, pulse rate curves and biomechanical parameters
have not yet been published. This study investigated the "50 m
saving a dummy" event during which the subject has to sprint swim for
25 m, dive for 2 m, and then pick up and tow a dummy for
approximately 25 m.

2 Methods

A total of 17 life guards and swimmers were selected to act as subjects for this study. The mean age of the group was 21.6 ± 2.3 years.

Blood samples, for the determination of lactic acid concentration, were taken from the lobe of the ear at rest and then four times after a maximum effort (1st, 3rd, 5th and 7th minute during recovery). For statistical treatment these five samples were indicated as lactate 1-4 and lactate R (rest status) in order to calculate the average values and standard deviations. A P value of < 0.05 was considered significant.

Heart rate was recorded and stored by a Sporttester PE 3000 S Unilife during swimming/lifesaving and during recovery (7th minute after swim) at intervals of 5 seconds. For statistical treatment three dominant peaks of heart rate were selected during the event from the stored data:

Heart Rate 1: Maximum level during sprinting   (HR 1);
Heart Rate 2: Minimum level during diving   (HR 2);
Heart Rate 3: Maximum level during dummy towing (HR 3).

Drag forces were measured during tethered swimming by means of a strain gauge load cell fixed between the traction rope and a gondola driven above the surface of a 50 m indoor pool. On top of the gondola, the facilities for measurement were installed. Drag forces were measured using an extended back layout position (passive steady state), dressed with lifesaving clothes, and transporting the dummy. The time of registration needed was 20 seconds; force values being sampled at a rate of 50/s.

3 Results and discussion

3.1 Lactate acumulation
The mean data of the lactate concentration levels of the subjects showed an increase from lactate 1 (sampled after 1 min recovery) to lactate 2 (sampled after 3 min recovery) and then a decrease to the third and fourth samples (P < 0.01). Table 1 illustrates these findings and shows that during the event "50 m saving a dummy", the utilization of anaerobic energy sources is predominant.

The curves of the lactate samples 1 to 4 show a similar trend for males and females (Fig. 1). This trend of lactic acid concentration was comparable to the results of competitive swimmers on sprint distances. In comparison men had higher levels in all lactate values.

3.2 Heart rate
The trend of heart rate is a further indication of actual performance, and combined with lactic acid trends it is possible to control training load norms. During "50 m saving a dummy" the heart rate curve for the values HR 1-3 shows three peaks (Fig. 1). For all subjects the mean heart rate decreased clearly during the dive to pick up the dummy (HR 2) after the peak heart rate from sprinting (HR 1). During the tow of the dummy, heart rate increased to a new peak

Table 1. Blood lactate (BLa) levels and significance levels

	n	x̄	SD	BLa1	BLa 2	BLa 3	BLa 4
Lactate 1	17	8.06	± 2.36	–	–	–	–
Lactate 2	17	9.19	± 2.66	0.01	–	–	–
Lactate 3	17	8.57	± 2.37	NS	0.05	–	–
Lactate 4	17	7.88	± 2.51	NS	0.01	0.05	–

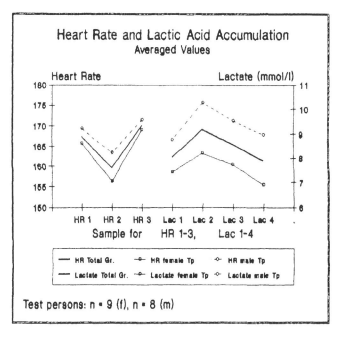

Fig. 1. Heart rate (HR 1-3) and lactate curves (Lac. 1-4) during
"50 m saving a dummy" (mean values).

value (HR 3). Male subjects reached a higher heart rate than female.
    Statistical analysis showed a significant difference between HR 2
compared to HR 1 and HR 3 values (Table 2). Thus the heart rate
showed a v-shaped pattern in the curve trend for males and females.
    The considerable increase of heart rate to a new maximum after
diving was expected because of the continued time of swimming, and
furthermore, the technique of swimming and body position were
changed. Individual subjects achieved values of 191 beats/min (male)
and 186 beats/min (female).
    In spite of this high level of individual values the mean heart
rate values did not reach the limit of maximum capacity. Bradycardia
during the dive and the fact that the propulsion results only from
kicking may be responsible for this. Female heart rates increased to
a higher HR 3 level. It may be that they needed more effort to
transport the dummy than men. The difference between the final
maximum level and the diving peak was 13 beats/min (female) and

Table 2. Heart rate (HR) and significance levels

	n	x̄	SD	HR 1	HR 2	HR 3
Heart rate 1	17	167.4	± 12.98	–	–	–
Heart rate 2	17	159.6	± 12.75	0.01	–	–
Heart rate 3	17	170.1	± 10.82	0.05	0.01	–

8 beats/min (male).

3.3 Drag forces

The objective of this research was to determine the level of drag forces during tethered swimming using different added loads. The speed of $v_{constant} = 1.2$ m/s is similar to the speed during the 50 m event.

During tethered swimming in an extended back layout position (passive) drag forces reached a level of x = 80 N for males. Because of extra loads, drag forces increased by 19% up to x = 95 N (dressed with lifesaving clothes) and by another 11% (x = 105 N) in towing the dummy. For females the increase in drag forces was more evident; 62 N in passive back layout position, 80 N dressed with lifesaving clothes (29% increase) and 112 N (40% increase) whilst towing the dummy (Fig. 2). All values are mean and valid for constant speed.

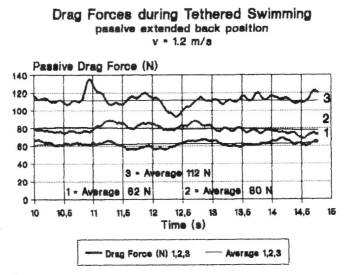

Fig. 2. Passive drag forces: 1 = without extra load, 2 = plus clothes, 3 = plus transporting a dummy.

The increase of drag forces during transportation of the dummy was relatively small for the males due to the tethered swimming. If fluctuations in swimming speed are to be taken into account the force needed for transporting the dummy must have doubled during positive acceleration, since the doubled mass has to be accelerated too (mass of dummy was similar to human mass).

This fact was responsible for the females' results. The female swimmer lost the balance of her body position during tethered swimming, so that her body, including the dummy, had a velocity fluctuation relative to the constant speed of the trailing device. These accelerations caused the higher level of drag forces, due to the inertia of the mass keeping its kinematic status. To change this status, the subject produced a higher level of drag forces (approximately 40%). Female subjects did not have enough power to keep the dummy in a steady state position.

4 Conclusions

Lactate accumulation and heart rate trends in life-saving are comparable to those results produced by competitive swimmers. Therefore life-saving training and events are endurance predominant in a similar way, but with evident increased drag forces in life-saving compared to swimming. Lifeguards therefore need a similar endurance training to influence the lactic acid threshold and to tolerate the increase of lactate accumulation.

Because of the character of a life-saving medley event, repeated performance is required and recovery enhancement following a maximal competition effort is necessary. The clearance of blood lactic acid between the events is one essential element of post exercise recovery.

During the tow, the dummy should be kept in a streamlined position without any movement to avoid added water resistance. Because of their own propulsive movements the lifeguard causes intracyclic fluctuations of speed with increased drag forces. These effects will be studied in a future research project.

5 References

Hollmann, W. and Hettinger, T. (1980) **Sportmedizin – Arbeits- und Trainingsgrundlagen.** F.K. Schattenauer-Verlag, Stuttgart, New York.
Kindermann, W., Simon, G. and Keul, J. (1978) Dauertraining – Ermittlung der optimalen Trainingsherzfrequenz und Leistungs-fähigkeit. **Leistungssport,** 8, 34-39.

PART EIGHT

MEDICAL CONSIDERATIONS

SWIMMING vs GYMNASTICS: WHAT IS BEST TO REHABILITATE BOYS WITH EXERCISE-INDUCED ASTHMA (EIA)

F. DROBNIC[*], A. CASTELLO[+] and J.I. SIERRA[^]
[*]Centre d'Alt Rendiment, Sant Cugat del Vallés; [+]Centre d'Alt Rendiment Esportiu, Esplugues del Llobregat; [^]Hospital San Juan de Dios, Barcelona, Spain

Abstract
The main purpose of this study was to investigate whether the prep-ubertal boy with exercise-induced asthma (EIA) is able to participate in sports, provided some preventive measures against bronchoconstriction (BC) are taken. A further objective of the research was to determine whether swimming or gymnastics helped improve EIA to a greater extent. After a two-month training in swimming or gymnastic exercises (3 hours/week) all subjects underwent an aerobic test on a bicycle ergometer. Both groups improved their physical condition assessed by the determination of maximal oxygen uptake. The course of the illness did not show any variation although there was an improvement in subjective well being. From this study it can be concluded that the child with EIA can and should be encouraged to participate in sport.
Keywords: Exercise-induced Asthma, Aerobic Training.

1 Introduction

The asthmatic boy has been considered to possess a handicap with regard to performing physical activity even of a moderate intensity. This is the result of an over-protective attitude of parents, friends, teachers and, in some cases, the family general practitioner. A review of the literature shows that some authors have investigated the relationship existing between the physical activity programme, physical fitness and the asthmatic's response. Whereas a beneficial effect on work capacity has been shown by most of them, the effects on the course of the illness are less clear. However, it is generally agreed that training programmes do not negatively influence the course of asthma.

It is worthy of mention that in the Los Angeles Olympic Games, 41 USA medals were won by athletes with bronchial hyper-reactivity (BH) (11.2% of all medallists).

Asthma is an illness which is characterised by increased variations of the resistance to airflow over short periods of time (Scadding, 1983), and the symptoms are manifested by recurrent coughing or dyspnoea attacks separated by free intervals. The obstruction of the airways and the symptoms are completely or partially reversible with treatment by bronchodilators or steroid drugs (Godfrey and Bar-Yishay, 1985). Exercise produces a dilation of bronchial airways during the first seconds in the asthmatic. This bronchdilation is maintained during the exercise period. When exercise is stopped bronchoconstriction (BC) results in a decrease of ventilatory function (5-20 minutes post-exercise). The duration and intensity of the exercise is related to the degree of the BC. Furthermore, there is a period free from BC during the first to the third hour post-exercise. This is mainly due to the resynthesis of the mast cell mediators. The administration of sodium cromoglycate and/or sympathomimetic drugs by aerosol is enough to prevent the crisis. In the same way, the probability of a crisis is substantially reduced when working in humid and hot climatic conditions.

2 Methods

Twelve boys with EIA (FEV$_1$ < 20%) who attended the Hospital de San Juan de Dios de Barcelona and 12 healthy boys (without EIA) of the same age (12 $\pm$ 1 years), social class, number of physical activity hours (< 3), free of respiratory dysfunctions, gave their written consent to participate in the research.

The maximal oxygen uptake values were obtained using a Minhard bicycle ergometer. The exhaled air was analyzed by an Oxycon 4 ergoanalyzer. The ventilatory volume ($\dot{V}E$) and the breath frequency (BF) were registered by a membrane pneumotachometer. The boys' heart rate was monitored by ECG (Hellige) and blood pressure was taken every three minutes.

Force spirometry was taken at 3, 5, 10, 15 and 20 min post-exercise for FEV$_1$ and FVC.

Following the exercise test, the EIA patients and controls had to go through a swimming or gymnastic aerobic programme. The EIA patients were advised to warm-up properly and take the prophylactic drug before every training session. The programme consisted of interval exercises (< 5 min) and was performed at a submaximal level.

3 Results and discussion

Table 1 shows that both 8-week training periods resulted in improvements in the physical fitness status of the groups. Significant improvements were particularly apparent with respect to $\dot{V}O_2$max in all groups, with $\dot{V}E_{max}$ in the gymnastic group, and with O_2 pulse in the 'normal' swimming group. Although the maximum work intensity achieved was not significantly elevated, it would nonetheless appear that some central and peripheral adaptation has occurred. In spite of the fact that there were no significant differences between the swimming and the gymnastics groups, those boys who used swim training improved their aerobic capacity by approximately 6% whilst those who underwent gymnastics training improved by approximately 10%. This may be attributed to the mode of testing (i.e. bicycle ergometer), which is more closely related to gymnastic type events than to swimming.

The data on spirometry (Table 2) showed that the training programmes did not lead to an improvement in respiratory parameters for the EIA groups. This is in accordance with the findings of Oseid et al. (1978), Graff-Lonnevig et al. (1980) and Zawadsky et al. (1988), but contrary to findings by Henrikssen and Nielksen (1983), Svenonius et al. (1983) and Haas et al. (1987).

Table 1. Mean fitness data for the groups before and after an 8-week training programme of either swimming or gymnastics

Training	Swimming group				Gymnastics group			
	Normal		EIA		Normal		EIA	
	Before	After	Before	After	Before	After	Before	After
$\dot{V}O_2$ max (ml/min)	1988	2116**	1788	1893*	2166	2243*	2071	2178**
$\dot{V}E_{max}$ (l/min)	65	70	54	58	82	86*	61	68**
O_2 pulse	10.4	11.2*	9.5	10.0	11.5	11.9	11.2	11.5
Heart rate max.	192	190	188	190	191	190	187	190
Work (watts)	148	152	129	134	154	157	1456	149

$*P < 0.05$; $**P < 0.01$

Table 2. Mean ventilatory responses of the EIA group before and after an 8-week training programme of either swimming or gymnastics

	EIA before training	EIA after training
FVC	73.9	74.2
FEV_1	83.3	84.8

The disparity in the results may be as a consequence of the illness itself. Asthma is a very changeable illness both in its manifestations and development. It is difficult not only to assess the exact evolution of asthma but also to know whether the modified factors being controlled are those that really affect the quality of the illness or not. The reasons for this difficulty are, firstly, there are a large number of factors that cause it, and secondly that there are many different variables to be taken into account when evaluating it. An increase in physical fitness normally involves an increase in minute ventilation, and consequently an improvement of respiratory muscle condition. Thus, although bronchial hyper-responsiveness may not change, respiratory musculature may be better prepared against further asthma attacks.

4 Conclusions

A three-hour activity programme for two months improves the physical condition status of all subjects assessed by $\dot{V}O_2$ max. There were no significant differences between sport or healthy status groups. The course of the illness did not show any variation but there was an improvement in the subjective well being.
    From this study it can be concluded that the child with EIA can and should be encouraged to practise sport in order to achieve a

further development of psychomotor activity, provided some preventive measures are taken.

5 References

Godfrey, S. and Bawr-Yishay, E. (1985) Exercise-induced asthma, in **Bronchial Asthma** (eds E.A. Weiss, M.S. Segal and M. Stein), Little Brown, pp. 500-507.

Graff-Lonnevig, V., Bevergard, S., Eriksson, B.O., Kraepelian, S. and Saltin, B. (1980) Two years' follow up of asthmatic boys participating in a physical activity programme. **Acta Paediatr. Scand.**, 69, 347-352.

Haas, F., Pasierski, S., Levine, N., Bishop, M., Axen, K., Pineda, H. and Haas, A. (1987) Effect of aerobic training on forced expiratory airflow in exercising asthmatic humans. **J. Appl. Physiol.**, 63, 1230-1235.

Henrikssen, J.M. and Nielksen, T. (1983) Effect of physical training on exercise-induced bronchoconstriction. **Acta Paediatr. Scand.**, 72, 31-36.

Oseid, S., Kendall, M. and Selbekk, R. (1978) Physical activity programs for children with exercise-indiced asthma, in **Swimming Medicine IV** (eds B. Erikson and B. Furberg), University Park Press, Baltimore, pp. 42-51.

Scadding, J.G. (1983) Definition and clinical categories of asthma, in **Asthma** (eds T.J. Clarck and S. Godfrey), pp. 1-11.

Svenonius, E., Kautto, R. and Arborelius, M. Jr. (1983) Improvement after training of children with exercise-induced asthma. **Acta Paediatr. Scand.**, 72, 23-30.

Zawadsky, D.K., Lenner, K.A. and McFadden, E.R. Jr. 91988) Effect of exercise on non-specific airway reactivity in asthmatics. **J. Appl. Physiol.**, 64, 812-816.

ALTERATION OF LYMPHOCYTE SUBSETS DURING A COMPETITIVE SWIM TRAINING SESSION

H.M. NEISLER, M.H. BEAN, W.R. THOMPSON and M. HALL
Naval Aerospace Medical Research Laboratory, Pensacola, FL. and
University of Southern Mississippi, USA.

Abstract
Lymphocyte subsets across an entire training season were studied in
17 male collegiate competitive swimmers. Pre- (PRE) and post-workout
(PS) samples were collected on seven occasions during the season.
Neither height, weight, % body fat, haematocrit nor haemoglobin
changed significantly across the PRE samples. Significant changes
across time occurred in all PRE leukocyte, absolute lymphocyte, T-
cell, B-cell, T-4, T-8, T4+2H4+, T4+4B4+ and NKH1 counts. Moreover,
the pattern of these PRE to PS samples changed significantly after
initial adaptation, during the period of greatest training stress,
and again during taper. Increases in self-reported physical and
psychological stress paralleled decreases in T4+4B4+ and NKH1 cells
and a plateau in performance.
Keywords: Swimming, Lymphocytes, H/S Ratio, Natural Killer Cells.

1 Introduction

Running and cycling have represented the predominate forms of
exercise used to study both hormonal and peripheral blood cellular
changes. From these studies, leukocyte populations are known to
change quantitatively and in distribution among the various populations during periods of stress and during exercise. Leukocytes,
moreover, increase to a greater degree than can be accounted for by
exercise-induced haemoconcentration alone, the highest levels occurring in the immediate post-exercise period. This increase is predom-
inantly a granulocytosis, but an increase in the absolute number of
lymphocytes in the circulation also occurs.

Cross-sectional studies of acute exercise at different levels of
training show that within the lymphocyte population there is a
proportional decrease in T-cells with an increase in non T-cells,
including B-cells (Edwards et al., 1984). These lymphocyte sub-
populations were enumerated by direct fluorescent microscopy which is
less accurate than flow cytometry. The decrease of T-cells was
accounted for by a reduction of T-helper/inducer cells and a proportional increase of T-suppressor/cytotoxic cells (Hedfors et al.,
1983). A more recent study (Deuster et al., 1988) using flow
cytometry again demonstrated a decreased T-cell response with a
rearrangement of the T-helper to T-suppressor cell ratio (H/S).

These studies have traditionally involved a single bout of
exercise or a brief short-term protocol. The significance of these

short-term changes is unknown (Nash, 1986). The effects of long-term physical conditioning on lymphocyte populations received little attention until recently (Neisler, 1989).

2 Method

Seventeen self-selected male Varsity swimmers ($\bar{X}$ age 19.7 $\pm$ 1.3 years) volunteered for this study following an oral presentation, written consent and medical history. Each subject had been on reduced or no training schedule for the prior three week period. Blood samples were obtained in the early morning before training by a single, non-traumatic venipuncture. A second sample was obtained within three minutes of completion of the swim training session on all dates. The samples were processed identically by the same researcher. Flow cytometry samples were prepared with a Coulter Q-PREP[R] Immunology Workstation. Complete blood count and differential were performed on a Coulter EPICS C Laser Activated Fluorescent Flow Cytometer using two-colour Coulter CYTOSTAT[R] monoclonal antibodies as follows: T4/T8, T11/B1, T8/NKH1, T3/I3, 4B4/T4, and T4/2H4. All results were expressed as percentages from which absolute sub-populations were calculated as follows: (total lymphocytes/cm^2 *% lymphocytes*% sub-population = absolute number of sub-population).

Water temperature was maintained at 28°C throughout the training season. Training sessions and intervening competitions were established by the coaching staff and were not modified to accommodate the study. Total weekly yardage increased from 16 750 in August to 69 950 in January with a slight reduction in late November and a full taper in February. Subjects exercised simultaneously as a group and all PRE and PS samples were each obtained within a 5 min period.

3 Results and discussion

Three subjects were dropped from the study because of injury or loss from the University. Among the remaining 14 subjects, there was no significant change in the percentage body fat, haematocrit or haemo-globin. The means of pre-exercise absolute numbers per cm^2, SE and percentage change from pre- to post-exercise sub-populations are given in Table 1. Changes across time occurred in all PRE leukocyte, absolute lymphocyte, T-cell, B-cell, T-4, T-8, T4+2H4+, T4+4B4+ and NKH1 counts. While the subjects were not haematologically a homogeneous group at the beginning of the season, as the season progressed, the pre-exercise NKH1 T4+4B4+ cells decreased both in absolute number, and in range across the subjects. This decrease in NKH1 cells resulted in 10 subjects dropping below a clinically normal range compared with only five below range as the season began. Likewise, the decreased T4+4B4+ cells resulted in 13 below clinical range post-season compared with 10 pre-season. Similarly, the season began with only four swimmers below the mean of 1.7 for normal helper-suppressor cell ratio, but ended with seven of the 14 below clinical mean values. The marked reduction of these cells in weeks 9, 20 and 26 parallel increased self-reported physical and psychological stress, upper respiratory infections and a plateau in performance. While the decreased performance cannot be attributed to

Table 1. Pre-exercise mean, SE, and Pre- to Post- % change per cm^2

	Week	3	9	14	20	21	26	27
T11	PRE	2018	1534	2376	1935	1738	1835	1546
	SE	128	115	130	87	93	178	85
	PS-PRE %	- 4	+28	+ 3	-10	- 4	-26	-14
T4	PRE	1272	962	1437	1153	972	1149	886
	SE	96	57	80	74	63	94	56
	PS-PRE %	-18	+ 6	- 4	- 1	+ 5	-15	- 5
T8	PRE	639	617	879	780	620	707	547
	SE	42	45	68	58	45	65	36
	PS-PRE %	+ 1	+40	+17	- 9	- 1	-21	- 3
H/S	PRE	2.03	1.65	1.74	1.58	1.66	1.68	1.66
	SE	0.12	0.14	0.14	0.14	0.13	0.13	0.11
	PS-PRE %	- 13	- 22	- 10	+ 12	+ 9	+ 9	- 2
NK	PRE	158	54	113	94	96	108	86
	SE	34	12	19	15	18	21	15
	PS-PRE %	+23	+111	+45	+31	-20	-43	- 3
T4+2H4	PRE	756	444	852	650	568	628	489
	SE	64	55	79	67	53	71	40
	PS-PRE %	- 1	+56	- 7	+ 3	0	-15	- 1
T4+4B4	PRE	240	87	338	184	184	114	165
	SE	41	19	29	17	10	11	16
	PS-PRE %	+20	- 3	+22	+19	- 9	-31	-24
BI	PRE	366	322	448	361	283	358	281
	SE	43	48	65	48	35	51	37
	PS-PRE %	-11	+ 1	+21	-11	5	-15	- 9

the alterations in lymphocyte populations, their change may be indicative of the cumulative effects of training and competition with simultaneous academic stresses.

The lymphocyte response to exercise changed significantly after initial adaptation, during the period of greatest training stress, and again during taper. Of greatest interest is the dramatic change in the pattern of T8 cells and NKH1 cells which increased following exercise early in the season, but decreased following exercise after the midpoint of the training season. Likewise, the helper-suppressor cell ratio reversed its post-exercise pattern at the midpoint. Although every subject did not exhibit identical response magnitude, all subjects exhibited basically the same pattern of responses across the season. Since every swim training session was not identical, this raises the possibility that the alteration in response pattern for the T8 and NKH1 cells may be dependent on the exercise intensity. Were this the case, we would anticipate that the other lymphocyte populations would follow similar patterns within each exercise protocol. This did not occur. Moreover, the pre-exercise values for these and other sub-populations exhibited a narrower range among the subjects at the end of the season, than comparable pre-season values.

4 Conclusions

It is concluded, therefore, that there is a cumulative effect on the lymphocyte populations in addition to that of acute exercise. This cumulative effect depresses the lymphocyte sub-populations and moves their values away from the mean of normal clinical reference intervals. This longitudinal study across a single training season with subjects exercising simultaneously emphasizes the necessity of knowing not only the exercise protocol, but also the phase of training and intervening exercise habits of subjects when interpreting haematological data.

5 Acknowledgements

This study was conducted at Northeast Louisiana University and the University of Southern Mississippi with the assistance of the NLU swim team and J. Pittington. This study was supported in part by grants from Ortho Diagnostics, Puckett Laboratory and the Vice President for Research, University of Southern Mississippi. Dr. Neisler is currently a Postdoctoral Fellow at the Naval Aerospace Medical Research Laboratory, Pensacola, Florida, USA.

6 References

Deuster, P.A., Curiale, A.M., Cowan, M.L. and Finkelman, F.D. (1988) Exercise-induced changes in populations of peripheral blood mononuclear cells. **Med. Sci. Sports Exerc.**, 20, 276-280.

Edwards, A.J., Bacon, T.H., Elms, C.A., Verardi, R., Felder, M. and Knight, S.C. (1984) Changes in the population of lymphoid cells in human peripheral blood following physical exercise. **Clin. Exp. Immunol.**, 58, 420-427.

Hedfors, E., Holm, G., Ivansen, M. and Wahren, J. (1983) Physiological variation of blood lymphocyte reactivity: t-cells subsets, immunoglobulin production, and mixed-lymphocyte reactivity. **Clin. Immunol. Immunopath.**, 27, 9-14.

Nash, H.L. (1986) Can exercise make us immune to disease? **Physician Sportsmed.**, 14, 250-253.

Neisler, H.M., Bean, M.H., Pittington, J., Thompson, W.R., Johnson, J.T. and Smith, J.L. (1989) Alteration of lymphocyte subsets and endocrine response during 42 days of competitive swim training. **Med. Sci. Sports Exerc.**, 21 (Suppl.), S110.

ALTERATION OF PATTERNS OF ENDOCRINE RESPONSE DURING A COMPRETITIVE SWIM TRAINING SEASON

H.M. NEISLER, M.H. BEAN and W.R. THOMPSON
Naval Aerospace Medical Research Laboratory, Pensacola, FL. and
University of Southern Mississippi, Hattiesburg, USA

Abstract
Endocrine responses to swim training across an entire training season
were followed in 17 male collegiate competitive swimmers ($\bar{X}$ age
19.7 ± 1.3 years). Venous blood samples were collected immediately
before (PRE) and upon completion (PS) of seven typical early morning
swim workouts at intervals during the season. Serum cortisol (COR),
growth hormone (hGH), prolactin (PRO), thyroid stimulating hormone
(TSH), triiodothyronine (T3), thyroxine (T4) and T3 uptake (T3U) were
measured by radioimmunoassay or enzyme immunoassay procedures.
Neither height, weight, % body fat, hGH or T3 changed significantly
across the PRE samples but significant changes across time occurred
in all other PRE analytes. The pattern of PRE to PS COR, PRO and TSH
changed significantly during the period of greatest training stress
while the response of the other analytes remained relatively
consistent across the season. Increases in self-reported physical
and psychological stress paralleled alterations of COR, PRO and TSH.
These changes in pattern of PRE to PS analytes demonstrate the
importance of cumulative training effects when evaluating single
endocrine samples.
Keywords: Swimming, Thyroid Hormones, Growth Hormone, Cortisol,
Prolactin.

1 Introduction

Although the psychological and physical manifestations of overtraining or burnout are well known, a consistent predictive marker
has not been described. Mood disturbances, alterations in sleep and
eating patterns, and performance changes are well recognized signs of
chronic psychological or physical situational stress responses.
Biochemical and immune parameters have been monitored during physical
stress and psychic stress and show similarities between the two
states. Catecholamines, adrenocorticotropin (ACTH), cortisol, triiodothyronine uptake (T3U) and free thyroxine index (FTI) fluctuate
during physical and/or psychic stress as do prolactin and growth
hormone. These stimuli vary proportionally with exercise intensity
and most increase during exercise, but not in concert.
    The reduction of stress by chronic exercise appears to lower
corticosteroids (Watson et al., 1986) and post-race cortisol levels
have been found to correlate inversely with training mileage (Moorthy
and Zimmerman, 1978). Baron et al. (1985) observed that cortisol was

elevated in over-trained runners and that the cortisol response to insulin-induced hypoglycaemia was abnormally low. These authors demonstrated that the latter response was due to hypothalamic-pituitary dysfunction rather than adrenal exhaustion. The alterations of other pituitary hormones; e.g. prolactin and thyroid stimulating hormone, have received less attention.

The catecholamine response to near-maximal exercise tends to be reduced among competitively trained swimmers (Kirwin et al., 1988). It is of interest that chronic exercise can also produce depletion of catecholamines which may reach 30% of normal within two weeks of intensive exercise (Tomasi et al., 1982). Thus moderate exercise and stress have different and probably opposing effects on the immune system. Exhaustive exercise may be more like the response of stress while regular exercise training may alter the suppressive effects of stress on the immune system (MacKinnon and Tomasi, 1986). Until recently, however, most endocrine parameters have been measured independently and in single bout or short duration training protocols. This project provides a composite description of the effects of twenty-six weeks of competitive training and academic stress on representative endocrine hormones.

2 Methods

Seventeen self-selected, male Varsity swimmers ($\overline{X}$ age 19.7 $\pm$ 1.3 years) volunteered for this study following an oral presentation, written consent and medical history. Each subject had been on reduced or no training schedule for the prior three week period. Blood samples were obtained in early morning before training by a single, non-traumatic venipuncture. A second sample was obtained within 3 minutes of completion of the swim training session on all dates. Serums were frozen and stored in liquid nitrogen until assay. Cortisol, growth hormone, T3, T4 and T3U were assayed by RIA. Thyroid stimulating hormone (TSH) and prolactin were measured by enzyme immunoassay. All samples were processed identically by the same researcher.

Water temperature was maintained at 28°C throughout the training season. Training sessions and intervening competitions were established by the coaching staff and were not modified to accommodate the study. Total weekly yardage increased from 16 750 in August to 69 950 in January with a slight reduction in late November and a full taper in February. Subjects exercised simultaneously as a group and all PRE and PS samples were each obtained within a 5 min period.

3 Results and discussion

Three subjects were dropped from the study because of injury or loss from the University. Among the remaining fourteen subjects, there was no significant change in height, weight, % body fat, hGH or T3 across the PRE samples. Serum COR, PRO, T4, TSH and T3U each showed alteration in baseline values during the season. Moreover, there were significant changes in the pre- to post-exercise responses among these hormones. These data are presented in Table 1. Among these hormones, only T4 and TSH failed to show statistical interactions

Table 1. Mean, SE and pre- to post-exercise changes in hormones

Hormone / Week 3

Hormone / Week		3	9	14	20	21	27	28	
COR	PRE	23.9	21.0	22.8	21.8	21.7	20.6	14.6	µg/dL
	SE	0.6	1.6	0.7	1.5	1.1	0.7	0.6	
	PS-PRE %	-24.5	-33.4	15.5	-5.7	-19.1	.39.8	-19.2	
PRO	PRE	20.7	14.1	22.6	18.4	15.8	22.5	18.2	ng/mL
	SE	1.8	1.1	1.5	2.0	1.5	1.9	0.9	
	PS-PRE %	-24.9	-29.9	22.2	-12.5	-9.0	-43.9	-10.4	
TSH	PRE	2.7	1.5	4.9	3.5	2.5	2.7	2.2	µg/dL
	SE	0.3	0.2	0.4	0.5	0.3	0.4	0.3	
	PS-PRE %	-14.6	28.8	24.1	-9.3	29.3	27.8	47.4	
T4	PRE	8.5	6.8	8.1	6.9	7.3	8.7	9.1	µg/dL
	SE	0.5	0.6	0.4	0.5	0.4	0.4	0.4	
	PS-PRE %	-1.8	17.7	14.5	4.9	-1.4	3.4	-8.2	
T3	PRE	153.7	155.0	152.7	145.9	156.2	150.7	143.6	ng/dL
	SE	5.9	3.2	6.2	3.9	6.8	4.9	5.5	
	PS-PRE %	-0.1	3.9	2.3	0.9	-0.1	-0.6	3.1	
T3U	PRE	41.3	37.6	41.7	29.9	30.4	40.4	40.%	%
	SE	0.6	2.9	0.7	1.7	0.9	0.6	0.7	
	PS-PRE %	0.0	-5.8	-2.9	1.2	2.5	-1.1	-6.8	

among the swimmers across the season. This statistical interaction was the result of increasing heterogeneity of post-exercise responses among the team members as the season progressed. While responses were reasonably consistent early in the season, individual differences among the members began to emerge during the third sampling session. These individual changes are obscured when represented only as a mean and SE while the pattern of uniform changes emerges. In this respect it is interesting that the majority of team members reversed their PRO and thyroid hormone response to swim sessions during the course of the season. Two subjects failed to show an increase in both post-exercise cortisol and prolactin response during any of the sessions. One of these also maintained among the higher values for pre-exercise TSH and hGH with lower lymphocyte numbers than most of the other team members. He was perceived to be one of the hardest workers on the team, yet never seemed to live up to performance expectations. Samples obtained at the middle and end of the season present a different picture of the response to exercise protocols designed to elicit the same effort. These alterations and interactions among the hormonal patterns across the season reemphasise the importance of accurate training and baseline data when interpreting exercise induced hormonal changes.

4 Acknowledgements

This study was conducted at Northeast Louisiana University and the University of Southern Mississippi with the assistance of the NLU swim team and J. Pittington. This study was supported in part by grants from Hybritech, Organon Teknika and the Vice President for Research, U. Southern Mississippi. Dr. Neisler is currently a Postdoctoral Fellow at the Naval Aerospace Medical Research Laboratory, Pensacola, Florida, USA.

5 References

Baron, J.L., Noakes, T., Levy, W., Smith, C. and Millar, R. (1985) Hypothalmic dysfunction in overtrained athletes. **J. Clin. Endocr. Metab.**, 60, 803-806.

Kirwin, J.P., Costill, D., Flynn, M., Mitchell, J., Fink, W., Neufer, P. and Houmard, J. (1988) Physiological responses to successive days of intense training in competitive swimmers. **Med. Sci. Sports Exerc.**, 20, 255-259.

MacKinnon, L.T. and Tomasi, T.B. (1986) Immunology of exercise. **Ann. Sport. Med.**, 3, 1-3.

Moorthy, A.V. and Zimmerman, S.W. (1978) Human leukocyte response to an endurance race. **Eur. J. App. Physiol.**, 38, 271-276.

Tomasi, T.B., Trudeau, F.B., Czerwinski, D. and Erredge, S. (1982) Immune parameters in athletes before and after strenuous exercise. **J. Clin. Immunol.**, 2, 173-177.

Watson, R.R., Moriguchi, S., Jackson, J.C., Werner, L., Wilmore, J.H. and Freund, B.J. (1986) Modification of cellular immune functions in humans by endurance exercise training during beta-adrenergic blockage with atenolol or propranolol. **Med. Sci. Sports Exerc.**, 18, 95-100.

SERUM ERYTHROPOIETIN OF ELITE SWIMMERS TRAINING AT MODERATE ALTITUDE

D. ROBERTS and D.J. SMITH
Faculty of Physical Education, The University of Calgary, Calgary,
Alberta, Canada

Abstract
The hormone erythropoietin (EPO), released under hypoxic conditions,
acts to stimulate RBC production. Serum EPO, reticulocyte count
(retic), haemoglobin concentration (Hb) and percent haemocrit (Hct)
were monitored in 6 male world-ranked swimmers during and following a
3-week training camp at 1850 m. Serum EPO and retics were
significantly increased by day 19 and remained elevated 3 weeks post-
altitude. The Hb values were raised by 5% at the end of the test
period, and had retained this level 6 months later. There was a
difference in the EPO response by sprinters and endurance
specialists. Further work is required to elucidate the mechanism of
EPO response and its effects upon performance.
Keywords: Erythropoietin, Reticulocytes, Moderate Altitude.

1 Introduction

Red blood cell (RBC) production by the colony forming units-erythroid
(CFU-E) of the bone marrow is under the control of the hormone
erythropoietin (EPO) (Cline and Golde, 1979). In adult mammals the
primary site of EPO production is the kidney (Jacobsen et al., 1957).
Production and release of EPO is stimulated by any condition wherein
the oxygen utilization of the tissue exceeds oxygen supply
(Anagnostou et al., 1981). Thus, conditions such as decreased
barometric pressure, decreased tissue perfusion, decreased
haemoglobin (Hb) concentration, or hypoxia results in an increase in
circulatory EPO. The reverse of these conditions, or those
conditions which result in decreased Hb-oxygen affinity, such as
increased 2,3 DPG, have the opposite effect on EPO levels. In
addition, protein deprivation (Catchatourian et al., 1980) and
endotoxin exposure (Schade and Fried, 1976) suppress EPO production.
Several hormones have also been shown to have modulating effects on
either EPO production or the sensitivity of the CFU-E to EPO. Both
testosterone (Mirand et al., 1965) and angiotensin II (Fried et al.,
1982) have been shown to lead to raised levels of EPO.

Williams et al. (1981) have shown that endurance capacity is
improved by raised Hb levels. Unethical methods such as autologous
transfusions and exogenous EPO have allegedly been used by some
athletes as a means of increasing the RBC mass and obtaining
endurance performance improvements (Stray-Gunderson, 1988). Training
at altitude with an increased hypoxic stimulus may provide a natural

method of enhancing RBC production. However, no reports have previously been made describing the influence of training at moderate altitude (up to 2230 m) on serum EPO levels. The purpose of this investigation was to monitor the changes in serum EPO in a group of elite swimmers during and following a 3-week training camp at 1850 m.

2 Methods

2.1 Subjects
Subjects were six male elite Canadian swimmers competitive at the international level. Mean ($\pm$ SD) values for age, height and weight were 21.8 $\pm$ 2.0 years, 181.5 $\pm$ 3.5 cm, and 76.3 $\pm$ 4.8 kg, respectively. Informed consent was obtained and the rights and privileges of the subjects were respected in accordance with the Human Ethics Committee, The University of Calgary.

2.2 Procedures
Eight blood samples were collected over a 3-week training camp at 1850 m and a 3-week post-altitude period at the swimmers' normal training centre at 1000 m. On the day of testing, a blood sample was collected by venipuncture between 06:00 and 08:00 hours in view of diurnal variation (Wilde et al., 1989).

Whole blood on EDTA (7.5% solution) was analyzed for Hb and haematocrit (Hct) using standard methods. Smears for reticulocyte (retic) count were prepared from whole blood stained with new methylene blue. Serum EPO was analyzed using the Incstar EPO-Trac 125/RIA kit, a competitive binding disequilibrium radioimmunassay. Intra- and inter-assay imprecision and sensitivity were equal to or better than the manufacturer's reported values. Control values were determined from a single sample provided by each of 20 subjects normally residing at 1000 m.

2.3 Statistical Analysis
Intra- and inter-assay reliability values were calculated as test-retest coefficients of variation. One-way analysis of variance with repeated measures was followed by two-tailed paired t-tests for identification of significant mean differences ($P < 0.05$). All means are $\pm$ 1 standard deviation ($\pm$ SD) of the mean).

3 Results

Group means ($\pm$ SD) for the measured parameters are presented in Table 1. The Hb and HCt values were within the normal range. However, EPO values in the post-altitude period and retic values following day 9 at altitude were above the established normal limits (Table 1).

The Hb concentration increased by 7.4% over the period at altitude and was maintained at 5% over baseline values at the 42nd day following ascent to altitude. The Hct values were unchanged. A significant increase was observed in EPO with a 21% rise at day 19 and a continued rise to 40% on the 42nd day. The retic count was also significantly increased with a 188% rise in the first 9 days at altitude, and was maintained at a raised level of 75% throughout the

Table 1. Mean (± SD) values for the Hb, Hct, serum EPO and retic
count on elite male swimmers with a 3-week training camp at
moderate altitude

	Pre-Alt	Altitude				Post-Altitude			Normal
Day		2	9	14	19	28	34	42	
Hb	16.3	18.0	17.0	16.8	17.5	16.8	17.6	17.1	14.0–
(g/dl)	±0.6	±1.0	±0.9	±0.8	±0.9	±0.6	±0.9	±0.7	18.0
Hct	48.7	49.3	45.8	47.2	48.2	48.6	49.9	47.5	42.0–
(%)	±1.8	±3.2	±1.5	±2.6	±2.5	±2.2	±2.1	±1.5	52.0
EPO	–	14.4	12.2	13.0	17.4	15.9	19.1	20.2	13.5
(U/l)		±5.3	±5.7	±5.3	±3.5	±8.1	±9.0	±8.1	±2.8
Retic	–	0.8	2.3	1.3	1.6	1.4	–	–	< 1%
(%)		±0.7	±1.7	±0.5	±0.6	±0.3	–	–	

altitude and post-altitude periods.

The subjects could be divided into endurance (n = 4) and spring
(n = 2) specialists. A differing trend in EPO was observed between
the two types of training on day 9 and again on day 28 (Fig. 1). In
both of these cases, blood sampling occurred within 24 hours of a
specific endurance workout. No additional differences were observed
between the endurance and sprint swimmers for any other measured
parameter.

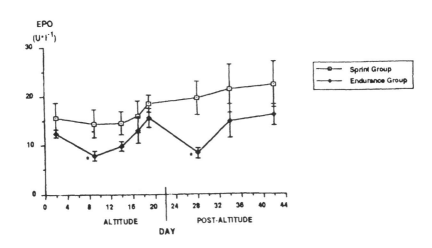

Fig. 1. Serum EPO concentrations (U/l) in elite endurance and sprint
trained swimmers with training at moderate altitude.

4 Discussion

Recent cloning of the human gene for EPO has allowed the manufacture of this hormone for clinical use in treating the severe anaemia associated with renal failure (Anagnostou et al., 1981). Only in 1979 was a radioimmunological assay developed by Sherwood and Goldwasser for use in the laboratory. These two events have renewed the study of the powerful effect of EPO on the stimulation of RBC formation, maturation, and release into the circulation.

In this study the EPO, rectic and Hb levels of elite swimmers training at 1000 m were observed to be within the normal range for sedentary subjects living at this same altitude. Following 19 days of exposure to moderate altitude (1850 m), significant increases in EPO and retics were observed. By this date, 67% of the EPO values and 83% of the retic values exceeded 2 SD values above the normal value.

There are few other reports of EPO values for athletes in the literature. Berglund et al. have published two studies (1988, 1989). The reported values for elite cross-country skiers and non-athletes living and training below 300 m (Berglund et al., 1988) were similar to the initial values found in the current study. However, the values reported by this same group for former endurance athletes and normal subjects in a blood letting study (1989) were considerably lower. The authors did not attempt to explain this discrepancy. The 25% increase in EPO levels following removal of 1350 ml of blood over 3 to 6 weeks was less than the 40% increase observed in the current study following training at altitude.

After reinfusion of autologous blood, Berglund et al. (1989) reported a 12% rise in Hb which dropped to a 5% increase over normal values within 4 weeks. Following the 3-week training camp at moderate altitude, a 5% rise in Hb was observed. Blood samples collected throughout the following season indicated that this rise in Hb was maintained 6 months later when the mean Hb level was measured at 17.6 ± 0.5 g dl. Improvements in endurance have been observed following training at similar altitudes (Mairbaurl et al., 1986) and with increased Hb levels (Williams et al., 1981). Further investigation is required to determine if these events are causal or merely coincident.

The data in this study were also examined for differences between athletes specializing in endurance and spring distances. On day 9 and day 28, a divergence in EPO was observed between the two groups (Fig. 1). On the 3 days prior to these dates, specific endurance sets at intensities of 85-90% of best event time were performed by the endurance group. However, no differences were observed between the endurance and sprint swimmers for retic count or Hb. While there does appear to be an influence of specific training upon EPO levels, much further work is required before the nature of this effect can be elucidated. Different mechanisms such as tissue hypoxia, vasoactive hormones, catecholamines and/or androgenic steroids may be involved to varying degrees in the control of erythropoeitic activity at and following exposure to moderate altitude.

5 Acknowledgement

This work was supported by a grant from the Alberta Sport Council.

6 References

Anagnostou, A., Fried, W. and Kurtzman, N. (1981) Haematological consequences of renal failure, in The Kidney (eds B.M. Brenner and F.C. Rector), W.B. Saunders, Toronto, pp. 2184-2212.

Berglund, B., Birgegard, G. and Hemmingsson, P. (1988) Serum erythropoietin in cross-country skiers. Med. Sci. Sports Exerc., 20, 208-209.

Berglund, B., Birgegard, G., Wide, L. and Pihlstedt, P. (1989) Effects of blood transfusions on some haematological variables in endurance athletes. Med. Sci. Sport Exerc., 21, 637-642.

Cachatourian, R., Eclerling, G. and Fried, W. (1980) Effect of short-term protein deprivation on hemopoietic functions of healthy volunteers. Blood, 55, 625-628.

Cline, M. and Golde, D. (1979) Cellular interactions in haematopoiesis. Nature 277, 177-181.

Fried, W., Barone-Varelas, J., Barone, T. and Anagnostou, A. (1982) Effect of angiotensin infusion on extrarenal erythropoietin production. J. Lab. Clin. Med., 99, 520-525.

Jacobson, L., Goldwasser, E., Fried, W. and Plzak, L. (1957) The role of the kidney in erythropoiesis. Nature, 179, 633-634.

Mairbäurl, H., Schobersberger, W., Humpeler, E., Hasibeder, W., Fischer, W. and Raas, E. (1986) Beneficial effects of exercising at moderate altitude on red cell oxygen transport and exercise performance. Pflüger Arch., 406, 594-599.

Mirand, E., Gordon, A. and Wenig, J. (1965) Mechanism of testosterone action in erythropoiesis. Nature., 206, 270-272.

Schade, S. and Fried, W. (1976) Suppressive effect of endotoxin on erythropoietin-responsive cells in mice. Am. J. Physiol., 231, 73-76.

Sherwood, J. and Goldwasser, E. (1979) A radioimmunoassay for erythropoietin. Blood, 54, 31.

Stray-Gunderson, J. (1988) Unethical alterations of oxygen-carrying capacity in endurance athletes. NIPS, 3, 241-244.

Wilde, L., Bengtsson, C. and Birgegard, G. (1989) Circadian rhythm of erythropoietin in human serum. Br. J. Haem., 72, 85-90.

Williams, M., Wesseldine, S., Somma, T. and Schuster, R. (1981) The effect of induced erythrocythemia upon 5-mile treadmill run time. Med. Sci. Sport Exerc., 13, 169-175.

A NUTRITIONAL ANALYSIS OF ELITE PRE-ADOLESCENT SWIMMERS

D.P. MACLAREN, J.E. HARTE and A.F. HACKETT
School of Health Sciences, Liverpool Polytechnic, England

Abstract
Information about habitual food intake of pre-adolescent children of
an elite swimming group and a non-active control group was systematically obtained. Thirty swimmers (15 male and 15 female, mean age
12.2 $\pm$ 0.9 years) trained an average of five times a week (approximately 9 h) and were competing at National level. The control group
(15 male and 15 female, mean age 11.9 $\pm$ 0.7 years) consisted of
normally active children. Measurement of weighed food intake was
conducted over three days. The total energy intake and the protein
intake for swimmers were significantly higher ($P < 0.05$ and $P < 0.001$
respectively), than those of the control group. No significant
differences were apparent between the groups for fat and simple and
complex carbohydrate intakes. When compared to recommended daily
allowances (RDAs), both groups were found to have significantly lower
fat intakes and significantly higher protein and total carbohydrate
intakes than normal ($P < 0.01$). Recommendations to the swimmers were
to increase carbohydrate intake and further reduce fat consumption so
that the possibility of lowered glycogen stores would be minimised.
Keywords: Carbohydrate, Energy, Fat, Nutrition, Protein, RDA.

1 Introduction

Training is perceived as the most important and effective way of
improving performance in sport. However, the contribution of
nutrition is often overlooked and not seriously considered despite
the mounting evidence linking body carbohydrate status and sports
performance (Costill, 1988). In their pursuit of excellence,
athletes subject their bodies to extreme levels of stress and undergo
strenuous training to achieve peak levels of fitness. This excess of
energy output needs to be balanced with an increase in energy input.

As the standards of sporting achievement are being set at ever
higher levels, the age of onset of rigorous training is being
lowered. Nutritional requirements of growing athletes have to be
carefully monitored owing to the energy demands not only for training
but for growth as well. Despite this fact, there is a relative
scarcity of literature pertaining to nutrition and the sporting
child. This study was undertaken in order to analyse the nutritional
intake of elite child swimmers and thereby make recommendations as to
the adequacy of their diet.

2 Method

Thirty pre-adolescent swimmers (15 male and 15 female, mean age 12.2 ± 0.9 yrs) from the City of Liverpool swim squad gave informed consent and took part in the study. On average the swimmers trained five times a week for a total of nine hours. A matched control group of 30 normally active children (15 male and 15 female, mean age 11.9 ± 0.7 years) was chosen from a Liverpool comprehensive school.

A weighed food intake was conducted over three days using electronic balances. A booklet gave guidelines for conducting the weighed food intake and provided space for storing the information. Parents and children were also given verbal advice on how to proceed with the study. One weekend day and two typical weekdays were chosen. On collection of the booklets, the food ingested was coded using food tables (Paul and Southgate, 1978) for application to the 'Daily D' computer program. Information was thus gained on macronutrients i.e. total energy (kJ), protein, fat and carbohydrate amounts (g) and percentage contributions.

Statistical treatment of data involved analysis of covariance (ANCOVA) on the total energy and the macronutrients both in terms of amounts and percentage contribution.

3 Results and discussion

Table 1 presents the mean nutritional data for swimmers, control groups and RDA values. The mean total energy intake was higher for both female groups when compared to the female RDA values, but only for the male swimmers when compared to male RDA values. The swimmers had a significantly higher energy intake than the control group ($P < 0.05$); the mean difference being 1412 kJ. Although data were not obtained on the energy expenditure during training, it can be estimated that a young swimmer may expend approximately 1200 kJ per hour (Brooks and Fahey, 1984), to provide a total of 2400 kJ for a 2-hour training session. Therefore 25% of the total energy intake of young swimmers was being used to replenish the energy used during two hours of training.

The data with respect to carbohydrates ingested show that although the swimmers consumed more carbohydrate in total than the respective control groups, the latter derived a greater percentage from complex carbohydrates. However, ANCOVA revealed that the only significant difference was between the male control group (55.06%) and the male swimmers (50.42%). If the swimmers did use up approximately 2400 kJ of energy and 60% of this energy was derived from carbohydrate, the swimmers should be ingesting a further 90 g of carbohydrates more than the control group. This patently had not occurred; the difference was +15 g for the female swimmers compared to the female control group and +24 g for the male swimmers compared to the male control group. The mean percentage of carbohydrate ingested by the swimmers was 50-51% of the total energy intake. Despite the fact that the total carbohydrate consumed was greater than that of the RDAs, the percentage contribution should be increased to at least 55% (better still 60%) of the total energy intake. The recommendation would be for swimmers to increase their carbohydrate intake by a further 90-100 g per day and this would lead to a greater percent

Table 1. Daily energy intake and contributions of the macronutrients

Sex	Subjects	Energy (kJ)	Protein (g)	Fats (g)	Simple CHO (g)	Complex CHO (g)	Total CHO (g)
Mean values:							
Female	RDA	8750.00	52.00	106.00			246.00
	Controls	9140.50	61.67	91.91	76.05	217.16	293.21
	Swimmers	9659.73	80.50	88.64	108.25	204.38	312.63
Male	RDA	10250.00	61.00	124.00			288.00
	Controls	9075.75	59.67	83.33	111.59	200.72	312.31
	Swimmers	10694.17	76.62	107.98	119.34	217.64	336.97
Percentage mean values:							
Female	Controls		11.47	37.21	13.31	38.01	51.33
	Swimmers		14.17	34.03	17.93	33.85	51.78
Male	Controls		11.18	33.97	19.67	35.39	55.06
	Swimmers		12.18	37.36	17.85	32.56	50.42

contribution of carbohydrates.

Analysis of variance revealed that the swimmers had a significantly larger intake of protein than the control group ($P < 0.001$). This finding was consistent with studies on preadolescent children and athletes (Hackett et al., 1984; Hickson et al., 1987). The percentage contribution of protein for the swimmers was below 12–14% and was above the RDAs. The mean protein consumption of the swimmers of 78.5 g represented a value of approximately 1.67 g/kg body weight per day. No further recommendations were needed since protein intake was deemed sufficient.

Fat intakes of all the groups were below RDA values and similar to those found in other studies (Bull, 1988; Hickson et al., 1987). The larger, though non-significant, fat intake of the swimmers may be attributed to the higher protein intake in the form of meat and dairy products.

Further data were obtained on the timing of meals and snacks (Figure 1). Results highlight the facts (1) that swimmers eat snacks in the hour prior to training, and (2) that swimmers eat a meal within the hour after training. Although the latter is recommended, particularly if the meal is high in carbohydrates, the former should not be encouraged due to the possible retention of food in the stomach whilst swimming and due to the possibility of 'rebound' hypoglycaemia (Costill et al., 1973).

4 Conclusion

In spite of the evidence supporting an apparent healthy diet of the elite pre-adolescent swimmers with respect to RDAs, recommendations were made in terms of an increase in complex carbohydrate ingestion (90–100 g per day), a reduction in fat ingestion for males in particular, no change in protein ingestion, and the elimination of snacks in the hour prior to training. Such a scenario should

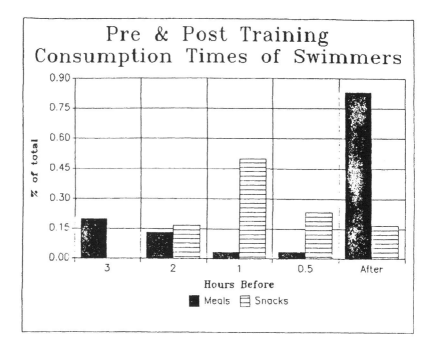

Fig. 1. Pre- and post- training food consumption times of swimmers.

minimise the possibility of lowered glycogen stores prior to training and 'rebound' hypoglycaemia during training.

5 References

Brooks, G. and Fahey, T. (1984) **Exercise Physiology: Human Bioenergetics and Its Applications.** John Wiley, New York.

Bull, N.L. (1988) Studies of the dietary habits, food consumption and nutrient intakes of adolescents and young children. **World Review of Nutrition and Dietetics,** 57, 24-74.

Costill, D.L. (1988) Carbohydrates for exercise: dietary demands for optimal performance. **Int. J. Sports. Med.,** 9, 1-18.

Costill, D.L., Bennett, A., Brahnam, G. and Eddy, D. (1973) Glucose ingestion at rest and during prolonged exercise. **J. Appl. Physiol.,** 34, 764-769.

Department of Health and Social Security (1981) **Recommended Intakes of Nutrients for the United Kingdom.** HMSO, London.

Hackett, A.F., Rugg-Gunn, A.J., Appleton, D.R., Eastoe, JK.E. and Jenkins, G.N. (1984) A two year longitudinal survey of 405 Northumberland children, initially aged 11.5 years. **Brit. J. Nutr.,** 51, 67-75.

Hickson, J.F., Duke, M.A., Risser, W.L., Johnson, C.W., Palmer, R. and Stockton, J.E. (1987) Nutritional intake from food sources of high school football athletes. **J. Am. Diet. Assoc.,** 87, 1656-1659.

Paul, A.A. and Southgate, D.A.T. (1978) **McCance and Widdowson's The Composition of Foods.** 4th edition. HMSO, London.

PART NINE

KINANTHROPOMETRY

GROWTH AND DEVELOPMENT CHARACTERISTICS OF ELITE FEMALE AGE GROUP SWIMMERS

A. BARZDUKAS, S. SPRY, J.M. CAPPAERT and J.P. TROUP
U.S. Swimming, International Centre for Aquatic Research, Colorado Springs, CO, USA

Abstract
There is a strong relationship between physiological development, performance, and general growth and maturation during adolescence. Thus the purpose of this study was to examine skinfold thicknesses, stature, weight, Tanner development scores, hand-wrist radiographs, age of menarche, and Androgeny index (3 x biacromal breadth - bicristal breadth) in elite female age group swimmers. Subjects were divided into three groups based on age and performance level. Group I (n = 49, age = 160.40 ± 2.93), Group II (n = 28, age = 184.36 ± 3.96), and Group III (n = 24, age = 196.43 ± 3.95 years) varied significantly in terms of all anthropometric factors, except height and sum of skinfold, and performance times. In summary, (1) the group as a whole, had biological ages which exceeded the mean chronological ages by approximately 7 months. The older girls were, as expected, more physically mature - heavier, leaner with higher androgeny indices.
Keywords; Skinfolds, Tanner, Development, Radiograph, Menarche, Androgeny.

1 Introduction

Physiological development in young female swimmers has been the focus of a number of studies during the last three decades (Åstrand et al., 1963; Cunningham and Eynon, 1973; Meleski et al., 1982; Bernink et al., 1983). Martinosov et al. (1984) suggested that performance improvement in adolescent female swimmers is directly related to increases in anthropometric and developmental factors associated with growth.

The purpose of this investigation, therefore, was to examine characteristic patterns of growth and development among elite female age group swimmers in the United States.

2 Methods

2.1 Subjects

One hundred and one (n = 101) elite female age group swimmers participated in this study. All swimmers were nationally ranked in the Top 10 in their respective events on the basis of competitive performance. Each swimmer signed an letter of informed consent.

All testing was conducted at the International Center for Aquatic Research during early season training camps in October and November.

Subjects were assigned a priori to one of three groups on the basis of age and performance level. Group age, select physiological and performance characteristics are presented in Table 1.

Table 1. Characteristics of elite female age group swimmers: mean ± SD

Group		Age (months)	Height (cm)	Weight (kg)	200 m freestyle (s)
I	(n = 49)	160.40*	168.48	52.54*	131**
		± 11.45	± 8.46	± 6.36	± 0.11
II	(n = 28)	184.36*	171.73	57.83	128
		± 3.96	± 6.05	± 6.29	± 0.23
III	(n = 24)	196.43*	168.77	59.11	126
		± 3.95	± 5.05	± 5.41	± 0.76

*P < 0.01; ** P < 0.05

2.2 Measurements

2.2.1 Biological age

Assessments of skeletal maturation were made using standard Health Examination Survey (HES) radiographic examination techniques. Hand-wrist radiographs were examined for "maturity indicators" to estimate skeletal maturation (Greulich and Pyle, 1959). Bone specific skeletal age assessments of the hand-wrist radiographs were averaged to estimate skeletal age.

2.2.2 Body mass index

Subjects were weighed on a balance beam scale and measured with a secured height anthropometer. Body mass index ($kg*m^{-2}$) was computed (Sallis et al., 1989).

2.2.3 Skinfold measurements

Skinfold fat thickness was estimated at nine skinfold (SF) sites using Lange Skinfold Calipers (Cambridge Scientific Industries Inc). The sites consisted of:

1. Biceps - midway between the elbow and the top of the shoulder on the front part of the upper arm;
2. Triceps - midway between the elbow and the top of the shoulder on the back of the upper arm;
3. Subscapular - along the diagonal line below the shoulder blade;
4. Midaxillary - directly below the armpit and across from the nipple.
5. Suprailiac - at a diagonal, 2.5 cm above the hip bone;
6. Abdomen - vertically, 2.5 cm to the right of the umbilicus;
7. Thigh - midway between the knee and the hip, on the front part of the upper leg;
8. Medial calf - in the middle of the belly on the inside of the calf;

9. Lateral calf - in the middle of the belly on the outside of the calf.

2.2.4 Estimated percentage body fat
Percentage body fat was estimated using the formula of Brozek et al. (1963): Fat = (4.570/Density - 4.142) × 100. Body density was determined using the formula of Meleski et al. (1982): Density = 1.08230 - 0.00046 × (Triceps SF + Subscapular SF + Suprailiac SF + Medial Calf SF).

2.2.5 Tanner development scores
Tanner development scores were assessed to estimate biological age and stage of maturation (Tanner, 1962). Females were evaluated on three measures: (1) pubic hair development (6 stages), (2) breast development (5 stages) and (3) axillary hair (underarm) development (3 stages). Males were also evaluated on three measures: (1) pubic hair development (6 stages), (2) genital development (5 stages) and (3) axillary hair (facial) development. Due to the personal nature of these evaluations, these data were collected via individual questionnaire using Tanner scale photographs and administered in a private setting.

2.2.6 Age at menarche
All data were gathered via questionnaire administered in a private setting. Menarche is defined as the first menstrual flow and the question was presented in these terms when data were collected regarding this maturational event.

2.2.7 Androgeny index
The androgeny index is defined as three times the biacromial breadth measurement minus the bicristal breadth measurement (Tanner, 1962). This scale is used to describe relative gender-specific somatotype.

2.3 Statistics
An ANOVA was used to evaluate group differences. A probability level of $P < 0.01$ was selected for statistical significance. Significance was localised using Tukey's post-hoc test. The Pearson product-moment correlation coefficient was calculated to determine the linearity of the relationship between selected variables.

3 Results

3.1 Age comparisons
Mean values ($\pm$ SD) of chronological and biological age are found in Table 2. Although there was no statistical difference, whole group mean biological ages exceeded mean chronological ages by approximately seven months. Tukey's post-hoc test revealed that significant differences between all groups for both chronological and biological age.

3.2 Body mass index
The ANOVA for Body Mass Index (BMI) revealed significant difference between groups (see Table 3). Tukey's post-hoc test indicated that Group I differed significantly from Group II for BMI.

Table 2. Chronological and biological ages of elite female age group
          swimmers

Age (months)	Group		
	I	II	III
Chronological	160.40*	184.36*	196.43*
	± 2.93	± 3.96	± 3.95
Biological	168.37*	189.43*	204.52*
	± 11.45	± 17.24	± 13.89

*$P < 0.01$

3.3 Body fat and skinfolds
The ANOVA and subsequent post-hoc analysis for body fat estimations
revealed differences between Group I and Groups II and III. There
were no statistically significant differences between groups for sum
of skinfold measurements (see Table 3).

Table 3. Body mass index, estimated percent body fat and sum of
          skinfold sites in elite female age group swimmers

Variable	Groups		
	I	II	III
Body mass index	18.54*	19.56*	10.49*
(kg/m^{-2})	± 2.02	± 1.39	± 1.34
Sum skinfolds	108.21	96.95	100.11
(mm)	± 21.99	± 23.32	± 22.96
Body fat	28.98*	17.56	17.53
(%)	± 2.12	± 2.24	± 2.31

*$P < 0.01$

3.4 Tanner development scores
The ANOVA for Tanner developmental stages revealed a significant
difference for all variables: pubic hair, breast and axillary hair.
Tukey's post-hoc analysis indicated that Group III differed
significantly from Group I for pubic hair, breast and axillary hair
development (see Table 4).

3.5 Age of menarche
The ANOVA for age of menarche indicated that there was significant
difference between groups. Post-hoc analysis revealed that Group I
differed from Groups II and III for age at menarche (see Table 5).

3.6 Androgeny index
The ANOVA for androgeny index indicated that there was significant
difference between groups. Tukey's post-hoc test showed that Group I
differed significantly from Groups II and III (see Table 5.

Table 4. Tanner development stages of elite female age group
swimmers

Tanner variable	Groups		
	I	II	III
Pubic hair	3.57*	3.89*	4.39
	± 0.79	± 0.58	± 0.66
Breast	3.22*	3.70	3.91
	± 0.59	± 0.67	± 0.73
Axillary hair	2.45	2.56	2.83*
	± 0.50	± 0.51	± 0.39

Table 5. Age of menarche and androgeny index values of elite female
age group swimmers

Variable	Groups		
	I	II	III
Age of menarche	12.07*	12.81	13.42
	± 0.81	± 1.23	± 1.09
Androgeny index	73.29*	77.73	76.54
	± 5.78	± 4.84	± 6.02

*P < 0.01

3.7 Relationship to performance

The Pearson product-moment correlation coefficient was calculated to
determine the relationship between selected variables and performance
(see Table 6).

Table 6. Product-moment correlations between physiological variables
and swimming performance for elite female age group
swimmers (r values)

Variable	BMI	Bio-Age	Age
200 m freestyle performance	0.86*	0.91*	0.79*

4 Discussion

In summary, the data show that the fastest elite female age group
swimmers were the heaviest and had the highest degree of biological
development (Tanner scores and skeletal age). Significant correlations were found between performance, BMI, biological age and chronological age. The strongest relationship with swimming performance
was found for biological age. Group III was also leaner and had
higher androgeny indices than the other two groups. These results
may be the result of the extreme physical training associated with
the training required for elite status as a swimmer.

Åstrand et al. (1963) reported a mean age of menarche of 12.88 for Swedish female swimmers. This value is similar to Group II data reported above. Interestingly, Group I reported age of menarche values were significantly lower than Group II and III. Thus, age of menarche was found to be decreasing with successive generations of swimmers. This phenomenon has also been reported in the general population (Malina, 1983). The data reported above did not differ from general population values (Malina, 1983).

Females gain adipose tissue early in adolescence and, unlike males, continue to gain in adiposity as adolescence continues. The data reported above suggest that Group II and III swimmers are past the adolescent growth spurt. Tanner development scores, however, indicated that the greatest degree of biological development occurs between Groups II and III.

5 References

Åstrand, P.O., Engstrom, L., Eriksson, B.O., Karlberg, P., Nylander, I., Saltin, B. and Thoren, C. (1963) Girl swimmers. **Acta Paediatrica, Suppl.**, 147.

Bernink, M.J.E., Erich, W.B.M., Peltenburg, A.L., Zonderland, M.L. and Huisveld, I.A. (1983) Body composition, biological maturation, and socioeconomic status of young talented female swimmers and gymnasts, in **Biomechanics and Medicine in Swimming** (eds A.P. Hollander, P.A. Huijing and G. de Groot), Human Kinetics Publishers Inc., Champaign, Ill, pp. 41-50.

Brozek, J., Grande, F., Anderson, J.T. and Keys, A. (1963) Densitometric analysis of body composition: Revision of some quantitative assumptions. **Ann. New York Acad. Sci.**, 110, 113-140.

Cunningham, D.A. and Eynon, R.B. (1973) The working capacity of young competitive swimmers, 10-16 years of age. **Med. Sci. Sport**, 5, 227-231.

Greulich, W.W. and Pyle, S.I. (1959) **Radiographic Atlas of Skeletal Development of the Hand and Wrist,**. 2nd edition, Stanford University Press, Stanford.

Malina, R.M. (1983) Menarche in athletes: A synthesis and hypothesis. **Ann. Human Biol.**, 10, 1-24.

Martinosov, E.G., Bulgakov, N.Z., Statkjawiczjenje, B.V., Filimonova, I.J. and Chebotarieva, I.V. (1984) Polowoj dimorfizm niekototych morfofunkcjonalnych pokazatelej i sportivnych dostizenij w plawanii. **Teoria Praktica Fiziczzeskoj Kultury**, 3, 16-18.

Meleski, B.W., Shoup, R.F. and Malina, R.M. (1982) Size, physique and body composition of competitive female swimmers 11 through 20 years of age. **Human Biol.**, 54, 609-625.

Tanner, J.M. (1962) **Growth at Adolescence.** 2nd edition. Blackwell Scientific Publications, Oxford.

Sallis, J.F., Patterson, T.L., Morris, J.A., Nader, P.R. and Buono, M.J. (1989) Familial aggregation of aerobic power: The influence of age, physical activity, body mass index. **Res. Quart. Exerc. Sport**, 4, 318-324.

DEVELOPMENTAL CHANGES IN MUSCLE SIZE AND POWER CHARACTERISTICS OF ELITE AGE GROUP SWIMMERS

A. BARZDUKAS, S. SPRY, J.M. CAPPAERT and J.P. TROUP
U.S. Swimming, International Center for Aquatic Research, Colorado
Springs, CO, USA

Abstract
There is a strong relationship between strength development and
general growth and maturation during adolescence. The purpose of
this study was to determine (1) the characteristic changes in muscle
size and power due to growth in elite swimmers and (2) how these
changes may affect performance. Measurements of leg and arm power,
four skinfold thicknesses and two circumferences were made on 101
female swimmers aged 13.4 to 16.4 and 84 male swimmers aged 14.4 to
17.5 years. Skinfolds and circumference measurements were combined
to provide estimates of the muscle/bone component of both the upper
and lower extremities. Subjects were divided into three groups based
on age and performance level. Group I (male, n = 32, age = 14.4 $\pm$
0.96; female, n = 49, age 13.4 $\pm$ 0.95), Group II (male, n = 28, age =
16.4 $\pm$ 0.58; female, n = 28, age = 15.4 $\pm$ 0.36), and Group III (male,
n = 24, age = 17.5 $\pm$ 0.61; female, n = 24, age = 16.4 $\pm$ 0.39) varied
significantly in terms of all anthropometric factors, except height,
power variables, and performance times. In summary, (1) the fastest
male swimmers were heavier and had higher power values and arm
muscle/bone component estimates, and (2) the fastest females had
higher power values, arm and leg muscle bone component estimates.
Keywords: Muscle/Bone Circumference, Skinfolds, Girths, Power.

1 Introduction

Physiological development in young athletes during adolescence has
been examined during the last three decades (Åstrand et al., 1963;
Malina, 1983). Martinosov et al. (1984) suggested that performance
improvement in adolescent female swimmers is directly related to
increases in anthropometric and developmental factors associated with
growth. Kunski et al. (1988) found significant correlations between
performance and body weight, lean body mass, lower extremity length,
and shoulder width in elite Polish junior swimmers.

The purpose of this investigation, therefore, was to examine
characteristic changes in muscle size and power in elite swimmers.
Also, the relationship between these changes and performance was also
examined.

2 Methods

2.1 Subjects

One hundred and eighty five (male, n = 84; females, n = 101) elite age group swimmers participated in this descriptive study. All swimmers were nationally Top 10 ranked in their respective events on the basis of performance. Each swimmer signed an letter of informed consent.

All testing was conducted at the International Center for Aquatic Research in the grounds of the United States Olympic Training Center in Colorado Springs, Colorado, during early season training camps in October and November.

Subjects were assigned a priori to one of three groups on the basis of age and performance level. Group age and performance characteristics are presented in Table 1.

Table 1. Age and performance characteristics of elite age group swimmers: mean ($\pm$ SD)

Group		Age (Yr)	200 m performance times (s)			
			Back	Brst	Fly	Free
I*	Males	14.44	139	158	139	122
	(n = 22)	($\pm$0.96)	($\pm$6.9)	($\pm$9.1)	($\pm$5.2)	($\pm$3.1)
	Females	13.37	152	167	147	131
	(n = 49)	($\pm$1.03)	($\pm$7.4)	($\pm$5.2)	($\pm$4.3)	($\pm$1.6)
II*	Males	16.39	132	148	130	117
	(n = 28)	($\pm$0.58)	($\pm$2.4)	($\pm$2.9)	($\pm$1.3)	($\pm$1.5)
III*	Males	17.51	126	144	128	115
	(n = 24)	($\pm$0.61)	($\pm$1.4)	($\pm$2.8)	($\pm$1.0)	($\pm$0.9)
	Females	16.37	141	160	139	126
	(n = 24)	($\pm$0.66)	($\pm$1.6)	($\pm$1.4)	($\pm$0.8)	($\pm$1.1)

Note: Back = backstroke, Brst = breaststroke, Fly = butterfly,
      Free = freestyle.
*$P < 0.05$, whole group differences.

2.2 Measurements

2.2.1 Muscle/bone circumference

Muscle/bone (MB) arm and leg components were estimated using a combination of skinfold thicknesses (S) and girth measurements (G) (Malina, 1989). Subcutaneous fat thickness was estimated at four sites using Lange Skinfold Calipers (Cambridge Scientific Industries Inc.). The sites consisted of: (1) biceps - midway between the elbow and the top of the shoulder on the front part of the upper arm; (2) triceps - midway between the elbow and the top of the shoulder on the back on the upper arm; (3) medial calf - in the middle of the belly on the inside of the calf; (4) lateral calf - in the middle of the belly on the outside of the calf.

Girths were measured at two sites: (1) relaxed upper arm - at the widest point, and (2) calf - around the widest part of the lower leg when the athlete stands with legs separated and weight balanced.

Muscle/bone areas (MBA) were estimated from the formulas (Malina, 1989):

    Arm MBA = G - 0.157*(S Bicep + S Tricep)
    Leg MBA = G - 0.157*(S Medial + S Lateral)

2.2.2 Power

Upper body power was measured using a Pacer 2A Biokinetic Swim Ergometer (Isokinetics Inc.). Each athlete completed a series of double arm pulls through a full range of motion, while prone, at four different settings (0, 3, 6, 9) on the swim ergometer. Power was calculated in watts as the highest average output of the three pulls.

Lower body power was measured using a Leg Power Machine (Takei & Company Ltd.). Subjects sat in a chair with legs flexed at the hip and knee with feet on a push platform. When given the start signal, the subjects fully extended their legs as fast as possible. Power was calculated in watts as the highest of four trials.

2.3 Statistics

A 2 x 3 ANOVA was used to evaluate sex and group differences. A probability level of $P < 0.05$ was selected for statistical significance. Significant variance was analyzed using Tukey's post-hoc test. The Pearson product-moment correlation coefficient was calculated to determine the relationship between variables.

3 Results

Mean values ($\pm$ SD) of body weights and heights are found in Table 2. Although there were no significant group differences in height for either males or females, significant differences occurred for body weights. Tukey's post-hoc tests revealed significant differences between Group I and Groups II and III for body weight.

Table 2. Mean ($\pm$ SD) body weights and heights for elite age group swimmers

Variable		Group		
		I	II	III
Height (cm):	Male	177.85	181.86	183.77
		($\pm$ 5.4)	($\pm$ 5.7)	($\pm$ 4.1)
	Female	168.48	171.73	169.77
		($\pm$ 8.5)	($\pm$ 6.1)	($\pm$ 5.4)
Weight (kg):	Male*	63.10	69.54	73.87
		($\pm$ 6.3)	($\pm$ 4.6)	($\pm$ 4.7)
	Female*	52.54	57.83	59.11
		($\pm$ 6.4)	($\pm$ 6.3)	($\pm$ 5.4)

*$P < 0.05$.

The ANOVA for Arm MBA revealed a significant difference for both male and female age group swimmers. Tukey's post-hoc test indicated that Group I differed significantly from Groups II and III for Arm MBA for both males and females. The ANOVA indicated a significant result for female Leg MB. Post-hoc analysis demonstrated that Group I differed from Groups II and III. There was no significant effect demonstrated for male Leg MB, however. The MBA results are shown in Table 3.

Table 3. Arm and leg muscle/bone circumferences in elite age group swimmers

Group		Arm MBA	Leg MBA
I	Male	24.3 ± 1.21*	33.16 ± 1.92
	Female	21.33 ± 0.95*	28.25 ± 0.87*
II	Male	26.5 ± 1.24*	33.03 ± 2.10
	Female	23.17 ± 1.01	29.96 ± 1.11
III	Male	27.81 ± 0.89	34.12 ± 1.54
	Female	23.33 ± 1.52	29.83 ± 1.67

*$P < 0.05$

Significant male and female group differences existed for leg and arm power measurements. Tukey's post-hoc test revealed that, for males, Group I, had significantly weaker legs and arms. For females, post-hoc analysis revealed that Group II was significantly stronger than Groups II and III for both arms and legs. Power results are shown in Table 4.

Table 4. Arm and leg muscle power in elite age group swimmers

Group		Arm (watts)	Leg (watts)
I	Male	391.50 ± 35.64*	891.63 ± 94.77*
	Female	234.70 ± 51.18*	567.83 ± 41.96*
II	Male	491.05 ± 40.15	1003.81 ± 72.49
	Female	327.05 ± 39.37	663.25 ± 55.28
III	Male	499.55 ± 52.87	1054.96 ± 79.24
	Female	310.27 ± 44.63	616.57 ± 29.80

*$P < 0.05$

Table 5, which shows the Pearson product-moment correlations between swimming performance (200 m freestyle) and power and muscle area measurments, demonstrates that increases in power and muscle mass are significantly related to swimming performance.

4 Discussion

In summary, the data show that the fastest swimmers were the heaviest, had the highest power values, and the largest arm MBA estimates. Additionally, the fastest female swimmers had the highest leg MBA estimates. Interestingly, although height increased with age, especially with males, there was no significant difference in height between groups for either sex. These findings suggest that increases in performance accompany increases in power and muscle.

Table 5. Product-moment correlations between selected physiological variables and swimming performance for elite age group swimmers (r values)

Variable	Arm MBA	Leg MBA	Arm power	Leg power
200 m freestyle performance:				
Male	0.84	0.65	0.89	0.73
Female	0.77	0.58	0.88	0.59

Huijing et al. (1988) found significant correlations between maximal body cross-section and active drag and a lower, but significant, correlation between body height and active drag. Overcoming drag is the most important factor in propulsion in swimming. Since the findings in the present study showed no significant difference in height between groups of elite adolescent swimmers, it may be speculated that the increases in power accompanying development may be substantial enough to overcome the concomitant increase in maximal body cross-section. The high correlations between power, muscle area and swimming perfomance for both males and females tend to support these findings.

Thus, the developmental changes undergone by elite age group swimmers during adolescence contribute significantly to concomitent increases in swimming performance. The greatest increases in muscle area and performance come following the adolescent growth spurt (Group II in males, pre-Group I in females, see Table 3). Gains in performance are significantly related to gains in power and muscle area. Therefore, the relationship between anthropometric variables and swimming performance bears continued study, especially with regard to biomechanical aspects of swimming technique.

5 References

Åstrand, P.O., Engstrom, L., Eriksson, B.O., Karlberg, P., Nylander, I., Saltin, B. and Thoren, C. (1963) Girl swimmers. **Acta Paediatrica, Supplementum** 147.

Huijing, P.A., Toussaint, H.M., Mackay, R., Vervoorn, K., Clarys, J.P., Groot, G. de, Hollander, A.P. (1988) Active drag related to body dimensions, in **Swimming Science V** (eds B.E. Ungerechts, K. Wilke and K. Reischle), Human Kinetics Books, Champaign, Ill., pp. 31-37.

Kunski, H., Jegier, A., Maslankiewicz, A. and Rakus, E. (1988) The relationship of biological factors to swimming performance in top Polish junior swimmers aged 12 to 14 years, in **Swimming Science V** (eds B.E. Ungerechts, K. Wilke and K. Reischle), Human Kinetics Books, Champaign, Ill., pp. 109-113.

Malina, R.M. (1983) Physical growth and maturity characteristics of young athletes, in **Children in Sport,** 2nd edition (eds R.A. Magill, M.J. Ash and F.L. Smoll), Human Kinetics Publishers, Champaign, Ill., pp. 73-96.

Malina, R.M. (1989) Unpublished lecture, Anthropometrics in Swimming

Meeting, Colorado Springs, Colorado.

Martinosov, E.G., Bulgakova, N.Z., Statkjawiczjenje, B.V., filimonova, I.J. and Chebotarieva, I.V. (1984) Polowoj dimorfizm niekototych morfofunkcjonalnych pokazatelej i sportivnych dostizenij w plawanii. **Teoria Praktika Fiziczeskoj Kultury,** 3, 16-18.

RELATION BETWEEN PHYSICAL CHARACTERISTICS AND UNDULATION IN THE BREASTSTROKE

V. COLMAN, D. DALY, S. DESMET and U. PERSYN
Instituut voor Lichamelijke Opleiding, K.U. Leuven, Leuven, Belgium

Abstract
In order to quantify undulation in breaststroke, five undulation
factors were constructed from body positions during the stroke cycle:
uphill in leg spreading, dome-shaped at the surface, S-shaped under
the surface, and uphill hydroplaning in the two recovery phases.
When international swimmers were placed in four groups, according to
a total undulation index, one continuum from flat to extremely
undulating was found in women. For men, two distinct groups were
observed: the majority very flat and the others extremely undulating.
When the mean percentile scores of women and men for each separate
undulation factor were presented in curves, the women showed higher
scores in the S-shaped and the uphill, hydroplaning body position.
Most of the individual curves of undulation factors were flat.
    The dome-shaped part of the undulation was related to good ankle
supination combined with outward hip rotation for women. Apparently,
the S-shaped and the striking uphill parts of the undulation in women
can be explained by more flexibility in lumbar cambering, even when
the hips were flexed. In men, a flat position was related to hip
inward rotation and ankle outward rotation and flexion.
Keywords: Breaststroke Swimming, Undulation, Physical
Characteristics.

1 Introduction

In a parallel study the breaststroke of an international woman
swimmer, who had drastically improved her performance after changing
from a flat to an extremely undulating pattern was described (Persyn
et al., 1992). This dolphin-like undulation became possible after
the rule change in 1987, allowing the head to dive under the surface.
    However, in this short period of evolution of the breaststroke it
is not yet possible to select the most appropriate pattern per
individual. It is not even known if international swimmers use a
continuum of flat to extremely undulating patterns or if some use an
asymmetric undulation, by taking only one typical body position:
dome-shaped (near the water surface) or S-shaped (under the surface)
or cambered (hydroplaning).
    To study these questions a method was developed to quantify
undulation in breaststroke swimming using both female and male
swimmers. Furthermore, relationships between undulation and physical
characteristics (body structure, flexibility and isometric strength)
were also investigated.

2 Methods

To study the degree of undulation a reference group of 16 female and
19 male international swimmers were selected (X̄ 100 m women 1.13'5",
male 1.05'5"). Six frames in one stroke cycle were digitised from
video recordings (Colman and Persyn, 1989) to compose five undulation
factors (defined in detail in Fig. 1):
  (a) Uphill body position in spreading the legs (I-II);
  (b) Most dome-shaped body position (one frame between kick and
pull, the turning point from up- to downhill) (III);
  (c) Most S-shaped body position (one frame during spreading of the
arms, the turning point from down- to uphill) (IV);
  (d) Cambered uphill body position in the first part of recovery
(V-VI);
  (e) Uphill body position in the second part of recovery (VI-I).
  The factors a, d and e refer to phases of uphill, hydroplaning
body position. One total undulation index is composed equally of
three essential parts (b, c and d-a). A mobility index is composed
of three essential parts (dome-, S-shaped and hydroplaning)(Fig. 1).
  Undulation was calculated from angles of the trunk with the
horizontal plane and from angles in body segments. The angles in
body segments, in the S-shaped and cambered position, which required
specific flexibility, were considered as mobility factors and were
combined in one total mobility index (Fig. 1).

DESCRIPTION		PATTERNS		FACTORS + INDICES	
STICK FIGURE	ANGLE	FLAT	UNDULATING	UNDUL.	MOBILITY
I. Begin leg spreading	1. Line shoulder-hip / horiz.	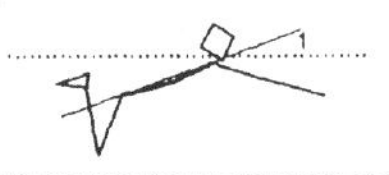	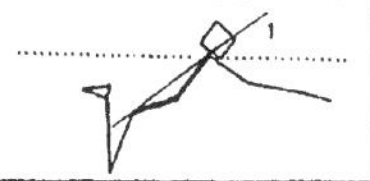	a. $\frac{1+2}{2}$	
II. Maximal leg spreading	2. Line shoulder-hip / horiz.	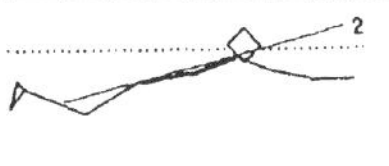	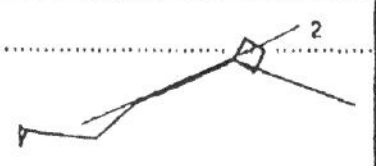		
III. Most dome-shaped position	Line should-hip 3. / leg 4. / arm	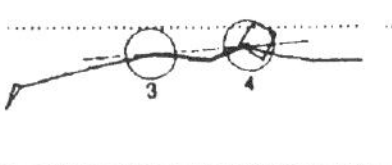	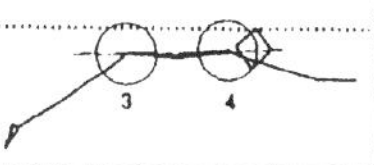	b. 3+4	
IV. 1/2 arm spreading or Most S-shaped	5. Knee extension 6. Hip flexion 7. Lumbar camber 8. Shoulder upw. extension	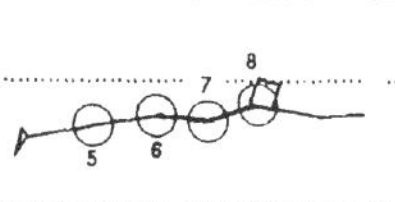	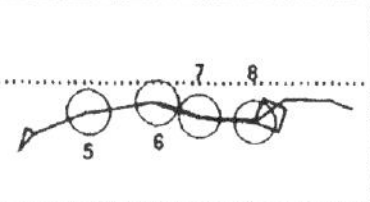	c. 6+7+8	5+6+7+8 +
V. Most cambered uphill position	9. Hip extension 10. Lumbar camber 11. Line shoulder-hip / horiz.	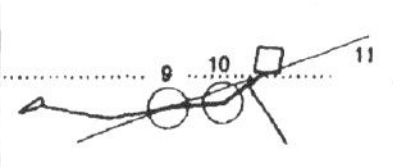	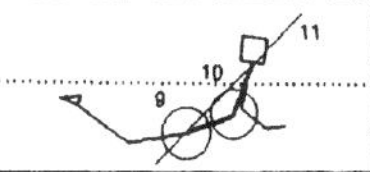	d. $\frac{11+13}{2}$ (e.$\frac{13+1}{2}$)	9+10 +
VI. Knee 90° recovery	12. Lumbar camber 13. Line shoulder-hip / horiz.	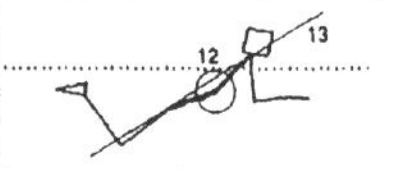	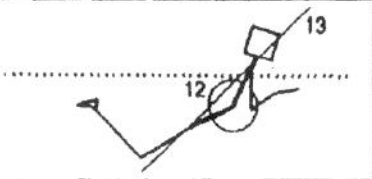		12

Fig. 1.   Description of the stick figures and angles used to
          compose undulation and mobility factors and indices.   An
          of only angles in body segments (5-10 and 12).

The undulation and mobility factors and indices were further correlated with physical characteristics (body structure, flexibility and isometric strength). In the Leuven Evaluation Center, the physical characteristics of swimmers have been measured for many years (Persyn et al., 1980, Vervaecke, 1983).

In order to increase the number of subjects for these correlation studies an additional 11 women and 7 men national swimmers were investigated ($\bar{X}$ 100 m performance of this additional group was for women 1.17'6" and for men 1.09'.

Correlation coefficients were obtained between the five factors and also between these factors and the physical characteristics of the swimmers.

3 Results and discussion

3.1 Identification of patterns
When the swimmers studied were placed in four groups, according to the total undulation index, one continuum from rather flat to extremely undulating was found in women (Fig. 2A). In men, however, two more distinct groups were observed. The majority remained very flat while the rest used rather extreme undulation. In order to visualise the two extreme patterns, the displacement of the body in relation to a fixed background is drawn in Fig. 2A for an 'experimental' swimmer.

When the mean percentile scores of each separate undulation factor for women and men were presented in curves, the women showed consistently higher scores, especially in the S-shaped and in the uphill, hydroplaning body positions during the entire recovery (Fig. 2B). What differences in body characteristics can cause these pattern differences?

When the individual curves of these international swimmers were drawn, most showed relatively stable scores (horizontal curves) for the five factors. The correlation between the dome-shaped and the S-shaped body position was 0.64 and between this S-shaped and the cambered, uphill body position, in the first part of the recovery, was 0.61 (P < 0.01). Could these differences in scores for the separate undulation factors, or the asymmetric undulation, which occur more frequently in individuals of a lower ability, be considered as a fault in technique?

3.2 Relation of physical characteristics with undulation and mobility
Body structure: in men, the flat pattern was used by tall subjects with a relatively large pelvis (Fig. 3: A and B) and in women, the undulating pattern was used by small and lean subjects (Fig. 3: A and C).

Isometric strength: in principle, a flat body position was maintained by a lateral paddle-like pull, which, in men, was related to a strong m. triceps (Fig. 3: 0). In principle, in the undulating pattern, the typical cambered, uphill body position (in the beginning of the recovery) was obtained by a propeller-like up-, down- and upward pull, which, in women, was related to a strong m. triceps and m. pectoralis (Fig. 3: 0, c and Q,d-e).

Flexibility: the cambered, uphill body position can only be

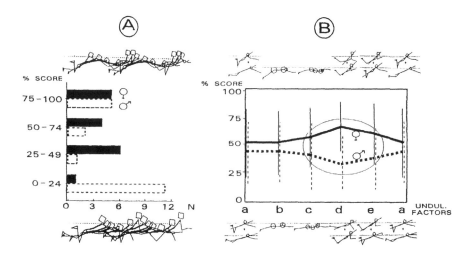

Fig. 2A.   Frequency diagram of the scores of the total undulation
           index, in four (25% score) groups, for women (n = 16) and
           men (n = 19) international level swimmers.
Fig. 2B.   Curves of the mean percentile scores of each separate
           undulation factor (and standard deviation) for women and
           men. For the total undulation index, as well as for each
           factor separately, a score 0 means least and 100 most
           undulation (or angulation), as seen in the stick figures.

maintained (in the recovery phases) due to lumbar camber. This
relation was found in men but not in women (Fig. 3: K-N, e, i and k).
This hydroplaning position, typical for women (Fig. 2B), was
maintained due to significantly more trunk flexibility than in men
(Fig. 3: K,i).

A dome-shaped uphill body position was obtained by a dolphin-like
bottomward kick, but, according to the rules, with the feet rotated
outward. This dome-shaped position was related to good ankle
supination and, for women, combined with outward hip and ankle
rotation (Fig. 3: F and H,b). Women, who undulate more than men,
were significantly more flexible in outward ankle rotation ($\overline{X}$ 8°) and
supination ($\overline{X}$ 11°). This allowed the soles of the feet to be kept
nearly horizontal, while rotated outward, at the end of the
bottomward spreading (similar to the tail position of a dolphin).

Specific lower limb flexibility appeared to be the prerequisite
for effective undulation. Indeed, this lower limb flexibility
(measured on dry land) was related to specific shoulder and trunk
mobility (Fig. 3: F and H,g and l). Specific shoulder and trunk
flexibility (measured on dry land) appeared to influence effective
undulation to a limited extent (Fig. 3: J-N, a-f). Thus, mainly
lower limb flexibility determined the degree of undulation.

A flat pattern was obtained by a horizontal kick, after
sufficient hip flexion in the recovery. A flat body position was
related to inward hip rotation and outward ankle rotation and outward
flexion (Fig. 3: E and G). This relationship was observed in men

		a	b	c	d	e	f(a-d)	g	h	i	j	k	l
		Uphill (leg spreading)	Dome-shape (glide)	S-shape (arm spreading)	Uphill camber (1° recovery)	Uphill (2° recovery)	Undulation index	Shoulder upward (arm spreading)	Lumbar camber (arm spreading)	Lumbar camber (begin recovery)	Hip extension (begin recovery)	Lumbar camber (knee 90°)	Mobility index
BODY STRUCTURE	**A. body height** ♀		-.39*	-.42**	-.50**		-.53***	-.37*				-.40*	-.48**
	♂		-.47**	-.39		-.51**	-.54**			-.47**			-.40*
	B. shoulder / hip width ♀									-.49**			
	♂		.41*		.53**	.38*	.41*	.38*		.41*		.47**	
	C. endomorphy ♀	.53**		-.53**	-.83***	-.73***	-.59**	-.56**				-.52**	-.68***
	♂	.42*											
	D. hand surface ♀	.47*	-.56**	-.58**			-.61**						-.62**
	♂									-.38			
FLEXIBILITY	**E. ankle flexion** ♀		-.46**										
	♂		-.50**	-.47**	-.52**		-.46**	-.46**			-.39*	-.38*	-.48**
	+		-.43**	-.35*	-.68***	-.43**	-.47**			-.33*	-.41**	-.33*	-.43***
	F. ankle supination ♀		.44**	.42**			.43**	.35*					.35*
	♂		.53**	.57***	.56***		.57***	.41*		.51**			.57***
	G. hip inw. rot. X ankle (flex. X outw.rot.) ♀♂	.44	-.47**		-.66***	-.64***	-.48**			.52**			
										-.48**		-.48**	
	H. hip outw. rot. X ankle supination ♀♂		.41**	.45**	.38*	.39*	.53***	.50**					.52***
		.46**	.39*					.44**				-.38*	.39*
	I. shoulder inward rotation ♀♂			.41*			.46*						.46*
	J. shoulder upward extension ♀♂ +								.55**				
	K. shoulder abduction ♀	.51*								.44*		.46*	
	♂		.36*			.38*			-.39*				
	+					.43*			-.55***	.53***			
	L. lumbar camber ♀♂					.51*			.36*				
	+		.54**		.47**	.47**	.50**					.57***	
	M. lumbar camber X shoulder upw. ext. J x L ♀	.52*				.71***		.48**	.55**	.44**			.47**
	+		.43*	.41*		.44*							
	N. lumbar camber X shoulder abduction L x K ♀	.54*				.67**					-.55**	.53** .52*	
	+				.41*	.41*			.46*	.46*		.42*	
ISOM. STRENGTH	**O. m. triceps** ♀		.61**			.46*		.41*					.63**
	♂		-.55**	-.51**	-.71***	-.65***	-.62***			-.44*		-.48**	
	P. m. latissimus + m. triceps ♀♂			-.39*				-.53**					-.58***
	Q. m. pectoralis ♀♂				.51**	.42**							
	R. hand flexors ♀♂		.36*	.51**			.41*	.39*		.35* .39*			.43*

Fig. 3. Spearman correlations of physical characteristics with
undulation and mobility factors and indices (women,
n = 24; men, n = 21) (***P < 0.01; **P < 0.05; *P < 0.1).

only, who remain flatter than women. Surprisingly, men were found to
be as flexible as women in inward hip rotation and ankle flexion.

Ankle flexion was required to keep the foot perpendicular to the
body's longitudinal axis. Outward ankle rotation was required to
keep the foot perpendicular to its out- and backward path, during the
spreading of the legs, and to function as a propeller blade, in the
beginning of closing the legs. Hip inward rotation, and some lateral
laxity in the knees, allowed for an optimal pitch and speed of the
soles in the propeller-like beginning of closing the legs.

4 Conclusion

The pattern analysis of international swimmers is an interesting basis to guide national swimmers. One hypothesis was that undulation is more effective (Persyn et al., 1980) and another that similar scores for each of the undulation factors (dome-, S-shaped and hydroplaning) should be strived for.

However, the body characteristics must be taken into account before any pattern change is suggested. Some body characteristics can be improved drastically by specific training: mainly upper limb strength and shoulder flexibility. When the lower limb flexibility allows a greater bottomward kick to be effective, it is advised to undulate more and to train, if necessary, for specific shoulder flexibility. In addition, it is hypothesized that an important performance improvement can be expected by an upper limb propeller action, combined with specific strength training.

Based on this strategy and the results in this study, a fault detection and advice system is being developed.

5 Acknowledgements

The data for this study were collected and processed with the help of D. De Bock, Y. Noppe and N. Hens.

6 References

Colman, V. and Persyn, U. (1989) PC seminars on sport technique and training, in **Learning and Optimalisation of Swimming** (ed W. Freitag), Mainz, pp. 69-110.

Persyn, U., Vervaecke, H., Hoeven, R. and Daly, D. (1980) Technical evaluation and orientation for skill in sprinting for competitive swimmers, in **Psychology of Motor Behaviour and Sport - 1979** (eds C.H. Nadeau, W.R. Halliwell and K.M. Newell), Human Kinetics Publishers, Champaign, Ill., pp. 714-728.

Persyn, U., Colman, V. and Van Tilborgh, L. (1992) Movement analysis of the flat and the undulating breaststroke pattern, in **Biomechanics and Medicine in Swimming** (eds D. MacLaren, T. Reilly and A. Lees) (this volume).

Vervaecke, H. (1983) **Somatische en motorische determinanten van de sprintsnelheid en van de bewegingsuitvoering bij elitezwemmers** (Somatic and motoric determinants of the sprint velocity and the movement of elite swimmers), Unpublished doctoral dissertation in Physical Education, K.U. Leuven, Leuven.

SOMATOTYPE PROFILE OF SOUTH AMERICAN SWIMMERS

J.C. MAZZA, P. COSOLITO, N. ALARCÓN, C. GALASSO, C. BERMUDEZ,
G. GRIBAUDO and J.L. FERRETTI
Biosystem Institute, Sports and Aerobic Activities Research Centre,
Rosario, Argentina

Abstract
Somatotype analysis was applied to 292 South American swimmers to
compare a general and multinational sample (SAS), with South American
Championship Finalist Swimmers (SACHS). Additionally, the somatotype
of the SACHS group was compared and evaluated during the Mexico
(1968) and Montreal (1976) Summer Olympic Games. The SAS group (149
males and 88 females) and SACHS group (29 males and 27 females) were
measured for somatotype (Heath-Carter) to determine Endomorphy (En),
Mesomorphy (Me) and Ectomorphy (Ec) components.
    The SACHS males were significantly older, heavier and taller than
the SAS group (P < 0.01); SACHS somatotype components were 2.4-4.7-3.1,
while SAS group registered 2.7-4.8-2.9 (significant difference, P <
0.05 - was found only for En). The SACHS females were older (P < 0.01)
than SAS, with no difference in weight and height. The SACHS
somatotype components were 3.1-3.8-2.9, and values for SAS were
3.9-4.0-2.7. The SAS group had the higher En component (P < 0.01).
    Analysis of both groups according to styles revealed differences (P
< 0.05) only in the En among free-stylers: SAS (both males and females)
had higher En value than the SACHS group. No difference was obtained
between SACHS and both Olympic samples (for males and females) for age,
weight, height, En, Me, and Ec components.
    According to these data, it is concluded that:
    (a) Fewer En components for SACHS groups (both males and females)
compared with SAS reflects a lower proportion of fat mass and,
consequently lower En/Me ratio.
    (b) The similarity in somatotype components between SACHS groups and
Mexico 1968 and Montreal 1976 samples (for both males and females)
would suggest that there are defined somatotype profiles related to
high-level performance in swimming.
Keywords: Olympic Swimmers, Performance, Physique, Kinanthropometry.

1 Introduction

Kinanthropometry has been considered by Ross et al. (1983) as a
quantitative link between structure and function, or between anatomy
and physiology, and is concerned with the application of measurements
to determine human size, shape, proportion, composition, maturation and
gross function in relation to growth, exercise, performance and
nutrition. It gives valuable information about the influence of
physical structure on athletic ability and at the same time, the

longitudinal evolution of such structure put under training effort and performance demands.

Kinanthropometric measurements applied to swimmers provide important information about anthropometric factors that might contribute to success in this specific sport. A review of previous work, embracing 60 references is contained in the "Kinanthropometric Aquatic Sport Project" proposal of Carter et al. (1989).

Some papers describe aquatic drag, buoyancy and somatic or body measurements. There are also several research reports that demonstrated a relationship between performance and physique.

The findings of several studies showed that swimmers have well defined physical characteristics and that differences exist according to the level of competition. Differences according to style, stroke, and distance events are not clearly established.

There are also previous studies which have applied kinanthropometry to South American swimmers. These have considered somatotype (e.g. Araujo, 1978; Araujo et al., 1978; Perez, 1977), or proportionality and anthropometric fractionation of body mass (Mazza et al., 1989).

Particularly, somatotyping represents a method to describe human morphology, consisting of a classification of total body shape expressed as a rating on sequential scales. The usefulness of somatotyping to describe athletes of different sports, has been demonstrated in studies such as those of Tanner (1964), Carter (1970), De Garay et al. (1974) and Stepnicka (1977).

The purpose of the present study is to describe somatotype profiles of swimmers (multi-national sample of the South American area), comparing two different groups: a general sample of South American swimmers (SAS) with South American Swimming Championship's finalists (SACHS) in a continental event (South American Swimming Championship, Medallin, Colombia – March 1988). Besides, somatotype profiles of SACHS were compared with those who were measured during Mexico and Montreal Olympic Games (Carter, 1982), in a combined sample (De Garay et al., 1974).

2 Methods

The sample included 292 South American swimmers (177 males and 115 fdemales). They were divided into two groups:- 237 South American swimmers in general (SAS: 149 males and 88 females) and 55 South American Swimming Championship's finalists (SACHS: 28 males and 27 females).

Both samples were measured in order to apply the Heath-Carter (1980) somatotype method for determining endomorphy (En), mesomorphy (Me) and ectomorphy (Ec) components. The landmarks, technical specifications and kinanthropometric instruments were as described by Carter (1980) and Lohmann et al. (1988).

Mean $(\overline{X})$ and standard deviation (SD) values for age, weight and height, and for all other components, were calculated. Significance on applying t-tests for two independent samples was set at a P value of 0.05.

The mean values of each sample (overall and by styles) were plotted on the somatochart, determining x and y coordinates, as in Heath-Carter's method. Additionally somatotype dispersion distances (SDD) among mean somatotypes (overall and by styles) were determined in order to calculate the difference between the means of two somatotypes (Carter, 1980; Hebbelinck et al., 1975) using the following formula:-

$$SDD = [3(x_1 - x_2)^2 + (y_1 - y_2)^2]^{\frac{1}{2}} \qquad (1)$$

The SDD is the distance between two somatoplots which have the coodinates (x_1, y_1) and (x_2, y_2). An SDD of 2.0 is the equivalent of the change by one component rating of 1 unit. This value of 2.0 was used as an empirical critical value for estimating the significance of the differences among the mean somatoplots of each group (no significant difference among somatoplots with SDD values below 2.0 (Hebbelinck et al., 1975).

3 Results

In Table 1 the statistical analysis and comparisons of age, weight, and height are shown. Somatotype ratings of SACHS and SAS males are also included.

Table 1. Somatotype ratings of SACHS and SAS males

Variables	SACHS (n = 28) $x \pm$ SD	SAS (n = 49) $x \pm$ SD	P
Age (years)	19.10 ± 2.84	16.19 ± 3.38	< 0.01
Weight (kg)	73.54 ± 7.10	65.16 ± 10.55	< 0.01
Height (cm)	181.26 ± 6.28	172.67 ± 8.93	< 0.01
Endomorphy (En)	2.37 ± 0.70	2.75 ± 1.02	< 0.01
Mesomorphy (Me)	4.70 ± 0.81	4.82 ± 0.82	NS
Ectomorphy (Ec)	3.12 ± 0.68	2.93 ± 0.87	NS

The SACHS males are older, heavier and taller than SAS males (P < 0.01). Besides, SACHS males have less En components than their counterparts (P < 0.05).

In Table 2, statistical analysis and comparison of age, weight, height and somatotype ratings of SACHS and SAS females are summarised. The SACHS females are older (P < 0.01) than SAS females, but no difference is established in weight and height. Similarly to males, the SACHS females have less En component than SAS subjects (P < 0.01).

Table 2. Somatotype ratings of SACHS and SAS females

Variables	SACHS (n = 27) $x \pm$ SD	SAS (n = 88) $x \pm$ SD	P
Age (years)	17.48 ± 3.42	15.49 ± 2.07	< 0.01
Weight (kg)	58.67 ± 7.15	57.15 ± 7.70	NS
Height (cm)	167.08 ± 5.81	165.01 ± 7.09	NS
Endomorphy (En)	3.15 ± 0.92	3.91 ± 1.23	< 0.01
Mesomorphy (Me)	3.82 ± 0.92	4.02 ± 0.74	NS
Ectomorphy (Ec)	2.94 ± 0.85	2.69 ± 0.86	NS

The respective x and y values are plotted on the somatochart for the two groups, and SDD calculated among the mean values.

According to somatoplot classification described by Heath-Carter, SACHS males are balanced mesomorph, similar to SAS males. Female groups, on the contrary, have different classifications: SACHS females belong to the central area, while SAS females are mesomorph-endomorph. Considering SDD, both values between male and female groups are less than 2.

To consider an analysis by styles for male groups, En, Me and Ec ratings were compared between respective groups. No significant differences ($P > 0.05$) in the En components were found between freestylers and other styles. No more differences for other components or styles were noted. Exactly the same conclusions were obtained for SACHS and SAS females.

Somatochart and SDD values between both groups (by styles), give useful information about the distance of somatoplots, preserving the component dominance concept, which is affected when we treat the components as independent variables. The plots and SDD for both groups are shown in Figures 1 and 2.

The SDD values between male groups do not register significant somatotype dispersion distances. It is not the same for female groups: SDD is higher than 2, between freestylers and backstrokers. Some of the results are probably affected by the small number of SACHS non-freestyle swimmers.

Finally, En-Me-Ec ratings between SACHS groups and a combined sample of male and female swimmers measured during the Mexico and Montreal Olympic Games were compared. Statistical analysis are presented in Tables 3 and 4. No difference was observed between respective

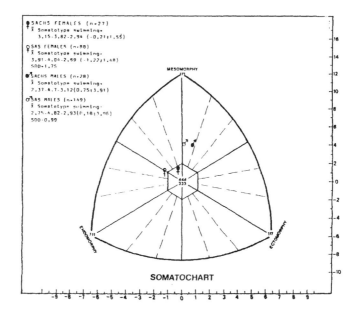

Fig. 1. Somatotype by styles SACHS (males and females).

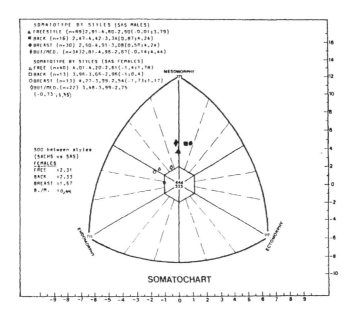

Fig. 2. Somatotype by styles SAS (males and females).

Table 3. Somatotype ratings of SACHS and Mexico-Montreal Olympic swimmers (males)

Components	SACHS (n = 28) x ± SD	Mexico-Montreal Olympic Swimmers (n = 97) x ± SD	P
En	2.37 ± 0.70	2.1 ± 0.60	NS
Me	4.70 ± 0.81	5.0 ± 0.80	NS
Ec	3.12 ± 0.68	2.9m ± 0.70	NS

Table 4. Somatotype ratings of SACHS and Mexico-Montreal Olympic swimmers (females)

Components	SACHS (n = 27) x ± SD	Mexico-Montreal Olympic Swimmers (n = 59) x ± SD	P
En	3.15 ± 0.92	3.20 ± 0.80	NS
Me	3.82 ± 0.92	3.90 ± 0.70	NS
Ec	2.94 ± 0.85	3.00 ± 0.90	NS

components in the groups in any component of somatotype. In Figure 3 somatoplots of both groups (males and females) and respective SDD values are presented. These do not reveal significant dispersion

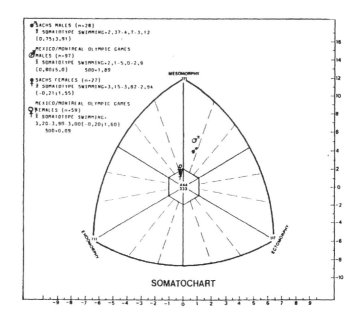

Fig. 3. Mean somatotype dispersion distance for the four samples,
         indicating Olympic Gamaes male and female data.

distances between the samples.

4 Discussion

When age, weight and height are considered, it is noted that while
SACHS males are older, heavier and taller than SAS, SACHS females are
older but not different in weight or height. These results agree with
typical individual height and weight-attained curves presented by Stini
(1984). While males continue growth development, increasing height and
weight between 15 and 19 years of age, females stabilize in these
variables for the same age period.

In reference to somatotype, only in endomorphy was a significant
result obtained; both male and female SACHS have less En ratings than
SAS groups. This revealed higher relative adipose tissue in SAS
groups. The SDD between both somatoplots was not significant.

A lack of endomorphic component in SACHS groups would be considered
representative of less percentage adipose tissue. These results are in
agreement with the previous conclusions, in which, applying
proportionality and fractionation of body mass, SACHS groups presented
a lower fat mass than SAS groups (Mazza et al., 1989). This affects
fat/muscle ratio, which would probably be related to a higher level of
performance. Other data reported previously relate positively between
lean body mass and performance level (Blanksby et al., 1916; Stager et
al., 1984). On the other hand, in our previous study, we concluded
that the SACHS group had higher muscle and less bone mass than the SAS
group (for both males and females). Considering that mesomorphy refers
to relative musculo-skeletal development per unit of height, it is

suggested that a similar mesomorphic component would reflect a relative compensation between muscle and bone contributions.

The relationship between fat mass and performance in swimming is still controversial. Previous studies related fat mass and buoyancy (more fat mass helps flotation and increases economy in swimming) (Von Dobeln et al., 1974); on the other hand, increased drag is related to a large body shape (as a consequence of higher fat mass) (Blanksby et al., 1989; Stager et al., 1984). Probably a higher En/Me ratio adversely affects muscular power output during swimming. This is in agreement with Carter and Yuhasz (1984) who reported: "when adiposity is low in athletes, fat-free mass is probably of greater functional significance than fat mass".

When both groups (males and females) were analysed by styles, the difference in En components reflected the predominance of free-stylers within the whole sample composition. The SDD between SACHS vs SAS somatoplots by styles revealed that male groups (SACHS and SAS) had a similar relative dominance (all SDD lower than 2). Exactly the opposite conclusion was obtained analyzing SACHS and SAS females (2 of 4 SDD are higher than 2).

Finally, no difference was found for anthropometric or somatotype variables between SACHS and the Mexico-Montreal combined sample. This reflects successful performance in swimming. Similar results apply to SDD values of somatoplots between both groups (males and females with values below 2.

5 Conclusions

Somatotype is a useful method of describing human morphology. Body structure and function are highly related and have an important influence in achieving top level performance.

Application of somatotype methodology to SACHS and SAS groups revealed less En components for SACHS groups (males and females) compared to SAS. It also reflected a lower proportion of relative adipose tissue, and could explain greater muscular power associated with higher competitive level. Finally, no difference between somatotype ratings for SACHS groups and the combined sample was found. This suggests there is a defined somatotype profile related to high-level performance in swimming.

6 References

Araujo, C.G.S. (1978) Somatotyping of two swimmers by the Heath and Carter method, in **Swimming Medicine IV** (eds B. Erickson and B. Furberg), University Park Press, Baltimore, pp. 188-189.

Araujo, C.G.S., Pavel, R.C. and Gomez, P.S.C. (1978) Comparison of somatotype and speed in competitive swimming at different phases of training, in **Swimming III** (eds J. Terauds and E.W. Beddingfield), University Park Press, Baltimore, pp. 329-337.

Blanksby, B.A., Bloomfield, J., Ponchard, M. and Ackland, T.R. (1986) The relationship between anatomical characteristics and swimming performance in a state age group championship competitors. J. **Swimming Res.**, 2, 30-36.

Carter, J.E.L. (1970) The somatotypes of athletes (Review). **Human**

Biol., 42, 535-569.

Carter, J.E.L. (1980) **The Heath-Carter Somatotype Method.** San Diego State University Syllabus Service, San Diego.

Carter, J.E.L. (1982) **Physical Structure of Olympic Athletes, Part I. the Montreal Olympic Games Anthropological Project.** S. Karger, New York.

Carter, J.E.L., Mazza, J.C., Ross, W.D. and Ackland, T.R. (1989) **Kinanthropometric Aquatic Sport Project. A Proposal for Kinanthropometric Study in Aquatic Sports (World Championships, Australia, 1991).** Presented to FINA Medical Committee, September 7-11, 1989.

Carter, J.E.L. and Yuhasz, M.S. (1984) Skinfolds and body composition of Olympic athletes, in **Physical Structure of the Olympic Athletes. Part II: Kinanthropometry of the Olympic Athletes. Med. Sport Sci. Vol. II,** (ed J.E.L. Carter), Karger, Basel.

De Garay, A.L., Levine, L. and Carter, J.E.L. (1974) **Genetic and Anthropometrical Studies of Olympic Athletes.** Academic Press, New York.

Hebbelinck, M., Carter, J.E.L. and de Garay, A.L. (1975) Body build and somatotype of Olympic swimmers, divers and water-polo players, in **Swimming III,** Int. Series of Sport Sci., Vol. 2, Proc. Second International Symposium on Biomechanics in Swimming (eds L. Lewillie and J.P. Clarys), University Park Press, Baltimore, pp. 285-305.

Lohman, T.G., Roche, A.F. and Martorell, R. (1988) **Anthropometric Standardization Reference Manual.** Human Kinetics Books, Champaign, Ill.

Mazza, J.C., Alarcón, N., Galasso, C., Bermudez, C., Cosolito, P., Gribaudo, F. (1989) Proportionality and anthropometric fractionation of body mass in South American swimmers. **Proc. VIII World FINA Medical Congress, London,** September 7-11.

Perez, B. (1977) Somatotype of male and female Venezuelan swimmers, in **Growth and Development Physique** (ed O. Eiben), Akademiai Kiado, Hungarian Academy of Sciences, Budapest, pp. 349-355.

Ross, W.D., Marfell-Jones, M.J., Ward, R. and Kerr, D.A. (1983) Kinanthropometry, in **Physiological Testing of Elite Athletes** (eds J.D. MacDougall, H.A. Wenger and H.J. Green), Movement Publications, Ithaca, New York, pp. 75-117.

Stager, J.M., Cordain, L. and Becker, T.J. (1984) Relationship of body composition to swimming performance in female swimmers. **J. Swimming Res.,** 1, 21-26.

Stepnicka, J. (1977) Somatotype of Czechoslovak athletes, in **Growth and Development Physique** (ed O. Eiben), Akademaiai Kiado, Hungarian Academy of Sciences, Budapest, pp. 357-364.

Stini, W.A. (1984) Kinanthropometry: An anthropological focus, in **Perspectives in Kinanthropometry, Vol. 1, Proc. The Olympic Scientific Congress** (ed J.A.P. Day), Human Kinetics Publisher, Champaign, Ill, pp. 5-23.

Tanner, J.M. (1964) **The Physique of the Olympic Athlete.** Allen and Unwin, London.

Von Dobeln, W. and Hamer, I. (1974) Body composition, sinking force and oxygen uptake of man treading water. **J. Appl. Physiol.,** 37, 55-59.

SKELETAL AGE OF WELL TRAINED YOUNG SWIMMERS

G.A. NICOLOPOULOS and S.K. CHATZICONSTANDINOU
Laboratory of Sports Medicine, Department of Physical Education and
Sport Science, Athens, Greece

Abstract
In this study the skeletal and chronological ages of 200 untrained
and 200 well trained male swimmers aged 7-19 years were compared. It
was found that when systematic swimming activity starts early in life
it can accelerate the rate of attaining biologica? maturity and the
appearance of the pubertal growth spurt.
Keywords: Swimming, Skeletal Age, Maturity, Growth

1 Introduction

It is acknowledged that chronological age is an imperfect indicator
of biological age during the process of gaining maturity. This may
apply particularly to subjects undergoing strenuous physical training
programmes during growth. The purpose of this study was to compare
skeletal and chronological ages of well trained young swimmers with
those of sedentary controls.

2 Methods

The skeletal and chronological ages of 200 well trained male swimmers
were compared to those of 200 males with no systematic participation
in swimming or other athletic activities. The latter acted as
sedentary controls. Both groups were divided into four sub-groups of
50 each, according to age, i.e. 7-10 years, 10-13 years, 13-16 years
and 16-19 years old. The definition of skeletal age was according to
the tables of Greulich and Pyle (1959) (Figs. 1 and 2).

3 Results and discussion

in the second group (10-13 years of age) the swimmers had a greater
advance in skeletal age in comparison to the sedentary control group
(p < 0.01). no significant differences were noticed in the other age
groups.
    the comparison between the differences of the average chronologi-
cal and skeletal age of swimmers, as they matured from the prepubescent to the late-adolescent age, gave the impression that in
younger groups swimmers matured skeletally earlier than the control

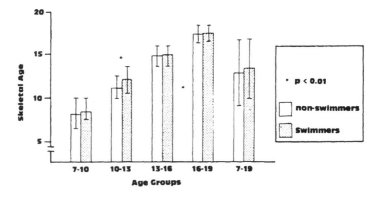

Fig. 1. Differences in average skeletal age between swimmers and
non-swimmers.

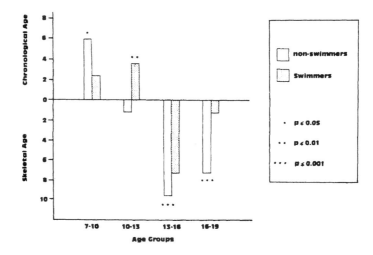

Fig. 2. Differences in average chronological and skeletal age
between swimmers and non-swimmers.

groups of the same age. It was noticed that after the growth spurt
of puberty, there is a tendency for the differences between the two
groups, swimmers and non-swimmers, to disappear.

Some delay in the skeletal age of swimmers was noticed in the late
adolescent subjects. Subjects with advanced skeletal age had greater
or faster growth in height compared to delayed skeletal age in all
swimmers and control groups studied. For example, advanced skeletal
age was combined with greater height (Fig. 3), greater body mass
(Fig. 4), longer upper and lower limbs, longer biacromial diameter as
well as greater chest and humeral circumferences.

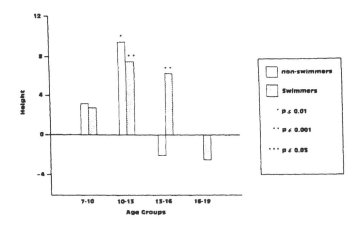

Fig. 3.   Differences between the average height in advanced
          and delayed skeletal age, in the four groups studied.

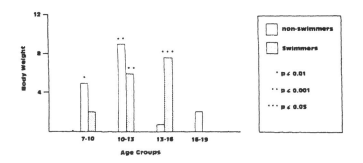

Fig. 4.   Differences of average body weight between advanced and
          delayed skeletal age, in the four groups studied.

The fact that increased physical activity can accelerate the
skeletal maturity of young persons has been noticed by other
researchers in swimming (Bugyi and Kausz, 1970) as well as in other
physical activities (Shephard et al., 1978; Malina et al., 1982).
Moreover, the skeletal age has been used as an indice of biological
maturity of young persons and has been correlated with several
anthropometric parameters (Bayley and Pinneau, 1952; Shephard et al.,
1968; Roche et al., 1971; Cumming et al., 1972; Shephard et al.,
1978).

4 Conclusion

In this comparison of maturation between swimmers and non-swimmers,
it was shown that if systematic swimming activities start early in
life, biological maturation is accelerated to a degree which is

statistically significant. Furthermore, swimming accelerated the
time of appearance of the pubertal growth spurt. After this
appearance the effect of swimming on maturity status was not in
accordance with age. By the end of adolescence, the final maturity
stage of both groups studied was chronologically similar.

5 References

Bayley, N. and Pinneau, L. (1952) Tables for predicting adult height
    from skeletal age: revised for use with the Greulich-Pyle hand
    standards. **J. Pediatr.**, 40, 423-441.
Bugyi, B. and Kausz, L. (1970) Radiographic determination of the
    skeletal age of the young swimmers. **J. Sports Med. Phys. Fit.**,
    10, 269-270.
Cumming, G.R., Garand, T. and Borysyk, L. (1972) Correlation of
    performance in track and field events with bone age. **J. Pediatr.**,
    80, 970-973.
Greulich, W.W. and Pyle, S. (1959) Radiographic Atlas of Skeletal
    Development of the Hand and Wrist. 2nd ed. Standford University
    Press, California.
Malina, R.M., Meleski, B.W. and Shoup, R.T. (1982) Anthropometric
    body composition and maturity characteristics of selected school-
    age athletes. **Pediatr. Clin. N. Amer.**, 29, 6,
Roche, A.F., Eyman, S.L. and Davila, G.H. (1971) Skeletal age
    prediction. **J. Pediatr.**, 78, 997-1004.
Shephard, R., Lavallec, H. and Rajic, M. (1978) Radiographic age in
    the interpretation of physiological and anthropological data, in
    Pediatric Work Physiology, Medicine and Sport, Vol. 11 (eds
    J. Borms and M. Hebbelinck), Karger, Basel, pp. 124-133.
Shephard, R. et al. (1968) The working capacity of Toronto school
    children. **Can. Med. Ass. J.**, 100, 560-566.

PART TEN

PSYCHOLOGICAL FACTORS

THE RELATIONSHIPS BETWEEN SELECTED PSYCHOLOGICAL PARAMETERS AND PERFORMANCE AMONG SWIMMERS AND DIVERS

R. STALLMAN, N. VIKANDER and N.P. FREIM
Norwegian College of Physical Education and Sport, Oslo, Norway

Abstract
One hundred and forty two swimmers and divers were ranked according to performance. Three self-report instruments from the Sport Psychology Consultation System (Rushall, 1985) were also administered to the subjects. Scores from these instruments were correlated with performance. In addition, for each instrument, the subjects were grouped in various ways (e.g. male vs female) and the scores were tested for group differences. The results showed low but significant correlations between performance and achievement motivation. No significant correlations were found between performance and self-control or locus of control. Significant group differences were found, however, between elites and sub-elites as well as between males and females, especially for achievement motivation.
Keywords: Achievement Motivation, Self Control, Locus of Control, Performance.

1 Introduction

Educators assume a direct relationship between motivation and achievement (or mastery). Harter (1981) has shown that this rela-tionship is complex. She demonstrated that achievement motivation is domain specific and identified separate domains of school, physical and social behaviour (Harter, 1982). Whether achievement produces motivation or motivation produces achievement is controversial. Most probably there is a circular relationship in which each element is the product and the producer of the other. When this circle is negative Seligman's (1975) "learned helplessness" is observed.

Both mastery and positive motivation are desirable in sport. Positive motivation implies security in that domain. Mastery or achievement refers both to concrete concepts (skills, knowledge) and less concrete concepts (perceived competence, cause and effect, cognitive self-control).

Motivation to achieve is, of course, vital to learning. However, that motivation must be directed in some way. There is a logical link between level of motivation and attribution. If an individual fails to receive or to understand feedback that he/she can attribute outcomes to his/her own actions, then we might expect motivation eventually to diminish. If one attributes outcomes to others or to powers beyond control, then the normal learning feedback loop is disturbed. Rushall (1983) reported greater attribution to one's own

actions (internal) among elite sportsmen than among sub-elites. With
cross-country skiers, longitudinal data showed that increases in
performance were paralleled by increases in internal attribution.

Once an individual understands the relationship between his own
actions and outcomes, there are tools to be acquired which can be
used in self-intervention to strengthen feedback, indeed to improve
the situation (outcomes). The key is to improve cognitive control
over emotional sensations, recognizing problems and solving them. In
other words, exercising self-control. Rushall (1985) reported
greater self control among elite sportsmen than among sub-elites but
suggests that these preliminary results required verification by
further research.

Participation in organized sport cannot be automatically assumed
to provide a positive experience (Roberts, 1984). Further understanding of cognitive and emotional aspects of sport are imperative
if we are to succeed in building programmes which emphasize human
qualities.

The purpose of this study was to examine more closely the relationships between certain aspects of achievement motivation, locus of
control, self-control and performance among swimmers and divers. The
Sport Locus of Control Scale (Stauss, 1975) assesses the degree to
which the sports person attributes the outcome of his/her actions to
him or herself (internal) as opposed to the extent to which outcomes
are attributed to others or to powers beyond control (external).

The Sport Self Control Schedule (Evans, 1985) evaluates four
different cognitive functions. The tendency to control emotional and
physiological sensations by cognitive processes, the tendency to seek
problem solving solutions to sport orientated problems, the tendency
to delay immediate gratification and general self-efficacy are
assessed. Diving is characterized by a competitive situation offering one chance to perform complex movements, each of which takes a
little over one second to perform. Chances to correct mistakes are
considerably less than in a swimming event which lasts longer. It is
commonly assumed that achieving optimal arousal levels is more difficult and more important in technical sports.

The Achievement Motivation Scale for Sporting Environments
(Rushall and Fox, 1980) provides the opportunity to assess the source
of motivation. It differentiates between the need to approach
success (positive motivation) as opposed to the need to avoid failure
(negative motivation). Sport situations are rich in the possibilities for one or the other to dominate. In addition, this instrument
allows for the differentiation between these tendencies in training
and in competition.

The working hypothesis was that each of the above generated scores
is correlated with performance and that differences exist between
elite and sub-elite sportsmen. Differences between males and females
were also tested.

2 Methods

One hundred and forty two swimmers and divers from 13-30 years were
tested. They were selected in a heterogeneous stratified sample
which included World Championship and Olympic finalists down to
moderately experienced club members. Ten clubs were represented from

both Norway and West Germany. Swimmers were ranked by the German Point Scoring table for performance while the divers were ranked by average score per dive over a series of important competitions. Swimmers and divers were treated separately for all correlational analysis but pooled for certain tests of group differences. Males and females could also be pooled where appropriate because of the manner in which they were ranked in performance. Each of the instrument's scores was tested for rank order correlation with performance and group differences were examined when comparing divers with swimmers, males with females and elites with sub-elites.

3 Results

Table 1 presents the correlation coefficients of each test score with performance. As can be seen, only scores from achievement motivation correlated significantly, though weakly, with performance.

Table 1. Rank order correlation with performance

Scores	Swimmers	Divers
Locus of control	.008	.046
Self-control	.277	.101
Total pos. motivation	.438*	.346*
Positive motivation – training	.389*	.321*
Negative motivation – training	.364*	.335*
Positive motivation – competition	.398*	.306*
Negative motivation – competition	.415*	.319*

*P < 0.05

In addition, the correlations between the various psychological parameters were examined. Scores from the locus of control instrument did not correlate significantly with the scores from the self-control instrument nor with any of the scores from the achievement-motivation instrument. Also, scores on the self-control instruments did not correlate significantly with achievement-motivation.

The Locus of Control (IE) Scale did not discriminate between any of the groupings within this sample and warrants no further discussion in this paper. None of the test scores discriminated between swimmers and divers. It was thus deemed appropriate to pool the divers and swimmers when comparing elites with sub-elites and males with females. Elites demonstrated significantly higher scores on self-control than sub-elites, suggesting an expected higher level of cognitive involvement. They also scored significantly higher on total motivation. When positive motivation for training and for competition were separated the elites scored significantly higher than their counterparts on both. Sub-elites scored higher on negative motivation (fear of failure) in training but elites showed greater negative motivation for competition.

When comparing females with males, the former showed higher self-control scores indicating greater cognitive involvement. Males, however, had higher total motivation. This implies a higher but more

Table 2. Group differences - significance level

	Self control	Total Motivation	Positive Training	Negative Training	Positive Competition	Negative Competition
Elite/Sub	.01 (E)	.01 (E)	.05 (E)	.05 (S)	.01 (E)	.05 (E)
Male/Female	.05 (F)	.05 (M)	.05 (F)	.01 (M)	.05 (M)	.01 (F)

(The letter after the significance level indicates the higher
 scoring group.)

poorly directed (or less disciplined) motivation for males. Most
interesting, however, were scores separating motivation for training
and competition. The girls were more positively motivated for
training while the boys were more positively motivated for competition. The boys on the other hand demonstrated greater negative motivation for training while the girls had greater negative motivation
for competition.

This close examination of the scores for achievement motivation
also revealed several unexpected results. There were six cases (n =
142), in which total negative motivation was higher than total positive motivation. These represent extreme cases. All were girls who
reflected higher negative motivation specifically in relation to
competition.

When the highest 25% and lowest 25% of scores for total motivation
were examined, nearly three times as many males as females were found
to lie in the highest quartile. Nearly three times as many females
as males were in the lowest quartile.

4 Discussion and conclusions

It would appear that motivation is generally higher among male
swimmers and divers and also among elites as opposed to sub-elites.
Indeed further sub-grouping showed male elites to be the most highly
motivated while the lowest scores were recorded by female sub-elites.
Motivation also correlated significantly with performance. Girls
were over-represented in all categories which scored high on negative
motivation relative to positive motivation.

Many individuals showed higher motivation for training than competition, especially girls and in general the younger subjects. Some
might consider this a problem and try to shift the focus to competition, hoping to improve performance. This may, however, imply a
healthy situation in training.

When the total sample was divided into sub-groups and even further
divided, the sub-samples are reduced in size. It is thus recommended
that caution be used in interpreting these results. The general
tendencies shown, however, confirm previous research and demonstrate
the need for further work. Where significant trends have yet to be
demonstrated, sample size or selection may offer an explanation.

It is the position of the authors that the results obtained confirm the previous research which indentifies rather large individual
differences and suggests that the role of cognitive processes in
determining performance has been under estimated.

5 References

Evans, L.E. (1985) A tool for measuring self control in athletes. Unpublished MS thesis, Lakehead University, Thunder Bay, Ontario, Canada.

Harter, S. (1981) A model of intrinsic mastery motivation in children: individual differences and developmental, in **Minnesota Symposium on Child Psychology** (ed A. Collins), volume 14, Erlbaum, Hillsdale, NJ.

Harter, S. (1982) The perceived competence scale for children. **Child Development**, 53, 87–97.

Roberts, G. (1984) Achievement motivation in children's sports, in **The Development of Motivation and Achievement** (ed J. Nichols), volume 3, JAI Press, London, pp. 219–250.

Rushall, B.S. (1983) Athlete psychological profiles. Useful measurement techniques, in **Sport for All, Proc., Int. Sports Science, Singapore.**

Rushall, B.S. (1985) **The Sport Psychology Consultation System, Manual.** School of Physical Education, San Diego State University, San Diego, California.

Rushall, B.S. and Fox, R.G. (1980) An approach – avoidance motivation scale for sporting environments. **Can. J. Sport Sci.**, 5, 39–43.

Seligman, M. (1975) **Helplessness: On Depression Development and Death.** Freeman Press, San Francisco.

Stauss, J. (1975) Source of reinforcement as a potential factor in women's sport involvement. Unpublished MSc thesis, University of South Carolina, Greensboro.

THE ATHLETE/COACH RELATIONSHIP IN COMPETITIVE SWIMMING: THE IMPLICATIONS OF PERSONALITY TYPE, TEMPERAMENT TYPE AND COACH EVALUATION

N.O. VIKANDER, R.K. STALLMAN and B. SOYLAND
Norwegian College of Physical Education and Sport, Oslo, Norway

Abstract
Personality profiles of 53 coaches and 163 competitive swimmers in Norway were mapped using the Myers-Briggs Type Indicator (MBTI). Distribution patterns of swimmers and coaches varied greatly indicating different recruitment and retention factors. Twenty of the coaches were evaluated by their swimmers using the Coach Evaluation Questionnaire (CEQ). The degree of coach/swimmer personality similarity was compared with CEQ scores using Spearman's rank order correlation. Significance was found (rho = 0.440) on an integrative measure but not on separate elements of personality. The CEQ scores indicate strong organizational skills but weaker human relations capacities. Results suggest a programme of self-development for coaches using MBTI/CEQ profiles as points of departure.
Keywords: Competitive Swimming, Myers-Briggs Type Indicator (MBTI), Personality Type, Temperament Type, Coach Evaluation Questionnaire (CEQ).

1 Introduction

Coaches experience problems and stresses warranting psychological services just as much as athletes (Hanin, 1989). Kroll and Gundersheim (1983) in a study of 93 male US high school coaches reported that the two most frequently cited stress factors in coaching were "disrespect from players" (42.8%) and "not being able to reach athletes" (20.7%). Personal relationships with athletes were cited four times more often than lack of technical expertise as reasons for leaving coaching.

From the athlete's side of the relationship, Vanden Auweele (1987) in a study of young Belgian athletes found that swimmers had poorer relationships with their coaches than track and field athletes. The explanation suggested was that swimming coaches had a more authoritarian style.

The relationship between athlete and coach appears, then, to be an issue of some importance; in spite of this little systematic research has been done. A helpful starting point would seem to be an investigation of the personality patterns of coaches and their athletes. What are the important factors in Methe personalities of coaches and in those of athletes for having an optimal relationship? Do similarities in personality lead to a more positive atmosphere? The Myers-

Briggs type indicator (MBTI) (Myers, 1962) is an appropriate instrument for personality mapping in sport since it offers "...information potentially useful to team building and better understanding of the coaching team". The MBTI has become the most widely used test of its kind and was developed on a normal, non-clinical population. Working within the MBTI framework Keirsey and Bates (1978) have developed an additional useful mode of analysis involving four basic temperament types.

To progress beyond simple personality comparisons, it is necessary to relate such profiles to measures of how in fact athletes and coaches view each other. Beginning with the athletes' perspective, one of the few robust instruments available is Rushall and Wiznuk's (1985) Coach Evaluation Questionnaire (CEQ). It measures how close the athletes' perception of their coach is to the established, researched characteristics of the outstanding coach.

The purpose of the study was to compare the patterns of swimmers and coaches on three major modes of analysis of MBTI data; to compile a profile of the coaches on the CEQ; and to investigate the relationship between MBTI and CEQ scores (in particular whether degree of personality consonance between coach and swimmer was related to CEQ performance.

2 Methods

The MBTI was administered to a sample of 53 swimming coaches and 163 competitive swimmers in Norway in 1989-90. Of the coaches 13 were female and 40 were male, while there were 80 female and 83 ma~le swimmers. The coaches and athletes ranged from club to international level. Twenty-one (19 males, 2 females) of the coaches were evaluated by their swimmers using the CEQ, with some swimmers relating to more than one coach (i.e. National Team athletes). The total number of CEQs completed was 204. Of the 21 coaches, 20 (18 males, 2 females) were in clubs/teams where both swimmers and coaches had completed the MBTI. The number of CEQs administered to these swimmers was 192.

Since simple frequencies and calculations of averages characterize the first two purposes of the study, comments here will be restricted to the third purpose. On each of the four polar dimensions (comprising the eight preferences) of the MBTI, the average of the unit distance between each swimmer and his/her coach was calculated for each club/team. In addition, an overall measure of MBTI similarity for each club/team was computed according to the average of these four scores. All coaches, then, were ranked on degree of similarity with their swimmers on five MBTI criteria. Spearman rank order correlations were carried out on these rankings compared to CEQ rankings. Finally, the average CEQ score of coaches whose Keirsey temperament type coincided with the "group average temperament" of their athletes was compared with the coaches whose temperament differed.

3 Results and discussion

3.1 The eight MBTI preferences (Table 1)

On the Extroversion:Introversion and the Sensing:Intuition dimensions the distribution pattern of coaches and swimmers is very similar. Compared to the general population figures (US data), however, the large numbers in both groups with the intuition preference suggests that innovative inclinations are rewarded in the swimming milieu more than in many other settings. The Judgement:Perception dimension shows a 15% difference between the two subject groups, with the coaches preferring the orderly "J" style nearly 2:1 over the impulsive "P" style preferred by half the swimmers (10% over the general population proportion). Room for spontaneity in training is likely to motivate these "P" swimmers. Finally, the Thinking:Feeling dimension exhibits a remarkable finding, a full 27% difference between the two groups. The swimmers are close to the 50:50 general distribution, whereas 83% of the coaches are "T" types. The impersonal, analytical style of the "T" coach is an advantage in the scienctific realm of sport, though an "F" preference is a strength in the human relations sphere.

3.2 The four temperament types (Table 2)

The most striking aspects of the temperament type distribution are the very large number of coaches in the "NT" category and their lack in the "SP" and "NF" groupings (in relation to both swimmers and the general population). Aside from being bureaucratic "SJs", Norwegian coaches, then, are likely to be cool, perfectionistic "NTs", leaving very few (23%) to match the 44% of the swimmers who are excitement-oriented "SPs" or sensitive "NFs".

3.3 The sixteen personality types (Table 3)

The atypical pattern for coaches continues in this mode of analysis. Sixty four percent are concentrated in just four personality types, the "Administrator", the "Fieldmarshal", the "Trustee" and the "Inventor" (compared to the general population's 31%). The swimmers, on the other hand, are more evenly spread with 46% found in their four most populous categories: "Administrator", "Journalist", "Seller" and "Inventor" (36% in general population). The first three types listed for the coaches contain 53% of S's and delineate practical, organizational and directive characteristics. The many "fieldmarshal" in particular bear comment since as Martin (1986) pointed out, independence and self-reliance are important characteristics of elite athletes. Of concern as well is that only one solitary "Pedagogue" was found among the coaches. Finally, it is interesting to note that not a single warm-hearted, conscientious "Seller" coach was found. Nearly one in ten of the swimmers is of this type and in the general population it shares the highest frequency spot (14%) with the "Administrator".

3.4 The Coach Evaluation Questionnaire (Table 4)

The 82% average score on the CEQ by the 21 coaches is comfortably above the 80% level indicated by the instrument's authors as the criterion for solid coaching performance. There were, however, five individuals who scored under 80%, four in the 70% range which is interpreted as requiring minor improvement effort, and one in the 60%

Table 1. Myers-Briggs Type Indicator: distribution of Norwegian swimmers and coaches on the eight preference dimensions (swimmers: N = 163; Coaches: N = 53).

Interaction with environment
The person's interest flows mainly to:

---

the outer world of actions, objects, and persons.	the inner world of concepts and and ideas.
E: Extroversion	I: Introversion
Swimmers: 71.2%	Swimmers: 28.8%
Coaches: 67.9%	Coaches: 32.1%
(Gen. pop. appr. 65%)	(Gen. pop. appr. 35%)

Information processing
The person prefers to perceive:

---

the immediate, real, practical facts of experience and life.	the possibilities, relationships, and meanings of experiences.
S: Sensing	N: Intuition
Swimmers: 60.7%	Swimmers: 39.3%
Coaches: 58.5%	Coaches: 41.5%
(Gen. pop. appr. 70%)	(Gen. pop. appr. 30%)

Decision making
The person prefers to make judgements or decisions:

---

objectively, impersonally, considering causes of events and where decisions may lead.	subjectively and personally, weighing values of choices, and how they affect others.
T: Thinking	F: Feeling
Swimmers: 55.8%	Swimmers: 44.2%
Coaches: 83.0%	Coaches: 17.0%
(Gen. pop. appr. 50%)	(Gen. pop. appr. 50%)

Organization
The person mostly prefers to live:

---

in a decisive, planned, orderly way aiming to regulate and control events.	in a spontaneous, flexible way, aiming to understand life and adapt to it.
J: Judgement	P: Perception
Swimmers: 49.7%	Swimmers: 50.3%
Coaches: 64.2%	Coaches: 35.8%
(Gen. pop. appr. 60%)	(Gen. pop. appr. 40%)

---

range where major efforts are recommended.

An analysis of the 36 CEQ item average scores shows that Norwegian coaches' area of excellence (90% score range) is primarily in the organizational sphere (items 24, 25, 27). Only the "Trust" item (13) could be viewed as a human relations item. The converse, however, is the case for the items scored below 80%. Five of the six 70% range items (all but 35) indicate lower than acceptable performance in human contact coaching tasks. In the 60% range where major behaviour

Table 2. Myers-Briggs type indicator: distribution of Norwegian swimmers and coaches on the Keirsey temperament types (swimmers: N = 163; coaches: N = 53)

Temperament	Type	Swimmers (%)	Coaches (%)	Gen. Pop. Est (%)
SJ	Sensing-Judgement	36.2	43.4	42
SP	Sensing-Perceptive	24.5	15.1	28
NT	Intuitive-Thinking	20.2	34.0	15
NF	Intuitive-Feeling	19.0	7.5	15

Table 3. Myers-Briggs type indicator: distribution of Norwegian swimmers and coaches on the 16 personality types (swimmers: N = 163 coaches: N = 53)

Personality	Type	Swimmers (%)	Coaches (%)	Gen. Pop. Est. (%)
ISTJ	"Trustee"	6.1	11.3	7
ISFJ	"Conservator"	3.7	5.7	7
ISTP	"Artisan"	4.9	5.7	5
ISFP	"Artist"	4.3	1.9	5
ESTP	"Promoter"	7.4	5.7	9
ESFP	"Entertainer"	8.0	1.9	9
ESTJ	"Administrator"	17.2	26.4	14
ESFJ	"Seller"	9.2	-	14
INFJ	"Author"	2.5	-	3
INTJ	"Scientist"	1.2	3.8	3
INFP	"Questor"	1.8	-	2
INTP	"Architect"	4.3	3.8	2
ENFP	"Journalist"	11.0	5.7	4
ENTP	"Inventor"	8.6	11.3	4
ENFJ	"Pedagogue"	3.7	1.9	6
ENTJ	"Fieldmarshal"	6.1	15.1	6

modification is called for, three of the five items (22, 8, 23) relate to "human quality" concerns. This scoring pattern is not surprising in view of the concentration of the coaches in the "T" and "J" preferences on the MBTI. Finally, cause for concern is generated by the low scores on items 16, 22 and 23 (X = 66.6%). These are the test items which focus on the athlete as a person. The importance of such a holistic coaching perspective has been emphasized by Martin (1986).

3.5 The relationship between personality/temperament and coach evaluation (Tables 5 and 6)

The Temperament: CEQ relationship was in the expected direction with coach/swimmer temperament consonance being reflected in the higher average CEQ score. However, the difference was slight and not statistically significant.

Turning to the four polar preference dimensions of the MBTI, the Spearman correlations with the CEQ are low order and non-significant,

Table 4. Coach Evaluation Questionnaire: evaluation of Norwegian swimming coaches by their athletes (excerpt) (Swimmers: N = 204; Coaches: N = 21)

Coach	Characteristics	Score (%)
Areas of excellence (scores of 90–100%)		
1	The coach is dedicated to the sport.	94.5
24	The coach provides training sessions that are organized.	94.1
13	I feel that I can trust the coach.	92.6
25	The coach is in command during practice.	90.4
27	The coach makes the best use of the time available for practice.	90.0
Minor improvement areas (scores of 70–79.9%)		
9	The coach gives attention to each athlete.	79.9
2	The coach is patient	79.8
35	The coach attends clinics and workshops to stay abreast of new coaching methods.	77.6
28	The coach interacts with each athlete at training.	77.4
17	The coach finds ways to make all the athletes feel good about themselves.	76.8
16	The coach is interested in me as a person.	72.2
Major improvement areas (scores under 70.0%)		
29	The coach encourages athletes to keep logbooks so they can measure their own improvement	68.6
22	The coach encourages social activities for the athletes	67.5
11	The coach's physical appearance sets a good example for the athletes.	67.1
8	The coach is strict	62.5
23	The coach is interested in the athlete's schoolwork or occupation.	60.0
Overall score		82.1
Range of club/team scores for coaches		69.3–87.8

though all are in the expected direction. The strongest correlation of 0.221 was exhibited on the Thinking-Feeling dimension. This was not surprising in view of the CEQ item analysis. The integrated measure of MBTI similarity demonstrated a significant 0.440 correlation with CEQ ($P < 0.05$). This indicates that personality similarity relates to coach evaluation scores. Moreover, this result provides support for the integrative theoretical perspective on the elements of personality structure (Silva, 1984).

Table 5. Keirsey Temperament consonance between Norwegian swimming coaches and the "group average temperament" of their athletes as related to CEQ scores

	Average CEQ score	Level of significance
Temperament consonance (N = 5)	82.48%	NS
No temperament consonance (N = 15)	81.19%	

Table 6. Spearman rank order correlation: Norwegian swimming coaches' degree of similarity with their athletes on Myers-Brigg Type Indicator personality dimensions compared with Coach Evaluation Questionnaire (CEQ) scores (Swimmers: N = 192; Coaches: N = 20)

	rho	Z
Extroversion-Introversion/CEQ	0.003	NS
Sensing-Intuition/CEQ	0.182	NS
Thinking-Feeling/CEQ	0.221	NS
Judgement-Perception/CEQ	0.077	NS
Overall measure of the four preference dimension/CEQ	0.440	0.027

4 Conclusions

What are the practical implications of this study? The CEQ profile can be used by the individual coach as a map in a programme of personal improvement. For a nation's sport associations, overall national CEQ profiles can guide coaching education. Personality information when shared among coaches and athletes can lead to greater understanding and appreciation of individual differences. Such information can be a point of departure in a self-development programme where core preferences are expanded into a growing repertoire enabling the individual to function more comfortably with diverse people in a variety of settings.

5 References

Hanin, Y. (1989) Applying sport psychology: international and cross cultural perspectives, in **Proceedings: First IOC World Congress on Sports Sciences,** US Olympic Committee, Dept. of Ed. Services, Colorado Springs, Co., pp. 359-363.
Keirsey, D. and Bates, M. (1978) **Please Understand Me: Character and Temperament Types.** Prometheus Nemesis Books, Del Mar, CA.
Kroll, W. and Gundersheim, J. (1983) Stress factors in coaching. Coaching Science Update, 47-49.
Martin, D. (1986) Psychological development and motor learning in boys and girls before and in puberty: conclusions for training.

Coaches' Resource Package, 1, 91-103.

Myers, I.B. (1962) **The Myers-Briggs Type Indicator.** Consulting Psychologists Press, Palo Alto, CA.

Rushall, B. and Wiznuk, K. (1985) Athlete's assessment of the coach – the Coach Evaluation Questionnaire. **Can. J. Appl. Sport. Sci.**, 3, 157-161.

Silva III, J. (1984) Personality and sport performance: controversy and challenge, in **Psychological Foundations of Sport** (eds J. Silva III and R. Weinberg), Human Kinetics Publishers, Champaign, Ill., pp. 59-69.

Vanden Auweele, Y. (1987) Personality diagnosis in young top level athletes, in **Proceedings of the 7th Congress of the European Federation of Sport Psychology, volume 2** (ed Wissenshaftlicher Rat Beim Staatssekretariat für Körperkultur und Sport der DDR), pp. 507-525.

EFFECTS OF SLEEP LOSS AND TIME OF DAY IN SWIMMERS

S.A. SINNERTON AND T. REILLY
Centre for Sport and Exercise Sciences, Liverpool Polytechnic, Byrom
Street, Liverpool L3 3AF, England

Abstract
The aim of this study was to examine the effects of partial sleep
deprivation (PSD) and time of day on swimming performance,
physiological and psychological variables. Eight swimmers (5 males,
3 females) aged 19-28 years were tested on 4 consecutive days,
morning (06:30 h) and evening (17:30 h), under conditions of normal
sleep and PSD (2.5 h a night). Measurements included grip and back
strength, lung function (VC and FEV_1), resting heart rate and mood
states. Swimming performances over 4 trials at 50 m and 1 trial at
400 m were also measured.
No effects of PSD were noted on grip (dominant hand), back
strength, heart rate, lung function, or swim times. Grip, back
strength, heart rate and oral temperature values were higher in the
evening than in the morning, values increasing by 4.1%, 7.9%, 5.5%
and 1.3%, respectively. A similar trend was noted in swim
performance; mean 50 m and 400 m times decreased by 1.9% and 3.6%
respectively from morning to evening.
Sleep loss affected mood states, with significant increases in
depression, tension, confusion, fatigue and anger and decreases in
vigour ($P < 0.001$). Results support the brain restitution theory of
sleep and indicate that the diurnal variation in swimming performance
is greater than any due to partial sleep loss.
Keywords: Circadian rhythms, Diurnal variation, Mood, Physiological
reactions, Swim performance.

1 Introduction

Sport competitors assume that sound sleep on a regular and habitual
basis is an essential part of preparing for top performances. Yet
there is no definitive standard as to what constitutes a good night's
sleep or convincing evidence that the assumption is correct. The
importance of sleep for the athlete can be established by studying
the effects of sleep loss. Besides any potential adverse effects on
subsequent performance, such experimental disruptions of sleep
impinge on the body's normal circadian rhythms.

Swimming performance has been shown to vary with time of day in
close accordance to the circadian rhythm in body temperature (Rodahl
et al., 1976; Baxter and Reilly, 1983). There have been no studies
on swimmers as to how sleep loss affects swim performance or its
circadian rhythm. Gross motor performances, such as muscular

strength and graded treadmill running, are well maintained in
conditions of three days of reduced sleep ration, whereas complex
skills such as choice reaction time are adversely affected after the
first night (Reilly and Deykin, 1983). The magnitude of the effect
is dependent on time of day (Reilly and Hales, 1987). These findings
are taken to support the brain restitution theory (Horne, 1988).

The aim of this study was to examine the effects of partial sleep
deprivation (PSD) and time of day on: (i) swimming performance;
(ii) cardiorespiratory variables and muscular strength; (iii) mood
states and subjective responses.

2 Methods

In order to determine the effects of sleep loss on swimmers, the
subjects were tested under two conditions, one of normal sleep
(control) and the other of partial sleep deprivation (PSD). Ten days
separated each condition. The 2.5 hours sleep during PSD was taken
from 03:00 h to 05:30 h, whilst being supervised. A counterbalanced
protocol was used to eliminate an effect of order of testing.

The testing procedure remained consistent for the morning and
evening sessions and from day to day during both conditions. Oral
temperature and resting heart rate were recorded on waking in the
morning and on arrival at the pool in the evening. Subjects
completed the Profile of Mood States (POMS) questionnaire before and
after each session. Assessments of sleepiness were made before,
during and after each session using the Stanford Sleepiness Scale
(Hoddes et al., 1973). Grip and back strength were measured using
Takeikiki Kogyo (Tokyo) dynamometers and vital capacity (VC) and FEV_1
were measured using a dry spirometer (Vitalograph, Buckingham).

Four all-out 50 m sprints and a 400 m swim followed a 400 m
warm-up. The timed swims were performed in front crawl. Perceived
exertion was rated using Borg's category-ratio scale (Borg, 1982) and
the 15-grade RPE scale (Borg, 1970) after each swim. Heart rate was
recorded over 20 s immediately following each swim. Results were
analysed using three and four-way ANOVA models. A value of $P < 0.05$
was taken to indicate significance.

3 Results

Oral temperature and resting heart rate increased significantly ($P <
0.001$) from morning to evening but were not significantly affected by
sleep loss. Values for vital capacity and FEV_1 showed no significant
variation. A 5.3% increase in maximum right hand grip strength in
the evening emphasised a significant effect of time of day ($P <
0.001$). Maximum and average left hand values also increased
significantly ($P < 0.01$). Average left hand grip strength values
were found to decrease with sleep loss ($P < 0.01$); the mean values of
the pre-exercise measures are given in Table 1. Back strength
(maximum and average) significantly increased from day 1 to day 4 ($P
< 0.001$, $P < 0.01$) and from morning to evening ($P < 0.01$).

The mean times for sprints 1, 3 and 4 decreased significantly from
morning to evening ($P < 0.01$). The first sprint showed the greatest
decrease of 2.2%. The mean times increased ($P < 0.001$) from sprint 1

to sprint 4, the greatest increase being from sprint 1 to sprint 2. No effects of PSD were noted in the sprint times (Table 2).

Time of day affected the stroke frequency (SF) of the sprints (P < 0.001) but not distance per stroke (d/S). The mean values of d/S decreased (P < 0.001) from sprint 1 to sprint 4 while SF remained unchanged. The mean times for the fastest sprint were found to decrease in the evening (P < 0.01). The fatigue index (indicating the percent fall in performance from first to fourth trial) remained unaffected by time of day and PSD. The effect of PSD on heart rate was non-significant, whereas increases occurred from morning to evening (P < 0.001) and from sprint 1 to sprint 4 (P < 0.001). The greatest increase of 7 beats min^{-1} was from sprint 1 to sprint 2. The 400 m swim times were found to vary from day 1 to day 4 and performance improved significantly in the evening (P < 0.001) by an average of 16.8 s. The split times also improved in the evening but the times increased from the first to the fourth 100 m (P < 0.001). Both SF and d/S during the 400 m decreased from the first to the fourth 100 m (P < 0.001). The stroke rate was significantly higher (P < 0.05) in the evening than in the morning (Table 2).

Perceived exertion increased from sprint 1 to sprint 4 (P < 0.001) for the arms, legs and breathing. Only the perceived exertion ratings for breathing were affected by sleep loss which increased the ratings (P < 0.001). During the 400 m swim only the ratings for the legs increased with PSD (P < 0.05).

The pre-exercise, post-sprints and post-exercise ratings of sleepiness (Table 1) increased with sleep loss (P < 0.001). Only the pre-exercise and post-sprints ratings were significantly lower in the evening (P < 0.001 and P < 0.05 respectively).

All the moods were affected by PSD (P < 0.001). Mood state ratings of anger-hostility, confusion-bewilderment, fatigue- inertia, depression-dejection and tension-anxiety increased whilst ratings of vigour-activity decreased from day to day as a result of sleep loss. Time of day did not significantly affect any of the mood states. Fatigue-inertia and vigour-activity increased, while mood state depression-dejection decreased following exercise (P < 0.01, P < 0.05 and P < 0.05 respectively).

4 Discussion

The diurnal variation in oral temperature is in agreement with previous findings (Reilly, 1987). Neither the variation in temperature nor the 5.5% increase in resting heart rate during the day was disrupted by sleep loss. Muscular strength variables showed increased values in the evening and only the left hand average and maximum grip strengths decreased as a result of sleep loss. The effect of sleep loss on the non-dominant hand grip strength may have been a result of increased fatigue and decreased motivation but was not replicated in the other strength measures.

The performance variables remained unaffected by sleep loss. The mean sprint and 400 m swim times showed a diurnal variation which predisposed towards an improved performance in the evening. The results from the performance measures indicate that PSD has no detrimental effects on swimming performance, whether during the short term 50 m sprints or the longer endurance-type 400 m swim. These

Table 1. Pre-exercise measures and subjective sleepiness (pre- and post-exercise)

		Day 1		Day 2		Day 3		Day 4	
		06:30	17:30	06:30	17:30	06:30	17:30	06:30	18:30
Oral temperature (°C)	C	36.7	37.1	36.6	37.2	36.7	37.1	36.7	37.1
	PSD	36.6	37.1	36.7	37.1	36.7	37.1	36.6	37.1
Resting heart rate (beats/min)	C	59	62	58	63	58	63	60	62
	PSD	60	64	59	63	60	63	60	62
Grip Strength (kg) (right,max)	C	30.9	32.4	31.2	33.4	29.3	32.8	31.1	31.4
	PSD	30.5	33.3	31.1	33.2	34.3	32.6	29.6	31.9
Grip Strength (kg) (left,average)	C	29.4	30.6	29.8	30.3	28.0	30.5	29.3	31.0
	PSD	28.4	29.5	28.3	29.3	29.0	28.3	27.9	29.5
Back Strength (kg) (Max.)	C	119.5	130.8	131.9	141.8	123.5	130.0	120.5	133.9
	PSD	113.8	129.4	131.9	137.3	121.5	128.1	122.4	138.3
Back Strength (kg) (average)	C	112.2	123.0	121.7	132.7	118.2	123.2	115.5	127.3
	PSD	109.6	123.0	126.0	130.4	115.0	121.7	116.3	127.1
Subjective Sleepiness Pre-exercise	C	2.38	1.88	2.38	2.00	2.63	2.13	2.50	1.75
	PSD	2.38	1.75	2.75	2.50	4.38	3.38	4.88	4.25
Subjective Sleepiness Post-sprints	C	2.38	2.00	2.13	2.25	2.25	2.00	2.5	1.75
	PSD	2.00	1.75	2.13	2.00	3.00	2.88	3.75	3.25
Subjective Sleepiness Post-exercise	C	2.25	1.88	2.00	2.25	2.25	1.88	2.25	1.88
	PSD	1.88	1.63	2.00	2.13	2.75	2.88	3.75	3.00

Table 2. Performance measures throughout the four days, morning and evening: C = controls

		Day 1		Day 2		Day 3		Day 4	
		06:30	17:30	06:30	17:30	06:30	17:30	06:30	18:30
Sprint 1(s)	C	40.23	39.57	40.38	39.62	39.73	38.94	40.69	38.34
	PSD	39.99	39.76	39.58	39.69	40.28	38.57	39.29	38.59
Sprint 4(s)	C	43.09	42.17	42.23	41.37	41.38	40.71	41.85	40.47
	PSD	42.60	40.95	42.26	41.48	41.36	41.55	42.01	40.42
Sprints 1-4(s)	C	42.00	41.10	41.22	41.10	40.72	40.22	41.10	39.69
	PSD	41.40	40.61	41.13	41.41	40.79	40.18	40.96	39.75
Stroke rate(sprints) (strokes/min)	C	77.0	79.2	77.6	79.2	79.3	80.6	80.0	82.6
	PSD	79.7	79.1	78.7	79.7	79.7	79.6	73.8	80.9
Heart rate(sprints) (beats/min)	C	130	133	132	130	128	133	127	135
	PSD	123	136	135	134	126	133	119	134
400 m swim(s)	C	473.8	450.1	461.0	449.5	454.6	438.0	455.3	436.1
	PSD	477.1	455.9	458.8	450.3	455.8	445.0	455.5	432.9
400 m swim(s) (split times)	C	114.44	112.59	114.94	112.44	113.53	109.63	114.00	109.25
	PSD	115.84	111.31	114.34	111.66	114.84	110.81	114.91	110.47
Fastest sprint (s)	C	40.07	39.51	40.21	39.35	39.11	38.82	39.81	37.96
	PSD	39.84	39.38	39.86	39.32	39.34	38.52	39.62	38.61
Stroke rate(400 m) (strokes/min)	C	61.0	62.1	60.0	60.6	59.5	62.7	61.9	63.1
	PSD	62.5	61.1	62.6	62.8	61.9	64.1	59.1	63.3
Finishing heart rate (beats/min)	C	154	150	144	149	146	146	138	154
	PSD	142	155	157	152	147	155	136	151

findings oppose the theory of sleep's tissue restitution function and suggest that physical performance may remain unimpaired by PSD.

Subjective sleepiness ratings were adversely affected by PSD after only one night. All the ratings were greatly affected after the second night of PSD. The pre-exercise ratings confirmed Horne's (1985) suggestion that sleepiness would be greatest in the morning with the mean values decreasing by 19% in the evening. This decrease was reduced to 11% following the sprints and 8.5% after testing, indicating that exercise helps to reduce subjective sleepiness.

All the mood states were substantially impaired by sleep loss and decrements were noted after one night of PSD. The mood states did not exhibit a diurnal variation but the ratings of depression-dejection and vigour-activity improved while those of fatigue-inertia were made worse by exercise. It seems that exercise is only partly beneficial in countering the deterioration in mental states due to sleep loss.

Although swimming performance was not impaired by PSD, decrements were observed in psychological measures such as perception of effort, subjective sleepiness and mood states. These may be attributed to impairment in cerebral restitution rather than tissue restitution. The pre-exercise and performance measures tended to follow the normal circadian rhythm in temperature, peaking in the evening. The time of day effect should be regarded as influential both in training and competition and persisted for at least three nights of PSD. Although swimmers should not lose sleep on a regular basis due to the dearousal effects, they need not be unduly worried when occasionally experiencing sleep loss. Present results show that they are capable of maintaining their physical performance, at least under non-competitive conditions.

5 References

Baxter, C. and Reilly, T. (1983) Influence of time of day on all-out swimming. Brit. J. Sports Med., 17, 122-128.

Borg, G.A.V. (1970) Perceived exertion as an indicator of somatic stress. Scand. J. Rehabil. Med., 2, 92-95.

Borg, G.A.V. (1982) Psychophysical bases of perceived exertion. Med. Sci. Sports Exerc., 14, 377-381.

Hoddes, E., Dement, W. and Zaroche, V. (1973) Development and use of Stanford Sleepiness Scale. Psychophysiol., 9, 150.

Horne, J.A. (1985) Sleep function, with particular reference to sleep deprivation. Annals Clin. Res., 17, 199-578.

Horne, J.A. (1988) Why we sleep. Oxford University Press. Oxford.

Reilly, T. (1987) Circadian rhythms and exercise. In: Exercise: Benefits, Limits and Adaptations (eds D. Macleod, R. Maughan, M. Nimmo, T. Reilly and C. Williams), E. and F.N. Spon, London, pp. 346-367.

Reilly, T. and Deykin, T. (1983) Effects of partial sleep loss on subjective states, psychomotor and physical performance tests. J. Human Mov't Stud., 9, 157-170.

Reilly, T. and Hales, A.J. (1988) Effects of partial sleep deprivation on performance measures in females. In: Contemporary Ergonomics 1988 (ed E.D. Megaw), Taylor and Francis, London, pp. 509-514.

Rodahl, A., O'Brien, M. and Firth, F.G.R. (1976) Diurnal variation
in performance of competitive swimmers. J. Sports Med. Phys.
Fit., 16, 72-76.

Index

This index uses keywords assigned to the individual chapters as its basis. The
numbers are the page numbers of the first page of the relevant chapter.